Brain Lesion Localization and Developmental Functions

Frontal lobes

Limbic system

Visuocognitive system

Fondazione Pierfranco e Luisa Mariani
Viale Bianca Maria 28
20129 Milan, Italy

Telephone: +39 02 795458
Fax: +39 02 76009582
e-mail: publications@fondazione-mariani.org
www.fondazione-mariani.org

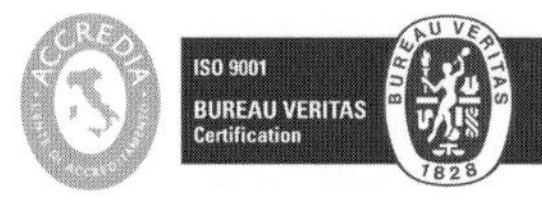

Fondazione con SGQ certificato

Brain Lesion Localization and Developmental Functions

Frontal lobes
Limbic system
Visuocognitive system

Remembering Ans Hey

Edited by

Daria Riva, Charles Njiokiktjien, Sara Bulgheroni

Mariani Foundation Paediatric Neurology Series: 25

Series Founder: Maria Majno

Associate Editor: Valeria Basilico

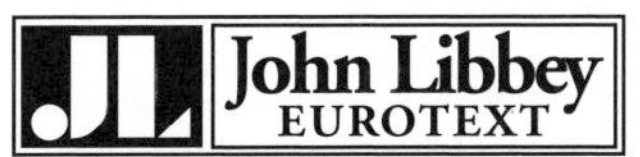

ISSN: 0969-0301
ISBN: 978-2-7420-0825-4

Cover design: Scriptoria (Fotolia). Abstract image by Costanza Magnocavallo.

Technical and language editor: Justine Cullinan.

Published by

Éditions John Libbey Eurotext
127, avenue de la République, 92120 Montrouge, France
Tél. : +33 (0)1 46 73 06 60
Fax : +33 (0)1 40 84 09 99
e-mail : contact@jle.com
www.jle.com

Contents

Limbic system

Visuocognitive system

Brain Lesion Localization and Developmental Functions, D. Riva, C. Njiokiktjien and S. Bulgheroni (eds.)

Chapter 1

Higher cognitive function processing in developmental age: specialized areas, connections and distributed networks

Daria Riva

Developmental Neurology Division, Fondazione IRCCS Istituto Neurologico 'C. Besta', via Celoria 11, 20133 Milan, Italy
driva@istituto-besta.it

Summary

This chapter deals with organization and architecture of brain functions in developmental age.
Starting from a brief history describing the alternate enunciation of localizationalist and associationist theories (with the description of classical disconnection syndromes), we conclude with the contemporary concept of brain organized in specialized areas strongly interconnected which form networks widely distributed throughout the brain. The highly specialized areas in the brain have territorially local connections and also moderately or very long connections. Any network malfunctioning may be due to damage to a connecting tract, or an area, or both.
The disconnection model has helped to develop the complex architecture of the neuron network on a vast scale, highly complex, consisting of nodes, hubs (*i.e.*, areas where numerous connections between associative areas converge), and connections; in this frame the brain uses not only serial, but also parallel processing methods to cope with the complexity of the higher mental functions. The results of these studies demonstrate that brain connectivity is arranged into what is called a *small world topology*, *i.e.*, small worlds organized in even smaller networks characterized by powerful local connections, but also connected remotely with other small worlds. This organization ensures a high level of local and global connectivity, enabling information to be circulated. The brain is a complex, dynamic system of functionally interconnected regions. Clinical studies and investigations on brain lesions have documented the increasingly complex characteristics of these circuits, and modern neuroimaging techniques have enabled us to see these networks and circuits expand, multiply and vary, and to shed light on their functional complexity and the related impairments, also in developmental age.

The whole is more than the sum of its parts
– Aristotle, (384/3 BC–322 BC)

The higher cognitive functions are the end-product of associative connections between cortical areas where sensory and motor processing takes place. These areas are highly specialized and work in synchrony, forming complex networks that are widely distributed throughout the brain. Lesions involving the cortical areas and/or the white matter cause specific neurobehavioural syndromes and/or impairments that stem from disconnection(s) occurring at one or more points within a network.

By the late 19th century, our understanding of normal brain functioning was based on two fundamental assumptions: that (i) functions are located in discrete areas of the brain; and (ii) these areas are connected by means of white matter pathways. The localization theory was first expounded in 1700 by Gall, a famous scholar of the anatomy of the brain, who also takes the credit for distinguishing between grey matter and white matter, arranged in ascending and descending tracts. Gall's theory envisaged an organologic system in which the brain was divided into 27 centers, each well localized and functionally specialized (*e.g.*, the center of love, the center of lies, and so on), and the variations and functional distinctions between these centers correlated simply with the dimensions of given cortical areas. A subsequent illogical jump led to the conviction that the dimensions of these cortical areas could be deduced from the external configuration of the skull. Such an exaggerated approximation considerably undermined the validity of the original intuition concerning localized functions, but nonetheless gave rise to two schools of thought: in England it paved the way to phrenology, while in France it was the starting point for localization studies, and those conducted by Broca (1824–1840), in particular.

The assumption of a localization of brain functions in different areas of the brain characterized the thinking in the late 19th century, at a time when Broca was studying a patient with a lesion involving the inferior frontal gyrus (still known today as Broca's area),who was unable to speak, but retained a fairly good verbal comprehension. It was Meynert (1833–1892) who recognized the crucial role of the connections between the cortical areas, and who classified the white matter pathways, dividing them into: ascending and descending projection pathways; commissural pathways, of which the prototype is the corpus callosum, which places homologous areas of the two hemispheres in communication, and the anterior commissure connecting the right and left amygdala, the right and left hippocampus, and the regions in this area; and above all into associative fibres, *i.e.*, white matter pathways that connect areas within the same hemisphere, creating complex functional networks, a few examples of which are the cingulate gyrus, the inferior longitudinal fasciculus, the inferior fronto-occipital fasciculus, and the arcuate fasciculus (well known for its role in language processing via the connection between Broca's area and Wernicke's area). In short, the associative and commissural tracts form what is called brain connectivity. This has become an important concept, especially in recent years, as a result of the growing tendency to interpret many neurodevelopmental syndromes, such as autism, ADHD, *etc.*, in the light of disconnectionist syndromes, *i.e.*, conditions in which the circulation of information does not function properly and the output is impaired (Catani & Ffytche, 2005). Brain connectivity is assured by the associative and commissural tracts and works in intricate patterns to integrate the regions of grey matter in functional sets of neurons. White matter consists of myelin, a mixture of lipids (70 per cent) and proteins (30 per cent) produced by the oligodendrocytes (Benarroch, 2009), which creates a concentric sheath all along the axon, leaving some unmyelinated tracts known as Ranvier nodes (Baumann, 2001). The principal function of myelin is to speed up the transmission of information: the conductivity, or conductance, of the myelinated fibers is approximately a hundred times greater than that of the unmyelinated axons. The myelination process continues after birth and up to 50 years of age, and then declines; it particularly concerns the connections between the tertiary associative areas, which are responsible for the multimodal integration of information coming from the sensory cortexes.

The advanced and rich cultural context of the turn of the century was also influenced by the works of Wernicke (1848–1904), who is considered the father of associationism and therefore necessarily of disconnectionism too. According to Wernicke, no mental process (apart from the primary sensory motor cortexes) can be localized in the cortex merely on the strength of an anatomo-functional correlation, as in the phrenological approach; instead, it is the product of mutual interactions that are the outcome of multiple connections passing through the associative fibres. Lesions of the associative tracts consequently cause disconnection syndromes, in which the network fails to function because of a disruption of these connections, giving rise to higher cognitive function disorders. Wernicke's tenacity in focusing on the associative fibres alone, rather than on the specialized areas as well, derives historically from his need to keep his distance from the phrenological theories.

Be that as it may, the historical and cultural scenario was ready for men of exceptional talent to succeed in describing the first disconnection syndromes. It is always worth emphasizing that there is always a logical sequence in the advances made in human culture and knowledge because they are the product of single individuals' insights: in this particular scenario, observing patients, adopting a strict test method, and correlating symptoms with a given lesion led to the identification of the disconnection syndromes, which paved the way for the original concept of the brain's being organized in distributed networks. In the framework of our current understanding, this organization of the brain can also be conceptualized using novel mathematical systems theories, and it can be demonstrated in healthy individuals as well with the aid of the latest neuroimaging techniques.

The following is a brief description of the four classic disconnection syndromes, as formalized during the associationism period of the Wernicke school.

Conduction aphasia was the prototypical syndrome described by Wernicke in his university dissertation, written when he was just 26 years old. Wernicke hypothesized that lesions of the associative tract connecting Broca's and Wernicke's areas cause a disconnection syndrome that is apparent from deficiencies of repetition and paraphasic language, but that leave comprehension and fluency intact. The paraphasias would correlate with the loss of a higher-order internal monitoring that would rely to some degree on the integrity of the connections between the Wernicke and Broca areas. This disconnection would be due to lesions involving the arcuate fasciculus. Lissauer (a pupil of Wernicke's) described cases of visual agnosia, *i.e.*, the inability to name an object caused by an interruption in the pathways between the visual area and the language area, or – in the case of apperceptive agnosia – of the areas enabling the object to be copied. Then Hugo Liepmann described cases of apraxia generated by disconnections between the posterior sensory areas and the areas governing hand movements, such that individual suffering from no form of paralysis and fully able to perform any motor action freely and deliberately, were incapable of completing actions on demand or by imitating others. There is also the pure alexia syndrome described by Joseph Jules Dejerine (1849-1917), which consists in the inability to read despite retaining the ability to write. Dejerine explained pure alexia as a disconnection syndrome, identifying the left angular gyrus as the site of the visual word center. This assumption stemmed from observing two patients, one with stroke of the angular gyrus who had lost the ability to read and write, the other a 68-year-old man with a posterior occipital white matter lesion who suffered from right hemi-anopsia and retained the ability to write, but was no longer able to read. These two cases prompted Dejerine to suggest that visual images of words are stored in the left superior angular gyrus. The identification of this center for visual images went beyond the restriction imposed by Wernicke's thinking, according to which function processing derived entirely from the connections, returning instead to the idea of specialized cortical areas.

It was during this period that Brodmann divided the cortex into discrete areas with different cell architecture characteristics (Brodmann, 1909).

With the subsequent ups and downs in the appeal of localizationism as opposed to associationism, and right up to holism, scientists ultimately lost interest in the controversy.

Much later on, Roger Sperry (an American neuropsychologist awarded the Nobel Prize in Physiology or Medicine in 1981) conducted studies on patients who had undergone corpus callosotomy for unilateral hemispheric epilepsy. These studies demonstrated a hemispheric functional specialization and therefore a localization in the brain of higher cognitive function processing.

In 1965, Geschwind published a famous article in *Brain* that spoke about disconnection syndromes in humans and animals in neo-associationist terms, as being caused by lesions involving the associative cortexes as well as the white matter fibres connecting these areas (Geschwind, 1965).

Geschwind based his scientific conclusions on two fundamental premises, *i.e.*, a myelination gradient and a gradient in the evolution of cross-modality associations. As far as the myelination gradient is concerned, there would appear to be areas of the brain where the white matter is already functioning at birth; Flechsig called these *primordial areas* in his myelogenic map of the human cortex (Flechsig, 1901). These areas are not directly connected to one another initially, but they become so later on, with the development of associative areas. The gradient in the evolution of cross-modality associations consists instead in the evolution of associative areas, which would evolve from primary into secondary and tertiary associative areas, based on increasingly complex levels of integration of multimodal information. In humans, there is no direct connection between the primitive sensory and motor areas (as there is in the rabbit, for instance), while the associative areas are directly connected to one another. With evolution, the associative areas have become increasingly integrated and plurimodal, as in the case of the inferior parietal lobe, and they become free of any integration in the limbic system.

Geschwind conceived brain functioning as relying on a much more widely distributed network than the small networks theorized in the earlier model, and he emphasized the importance of the specialization of the associative areas and of the cortical–subcortical connections. In the article in *Brain* in 1965, Geschwind described numerous disconnection syndromes including: sensory-motor disconnection syndromes relating to discontinuities between the sensory areas and the motor cortex and Broca's area; sensory-limbic disconnection syndromes relating to the connections between the limbic system and sensory areas; and disconnection syndromes (Wernicke's having to do with disconnections between the sensory areas and Wernicke's areas). These syndromes can thus derive from damage either to the white matter or to the associative areas, which represent the relay stations between the primary motor, sensory, and limbic areas. This concept has facilitated the publication of single case studies in the clinical setting, and the development of connectionist theories and, of course, the theory of distributed networks in the field of the neurosciences. Modern functional neuroimaging methods (PET, SPECT, volumetry, fMRI, DTI, *etc.*) are extremely useful when it comes to studying information processing in the localization of functionally specialized systems, and for analyzing white matter pathways, and identifying further functional specializations within the same fascicule.

Advances in the neurosciences have consequently given rise to the current model, defined as hodological and topological, in the sense that it studies pathways and localizations (Catani & Ffytche, 2005). There are specialized areas in the brain that have territorially local connections and also moderately or very long connections. Any network malfunctioning may be due to damage to a long tract, or an area, or both.

The disconnection model has helped to develop the complex architecture of the neuron network on a vast scale, including not only the networks foreseen in the Wernicke and Geschwind models, but also other, highly complex networks consisting of nodes, and hubs (*i.e.*, areas where numerous connections between associative areas converge), switching stations, divergences, feedbacks, connections, and permutations; and the brain uses not only serial but also parallel processing methods to cope with the complexity of the higher mental functions (Bassett & Bullmore, 2006).

In 1990, Mesulam suggested on theoretical grounds that Broca's area and Wernicke's area had connections that are far more widely distributed than those considered in the classical studies on aphasia (Mesulam, 1990), as recently demonstrated by functional resonance and tractographic studies (Mesulam, 2005). To give an example of how modern neuroimaging methods have contributed to a better definition of certain circuits/networks, it is worth mentioning the studies conducted by Catani *et al.* (2005), who re-explored perisylvian language connectivity using *in vivo* diffusion tensor magnetic resonance imaging tractography; they found that Broca's and Wernicke's territories are connected not only *via* the well-known direct pathway, but also through indirect pathways in the normal brain. The direct pathway runs medially and corresponds to the classical descriptions of the arcuate fasciculus. The indirect pathway passes through the inferior parietal cortex, running laterally, and comprises an anterior segment connecting the inferior parietal cortex (Geschwind's territory) to Broca's territory, and a posterior segment connecting Geschwind's and Wernicke's territories. The direct pathway would be responsible for repetition and consequently for processing the more phonological aspects of language, while the indirect pathways would be more involved in managing the semantic component in vocalization (the anterior segment) and comprehension (the posterior segment).

This model of two parallel pathways helps to explain the heterogeneous clinical presentations of conduction aphasia (Catani *et al.*, 2005).

Our better anatomo-functional understanding of the perisylvian language networks also enables us to describe hyperfunctioning conditions that are expressed by the onset of positive signs. A dysfunctioning of the indirect pathways during the generation and monitoring of inner speech would cause the acoustic hallucinations typical of schizophrenia, while hyperfunctioning of the direct pathway would be responsible for an excessive tendency for repetition expressed in the form of the echolalia seen in some neurodevelopmental disorders, such as autism (Wass, 2011).

The network connecting Wernicke's and Broca's areas consists of more than just two pathways (one direct and one indirect), however. In fact, Bernal and Ardila (Bernal & Ardila, 2009) used tractography to study the role of the arcuate fasciculus in conduction aphasia, and proposed a new language network model, emphasizing that the arcuate fasciculus connects posterior brain areas to Broca's area *via* a relay station in the premotor/motor areas (Brodmann's area 6), and consequently questioning the existence of a direct pathway. Electrocortical studies have also demonstrated that the arcuate fasciculus not only transmits information from the temporal to the frontal areas, but also in the opposite direction; the transfer of speech information from the temporal to the frontal lobe relies on two different streams, and conduction aphasia can occur in cases of cortical damage not extending to the subcortex. The information flow between

Broca's and Wernicke's areas therefore works both ways. In fact, in addition to a language that lacks fluency and is agrammatical, patients with Broca's aphasia often have morphosyntactic comprehension difficulties; patients with Wernicke's aphasia, on the other hand, may experience semantic or phonological paraphasias and have paragrammatical disorders.

The arcuate fasciculus serves an important purpose in language development by facilitating the repetition of phonological clues, and therefore helping in language learning and speech monitoring. The arcuate fasciculus may serve as an additional aid, facilitating repetition or monitoring speech at the phonological level. These theories suggest that the processes involved in speech production are the same as those participating in speech perception. In other words, the two-way transfer of information would indicate that, to some extent, information about language production is important to understanding language. It may have a dual role in speech as well, monitoring speech production and providing information on verbal output.

Understanding and defining all the components in a more distributed network may thus help us to understand the heterogeneity of certain clinical pictures.

The network connecting the areas responsible for language processing also involves the cerebellum, which projects contralateraly to the prefrontal cortexes, and Broca's area in particular, via the thalamus, receiving feedback from the pontis. A recent diffusion tensor imaging (DTI) study confirmed these cerebellar projections towards the prefrontal and posterior parietal cortexes *in vivo* using tractography (Jissendi *et al.*, 2008). We used fMRI to study ten healthy right-handed children from 7 to 15 years old and found that verbal fluency models activate Broca's area, Wernicke's area, the supplementary motor area of the left hemisphere, and the right cerebellar hemisphere, with a negative linear correlation between the cerebellar lateralization index and the frontal supratentorial lateralization index.

Finally, the part played by mathematical models in formulating and interpreting mental functioning should be mentioned. Numerical models enable us to investigate mathematical brain functioning hypotheses (graph theory) and then test them with the aid of neuroimaging methods, particularly using resting state fMRI. For this test, individuals have no active tasks to perform, no external afferences; they keep their eyes closed and their hands still; and remain simply in a state of rest, letting their minds wander, without thinking about anything in particular. The results of these studies demonstrate that brain connectivity is arranged into what is called a *small world topology*, that is, small worlds organized in even smaller networks characterized by powerful local connections, but also connected remotely with other small worlds. This organization ensures a high level of local and global connectivity, enabling information to be circulated (Gerloff & Hallett, 2010). This model supports the existence of super-specialized areas, since the small worlds are areas exhibiting a very strong cohesion with one another that process certain component parts of consciousness in a highly specialized manner, and that also have a far-reaching, distributed but integrated information processing capacity.

The brain's functional connectivity is also dynamic. The networks consist of nodes or hubs (where processing takes place), with links between these nodes that enable interactions and exchanges of information. In adults, resting state fMRI identifies activation particularly of the multimodal associative areas (precuneus/posterior cingulate cortex, medial PFC, anterior cingulate cortex, bilateral parietal lobe, and bilateral insula), while in children activation is more prevalent in the homomodal cortexes (the primary sensory and motor areas), and less so in the prefrontal cortex (Fransson *et al.*, 2011).

This functional connectivity is inter-hemispheric before it becomes intra-hemispheric: Nature initially creates the right conditions for the hemispheres to communicate with one another, then it enables the associative areas within the hemispheres to form connections. In children, the connections between the somatosensory areas and the subcortical connections are more strongly represented than the cortical connections, and there is a more limited hierarchical organization, but by the time they are 7–9 years old, their brains' organization into small worlds is much the same as in adults. Any disruption of their development or destruction of the brain's connectivity gives rise to a wide variety of neurodevelopmental disorders, such as autism, the whole complex picture of which is the outcome of such a distorted connectivity and a condition of functional underconnectivity (Uddin *et al.*, 2010).

In conclusion, the brain is a complex dynamic system of functionally interconnected regions. Clinical studies and investigations on brain lesions have documented the increasingly complex characteristics of these circuits, and modern neuroimaging techniques have enabled us to see these networks and circuits expand, multiply and vary, enabling us to shed light on their functional complexity and the related impairments and disconnection syndromes.

Graph theory has been used successfully to describe the organization of these dynamic systems. Recent resting state fMRI studies have suggested that the brain's inter-regional functional connectivity features a small-world topology, indicating an organization of the brain in highly clustered sub-networks (in which voxels are connected mainly with their direct neighbors), combined with a high level of global connectivity.

Within the complex network of multiple 'nodes' and 'links' inside the brain, the notion that only one place in the brain is responsible for anything is tantamount to phrenology. Nodes in large-scale neuronal networks usually represent anatomic regions, while links represent functional or effective connections. The brain requires an optimal balance between regional segregation and inter-regional, global integration of neuronal activity. So, for us to understand pathologic brain states, it seems crucial to ascertain what happens to brain network structure and function. Functional connectivity studies have consistently demonstrated impairments in numerous neurodevelopmental disorders, including autism (Shukla, 2010).

References

Bassett, D.S. & Bullmore, E. (2006): Small-world brain networks. *Neuroscientist* **12,** 512–523.

Baumann, N. & Pham-Dinh, D. (2001): Biology of oligodendrocyte and myelin in the mammalian central nervous system. *Physiol. Rev.* **81,** 871–927.

Benarroch, E. (2009): Oligodendrocytes susceptibility to injury and involvement in neurologic disease. *Neurology* **72,** 1779–1785.

Bernal, B. & Ardila, A. (2009): The role of the arcuate fasciculus in conduction aphasia. *Brain* **132,** 2309–2316.

Brodmann, K.(1909): Vergleichende Lokalisationslehre der Grosshirnrinde. In: *Ihren Prinzipien dargestellt auf Grund des Zellenbaues.* Leipzig: Johann Ambrosius Bart.

Catani, M. & Ffytche, D.H. (2005): The rises and falls of disconnection syndromes. *Brain* **128,** 2224–2239.

Catani, M., Derek, K.J. & Ffytche, D.H. (2005): Perisylvian language networks of the human brain. *Ann. Neurol.* **57,** 8–16.

Damoiseaux, J.S. & Greicius, M.D. (2009): Greater than the sum of its parts: a review of studies combining structural connectivity and resting-state functional connectivity. *Brain Struct. Funct.* **213,** 525–533.

Flechsig, P. (1901): Developmental (myelogenetic) localisation of the cerebral cortex in the human subject. *Lancet* **2,** 1027–1029.

Fransson, P., Aden, U., Blennow, M. & Lagercrantz, H. (2011): The functional architecture of the infant brain as revealed by resting-state fMRI. *Cerebral Cortex* **21,** 145–154.

Gerloff, C. & Hallett, M. (2010): Big news from small world networks after stroke. *Brain* **133,** 952–955.

Geschwind, N. (1965): Disconnexion syndromes in animals and man. *Brain* **88,** 237–94.

Jissendi, P., Baudry, S. & Balériaux, D. (2008): Diffusion tensor imaging (DTI) and tractography of the cerebellar projections to prefrontal and posterior parietal cortices: a study at 3T. *J. Neuroradiol.* **35,** 42–50.

Mesulam, M.M. (1990): Large-scale neurocognitive networks and distributed processing for attention, language, and memory. *Ann. Neurol.* **28,** 597–613.

Mesulam, M.M. (2005): Imaging connectivity in the human cerebral cortex: the next frontier? *Ann. Neurol.* **57,** 5–7.

Shukla, J. (2010): White matter compromise of callosal and subcortical fiber tracts in children with autism spectrum disorder: a diffusion tensor imaging study. *Am. Acad. Child Adolesc. Psychiatry* **49,** 1269–1278.

Uddin, L., Supekar, K. & Menon, V. (2010): Typical and atypical development of functional human brain networks: insights from resting-state fMRI. *Frontiers in System Neurosciences* **4,** 1–21.

Wass, S. (2011): Distortions and disconnections: disrupted brain connectivity in autism. *Brain Cognit.* **75,** 18–28.

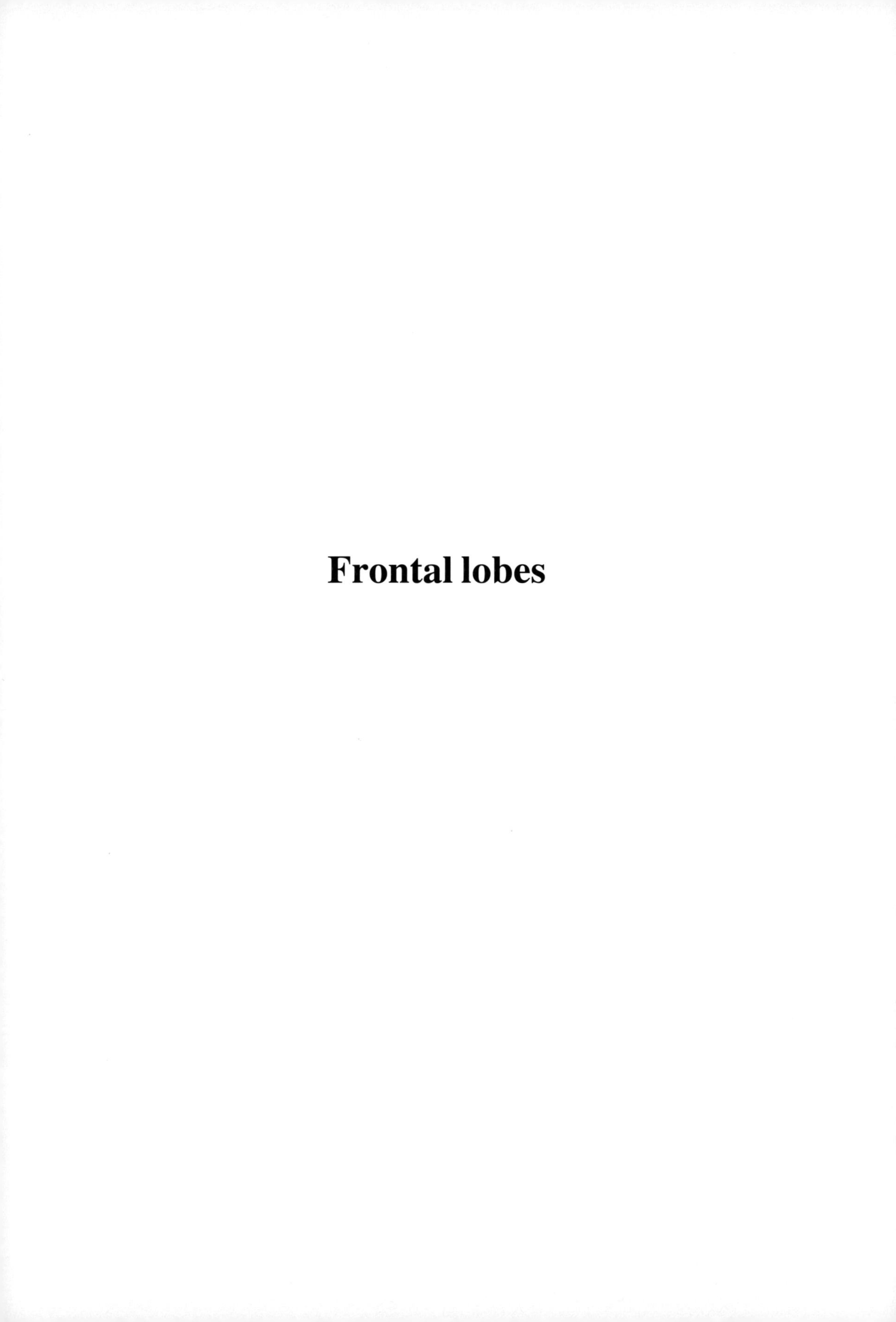

Frontal lobes

Brain Lesion Localization and Developmental Functions, D. Riva, C. Njiokiktjien and S. Bulgheroni (eds.)
© 2011 John Libbey Eurotext, pp. 11–18.

Chapter 2

Frontal lobes: anatomy, connections and functions

Alessandra Erbetta

Neuroradiology Department, Fondazione IRCCS Istituto Neurologico 'C. Besta', via Celoria 11, 20133 Milan, Italy
aerbetta@istituto-besta.it

Summary

The frontal lobes, which are the focus of the present article, comprise several architectonic areas in the human brain. Neuroimaging studies can provide some evidence about the anatomy and functional contribution of these areas by demonstrating overall increases in activity within particular regions in relation to various aspects of motor, language and cognitive processing.

In this analysis we consider frontal lobe anatomy and connections with other cortical regions and frontal lobe projections with basal ganglia, thalamus, and cerebellum and describe the clinical manifestations arising from frontal lobe lesions.

Introduction

The frontal lobe is not a single anatomic and functional brain region. Several lines of research, such as behavioural, electrophysiologic, clinical, and neuroimaging studies, have demonstrated that particular subregions within the frontal lobe are associated with specific motor and cognitive functions. Recent advancements in magnetic resonance (MR) techniques have provided a great deal of meaningful neurobiologic information, allowing non-invasive investigations into the brain, even in children. By means of powerful MR equipment and highly specialized methods it is now possible to employ MR neuroimaging techniques to map such important neurobiologic indexes as the brain functions themselves, detailed local neuroanatomic correlates of cortical organization, and brain functional, anatomic, and effective connectivity. The noninvasiveness of neuroimaging techniques permits their repeated use over time, which is crucially important to discern the temporal impact of any strategy of treatment. Voxel-based morphometry (VBM), an unbiased technique that is operator-independent, is designed to detect statistically significant differences in grey and white matter cerebral tissues between groups. Diffusion tensor imaging (DTI) is a technique that allows demonstration of fibre tracts *in vivo* in humans. The recent introduction of functional magnetic resonance imaging (fMRI) to investigate the functionality of brain physiology and pathology has substantially enhanced the possibilities of studying the workings of the human brain.

In this analysis we consider frontal lobe connections with other cortical regions and frontal lobe projections with basal ganglia, thalamus, and cerebellun and describe the clinical manifestations arising from frontal lobe lesions.

Review of the topic

The frontal lobe is considerably larger in humans than in the rest of the hominoids and constitutes the latest area of the brain to develop.

The landmarks separating the frontal lobe from the rest of the hemisphere are the central sulcus or Rolandic fissure, posteriorly, and the Sylvian fissure, laterally. The anterior, superior, and inferior boundaries are defined by their natural limits. The callosal sulcus constitutes the inferior boundary on the medial wall of the hemisphere (Nieuwenhuys *et al.*, 2008). Traditional classification systems divide the frontal lobe into the following areas: primary motor cortex, prefrontal cortex (extending from the frontal poles to the primary motor cortex, and including the frontal operculum, dorsolateral and superior mesial regions), orbitofrontal cortex (including orbitobasal and inferior mesial regions), and mesial regions containing the cingulate gyrus. These regions are tightly connected to each other, to other cortical regions, and to subcortical structures, such as the basal ganglia, thalamus, and cerebellum.

In the frontal lobe the primary motor region acquires myelin earlier than do the premotor and prefrontal regions. Fibres from and to associative areas of the prefrontal cortex continue to myelinate into the third and fourth decades of life. The prefrontal cortex is the latest brain structure to develop, both phylogenetically and ontogenetically.The time course of prefrontal maturation makes it possible that myelination is a basis for the gradual development of prefrontal functions, such as increased capacity of the working memory, regulation of attention, planning, and mental flexibility (Crespo-Facorro *et al.*, 1999).

Cortical regions

The *primary motor cortex* runs vertically between the Rolandic fissure and the precentral sulcus. It is the major source of corticospinal and corticobulbar pyramidal tracts (Fig. 1), and has been traditionally considered to control voluntary movement. The primary motor cortex is typically activated during finger-tapping tasks on fMR examination (Fig. 2).

The *inferior frontal gyrus* (IFG) is located in the frontal operculum. The anterior horizontal ramus and the anterior ascending ramus of the Sylvian fissure divide the IFG into the pars orbitalis, pars triangularis, and pars opercularis. The posterior portion (pars triangularis and pars opercularis) of the left IFG is the seat of Broca's area, which is dedicated to speech (Fig. 3). Functional imaging studies about language organization involving healthy subjects demonstrate activation of the pars triangularis in semantic tasks and the pars opercularis in syntax/phonology (Buckner *et al.*, 1995). The contribution of the right Broca's homologue to language includes prosody, discourse, and the processing of syntactic violations (Kaplan *et al.*, 2010; Nichelli *et al.*, 1995).

Projections from Broca's area to the superior temporal gyrus have been implied by a number of fMRI studies, suggesting functional connectivity (Binder *et al.*, 1887; Ford *et al.*, 2010), as well as by diffusion-weighted MRI, suggesting structural connectivity. Catani and colleagues (2005) demonstrated direct as well as indirect connections between Broca's and Wernicke's areas serving phonological and semantic functions, respectively. Functional and structural

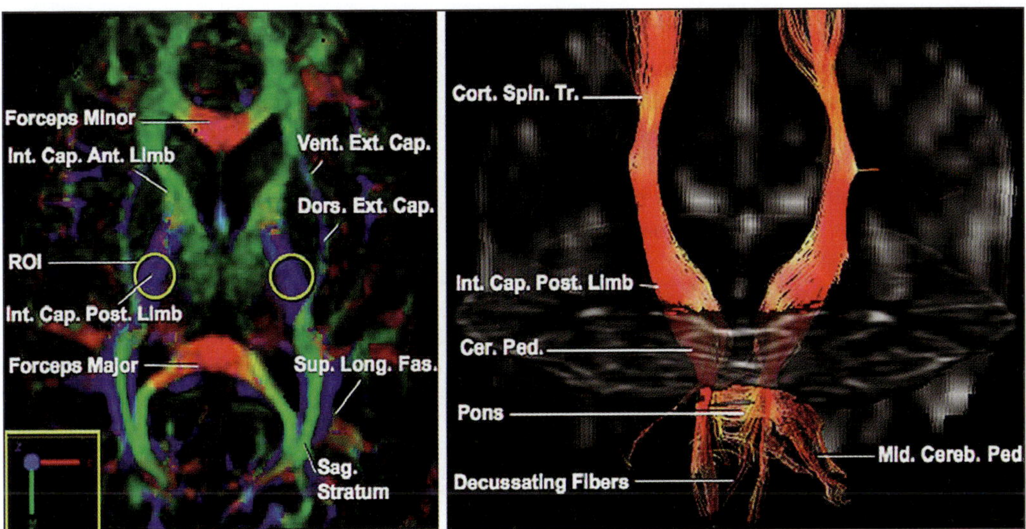

Fig. 1. Diffusion tensor imaging (DTI) in studying the corticospinal tract. The regions of interest (ROIs) are positioned in the posterior limb of the internal capsules.

connectivity of Broca's area with the medial frontal cortex were also investigated. Ford and colleagues (2010) showed connections with Brodmann's areas (BA) 9, 8, and 6 (both supplementary motor area [SMA] in caudal BA 6, and pre-SMA in rostral BA 6). Trajectories follow an anterior-to-posterior gradient, wherein the most anterior portions of Broca's area connect to BA 9 and 8, whereas the posterior Broca's area connects to pre-SMA and SMA.

The superior frontal gyrus (SFG) consists of the first large gyrus on the superior aspect of the lateral surface of the frontal cortex. It is a large frontal subregion that overlaps the superior margin of the hemisphere and extends onto the medial surface. The supplementary frontal eye field (BA 8), and BA 9 (involved in attention) are usually included in this gyrus. The supplementary motor area (BA 6) represents a rostral expansion of the frontal agranular motor cortex on the medial and superior walls of the hemisphere. The SMA is formed by two anatomically and functionally distinct areas: pre-SMA (rostral part) and the SMA proper (caudal part). The pre-SMA is involved in language, internal representation of time, and internal selection of movement, and it is activated during 'complex' tasks requiring selection of response. It is connected to the thalamus, caudate nucleus, and cerebellum. The SMA proper seems to be involved in motor functions and it is connected to the primary motor area, putamen, and globus pallidus.

The *middle frontal gyrus* (MFG) is usually defined as the lateral frontal cortex that lies between the SFG and IFG. The intermediate frontal sulcus splits the MFG into a superior and an inferior portion. The dorsolateral prefrontal cortex, involved in several critical cognitive functions, is partially located on the MFG and in SFG.

The *dorsolateral prefrontal cortex* (DLPFC) is a functional area. It is located in the upper and lateral aspects of the prefrontal cortex. It receives connections from the parietal and temporal lobes, which convey information regarding location, objects and their meaning, and the face and emotional status of others. The dorsolateral prefrontal areas play a role in the control, regulation, and integration of cognitive activities. It mediates attention and focus, controls distractibility, maintains focus of the cognitive set as well as flexible shifts of the cognitive set

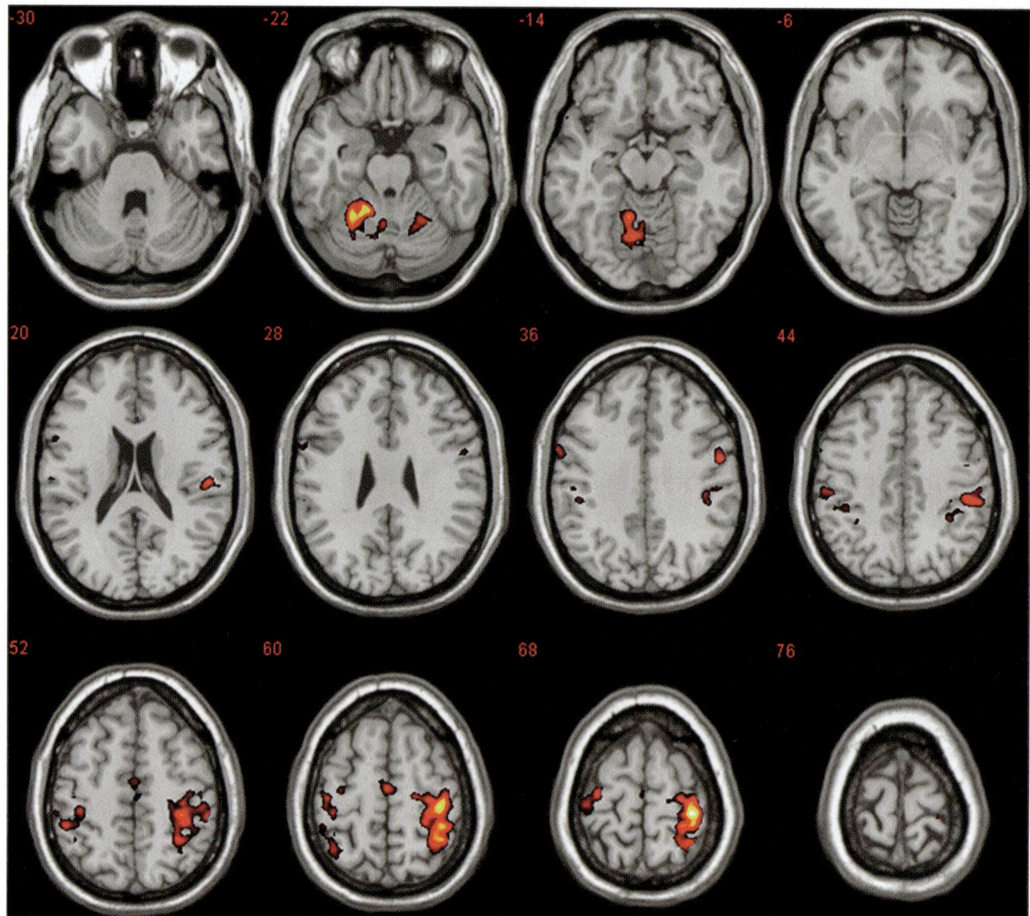

Fig. 2. fMRI study shows activation of the primary motor cortex on the left side during a finger-tapping task for the right hand in eight right-handed volunteers. Note also the activation of the right cerebellum and the caudal or SMA proper.

when required, and is involved in memory and generating fluent verbal and nonverbal activity. The DLPFC also plays an important role in working memory, which refers to the ability to retain information so that it can be used for a few seconds.

The *anterior and superior cingulate gyrus* is located in the medial surface of the frontal lobe. It has extensive and anatomic connections to the prefrontal, orbitofrontal, and parietal neocortex, and receives projections from ventral tegmental areas of the midbrain and anterior pole of thalamus. It is a part of the limbic system and it is involved in several psychological functions such as motivation, attention, and emotion (Mesulam, 1981). Subcallosal regions of the cingulate gyrus, which are most directly connected to the orbitofrontal cortex, are more involved in the regulation of autonomic nervous system functions. Supracallosal regions of the cingulate gyrus appear to activate during more effortful activities during the early stages of learning or when increased attention and arousal are required. Given its central role in attention, arousal, emotion, and motivation, it is not surprising that damage to the cingulate circuit results in decreased motivation, apathy, monosyllabic verbal responses, poor attention, and hypokinesia.

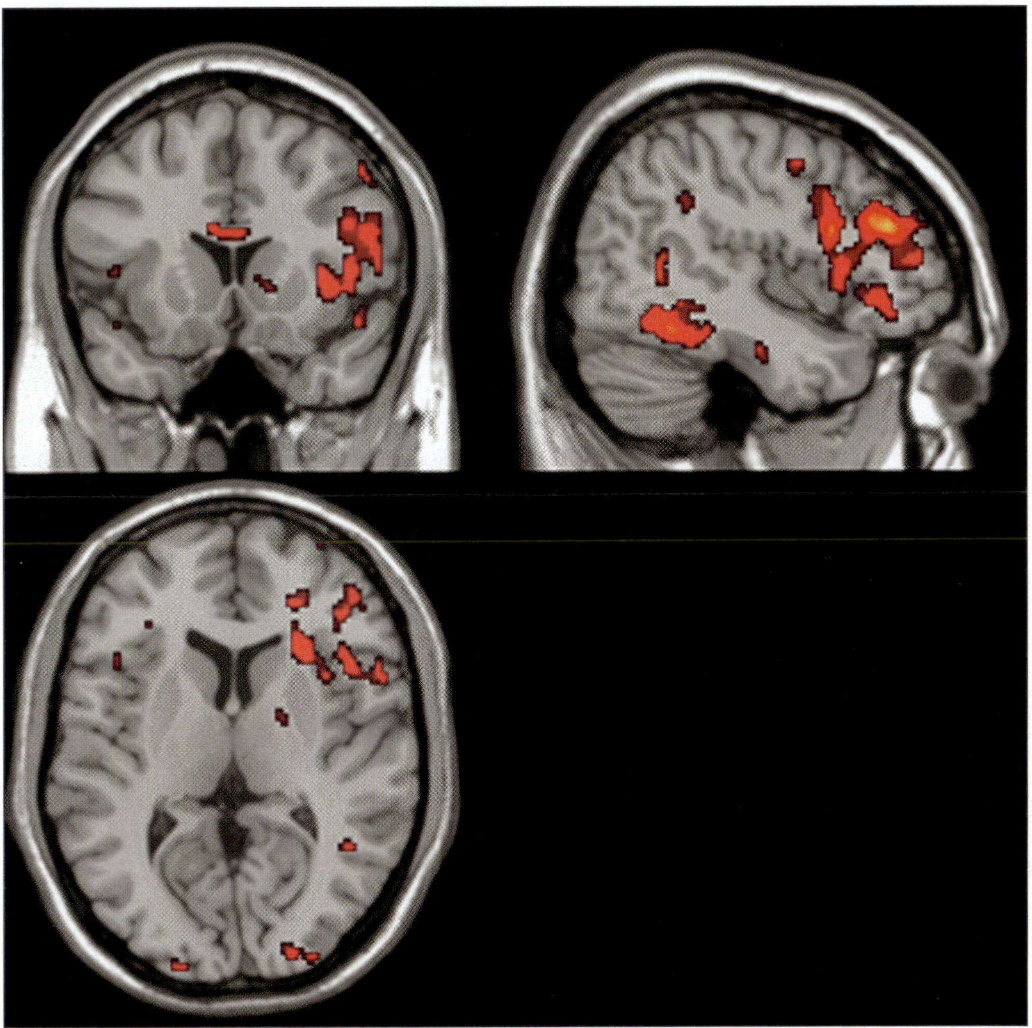

Figure 3. fMRI study shows activation of the IFG in a group of right-handed volunteers during an overt verbal fluency task.

The *straight gyrus* (SG) lies along the ventromedial margin of the frontal lobe medial to the olfactory sulcus. Animal studies have reported that the SG is a part of the anterior limbic system and is specifically connected to auditory cortex neurons in the convexity of the superior temporal gyrus.

The *orbitofrontal cortex* is a large cytoarchitectonically heterogeneous region of the ventral prefrontal cortex. It is considered to be a component of the limbic system and it is involved in two subcircuits. The lateral orbitofrontal subcircuit projects to the ventromedial caudate, globus pallidus/substantia nigra pars reticulata, ventral anterior nucleus of the thalamus, and back to the medial orbitofrontal cortex. The medial orbital subcircuit follows a similar pathway, but initially projects to the ventral striatum. These circuits integrate emotional and autonomic information and memories into behavioral programs. They are involved in the modulation of social behavior, including aspects of empathy, morality, self-monitoring, and social restraint.

Associative pathways

The *cingulum* is a medial associative bundle that runs within the cingulated gyrus all around the corpus callosum. It contains fibres of different length, the longest of which runs from the anterior temporal gyrus to the orbitofrontal cortex. The short U-shaped fibres connect the medial frontal, parietal, occipital, and temporal lobes and different portions of the cingulated cortex. The cingulum is part of the limbic system and is involved in attention, memory and emotions (Catani & Thiebaut de Schotten, 2008).

The uncinate fasciculus is a ventral associative bundle that connects the anterior temporal lobe with the medial and lateral orbitofrontal cortex (Catani *et al.*, 2002). This fasciculus is considered to belong to the limbic system, but its functions are poorly understood. It is possible that the uncinate fasciculus is involved in processing emotions as well as in memory and language functions (Catani & Mesulam, 2008).

The *inferior fronto-occipital fasciculus* is a ventral associative bundle that connects the ventral occipital lobe and the orbitofrontal cortex. In its occipital course the inferior fronto-occipital fasciculus runs parallel to the inferior longitudinal fasciculus. On approaching the anterior temporal lobe, the fibres of the inferior fronto-occipital fasciculus gather together and enter the external capsule dorsal to the fibres of the uncinate fasciculus. The functions of the inferior fronto-occipital fasciculus are poorly understood, although it is possible that it participates in reading (Catani & Mesulam, 2008), attention, and visual processing. The inferior fronto-occipital fasciculus may only exist in the human brain (Catani & Thiebaut de Schotten, 2008).

Arcuate fasciculus is a lateral associative bundle composed of long and short fibres connecting the perisylvian cortex of the frontal, parietal, and temporal lobes. The short fibres lie more laterally than the long fibres. The arcuate fasciculus of the left hemisphere is involved in language (Catani & Thiebaut de Schotten, 2008; Catani & Mesulam, 2008) and praxis. The arcuate fasciculus of the right hemisphere is involved in visuospatial processing and some aspects of language, such as prosody and semantic functions (Catani & Thiebaut de Schotten, 2008).

Frontal-subcortical circuits

Neuroanatomic, electrophysiologic, and neuroimaging studies show that there are multiple parallel loops, or circuits, in the corticostriatal system, each of which comprises a parent cerebral cortical area (motor, association, or limbic cortex) that projects in a topographically arranged manner to nuclei of the basal ganglia, which project in turn via the thalamus back to the cortical region of origin (Lehericy *et al.*, 2004). Each of these segregated loops supports distinct domains of behaviour. Sensorimotor and parietal intramodality sensory association cortices project predominantly to the dorsal and mid-sectors of the putamen. Association areas in prefrontal cortices project preferentially to the caudate nucleus. Orbital and medial prefrontal cortices and the cingulate gyrus project to the ventral striatum (Lehericy *et al.*, 2004).

The major behaviour-cognitive syndromes that arise from basal ganglia lesions such as working memory, strategy formation, cognitive flexibility, obsessive-compulsive disorder and apathy, reflect the anatomic connections with the cerebral cortex.

Deficits in executive function and spatial cognition caused by lesions of the rostral head of the caudate nucleus reflect the connections with the dorsolateral prefrontal cortex (DLPFC), which is concerned with personal and extra-personal space.

Limbic behaviours, such as disinhibition, irritability and obsessive-compulsive disorders, result from lesions of the ventral striatum, reflecting connections with the medial prefrontal and anterior cingulate gyrus.

Extrapyramidal motor syndromes result from lesions of the dorsal and mid-regions of the putamen, which receive afferents from motor cortex. Motor and behavioural consequences of pallidotomy are also determined by the location of the lesion. Rostral and dorsomedial globus pallidus internus (GPi) lesions (linked to prefrontal cortical areas 9 and 46) produce impaired semantic fluency, impaired mathematical ability, and memory interference. Posterior and ventrolateral regions of GPi (linked to motor cortical areas) have a beneficial impact on bradykinesia, but no influence on cognitive performance (Schmahmann & Pandya, 2008).

Frontal-cerebellar circuits

The role of the cerebellum in modulating motor functions of the brain has been established. The cerebellum is now recognized as playing an important role in regulating such processes as language, visuospatial organization, memory and planning, emotional response, and personality (Riva *et al.*, 2000; Schmahaman, 1997; Van Dongen *et al.*, 1994). Some cognitive deficits that occur after damage to the cerebellum bear a strong resemblance to the pattern deficit that occurs after a lesion to the prefrontal cortex. The DLPFC and cerebellum are activated at the same time during performance of a number of different types of cognitive tasks. Neuroanatomic and neuroimaging studies (Jissendi *et al.*, 2008) reveal that the DLPFC projects to the neocerebellum and receives projections from the neocerebellum, via dentate nucleus, brainstem, and anterior thalamus. The prefrontal areas identified to receive direct output from the dentate nucleus are BA 9 and BA 46. These areas have been reported to be involved in working memory performances.

Conclusions

In this analysis we have considered frontal lobe anatomy, functions, and connections with other cortical regions and frontal lobe projections with basal ganglia, thalamus, and cerebellum, and we describe the clinical manifestations arising from frontal lobe lesions. Neuroimaging research continues as the pre-eminent technique for evaluation of the frontal lobe. MRI technique allowed quantitative measurement of frontal volume, facilitating studies on the role of the frontal cortex or white matter lesions in the pathogenesis of a wide variety of motor, language, cognitive, and behavioural syndromes. fMRI is a powerful tool that has dramatically changed research into the frontal lobes by allowing noninvasive evaluation *in vivo*. Another exciting development with fMRI has been the mapping of networks activated with cognitive tasks or during rest. Understanding the frontal lobes will lead to advances against a wide variety of neurologic and psychiatric conditions.

References

Binder, J.R., Frost. J.A., Hammeke, T.A., *et al.* (1997): Human brain language areas identified by functional magnetic resonance imaging. *J. Neurosci.* **17,** 353–362.

Buckner, R.L., Raichle, M.E. & Peterson, S.E. (1995): Dissociation of human prefrontal cortical areas across different speech production tasks and gender groups. *J. Neurophysiol.* **74,** 2163–2173.

Catani, M. & Mesulam, M. (2008): The arcuate fasciculus and the disconnection theme in language and aphasia: history and current state. *Cortex* **44,** 953–961.

Catani, M. & Thiebaut de Schotten, M. (2008): A diffusion tensor imaging tractography atlas for virtual in vivo dissections. *Cortex* **44,** 1105–1132.

Catani, M., Howard, R.J., Pajevic, S., *et al.* (2002): Virtual in vivo interactive dissection of white matter fasciculi in the human brain. *NeuroImage* **17,** 77–94.

Catani, M., Jones, D.K. & Ffytche, D.H. (2005): Perisylvian language networks of the human brain. *Ann. Neurol.* **57,** 8–16.

Crespo-Facorro, B., Kim, J.J., Andreasen, N.C., *et al.* (1999): Human frontal cortex: and MRI-based parcellation method. *NeuroImage* **10,** 500–519.

Ford, A., McGregor, K.M., Case, K., *et al.* (2010): Structural connectivity of Broca's area and medial frontal cortex. *NeuroImage* **52,** 1230–1237.

Jissendi, P., Baudry, S. & Baleriaux, D. (2008): Diffusion tensor imaging (DTI) and tractography of the cerebellar projections to prefrontal and posterior parietal cortices: a study at 3T. *J. Neuroradiol.* **35,** 42–50.

Kaplan, E., Naeser, M.A., Martin, P.I., *et al.* (2010): Horizontal portino of arcuate fasciculus fibers track to pars opercularis, not pars triangularis, in right and left hemisphere: a DTI study. *NeuroImage* **52,** 436–444.

Lehericy, S., Ducros, M., Van de Moortele, P.F., *et al.* (2004): Diffusion tensor fiber tracking shows distinct cortico-striatal circuits in humans. *Ann. Neurol.* **55,** 522–529.

Mesulam, M.M. (1981): A cortical network for directed attention and unilateral neglect. *Ann. Neurol.* **10,** 309–325.

Nichelli, P., Grafman, J., Pietrini, P., *et al.* (1995): Where the brain appreciates the moral of a story. *NeuroReport* **6,** 2309–2313.

Nieuwenhuys, R., Voogd, J. & van Huijzen, C. (2008): *The Human Central Nervous System.* 4th ed. Berlin: Springer-Verlag.

Riva, D. (2000): The cerebellum contributes to higher cognitive and social behaviour in childhood: evidence from acquired cerebellar lesions. In: *Localization of Brain Lesions and Developmental Functions*, eds. D. Riva & A. Benton, pp. 151–60, Mariani Foundation Paediatric Neurology Series – IX. London: John Libbey & Company Ltd.

Van Dongen, H.R., Catsman-Berrevoets, C.E. & Van Mourik, M. (1994): The syndrome of 'cerebellar' mutism and subsequent dysarthria. *Neurol.* **44,** 2041–2045.

Schmahmann, J.D. (1997): *The Cerebellum and Cognition.* New York: Academic Press.

Schmahmann, J.D. & Pandya, D.N. (2008): Disconnections syndromes of basal ganglia, thalamus and cerebrocerebellar systems. *Cortex* **44,** 1037–1066.

Brain Lesion Localization and Developmental Functions, D. Riva, C. Njiokiktjien and S. Bulgheroni (eds.)

Chapter 3

Role of the parieto-frontal mirror system

Leonardo Fogassi

Department of Neurosciences, University of Parma, via Volturno 39, 43100 Parma, Italy; Italian Institute of Technology (RTM), University of Parma, Parma, Italy; Department of Psychology, University of Parma, Parma, Italy
leonardo.fogassi@unipr.it

Summary

In the last three decades the concept of the cortical motor system has changed deeply since neuroanatomic and neurophysiological investigations have demonstrated that this system includes reciprocal parieto-premotor connections responsible for sensorimotor transformation and that its neurons are not simply involved in the execution of movement, as previously maintained, but also code the goal of motor acts and actions. From this high-level motor organization cognitive properties emerge, such as action understanding. Many studies have shown that this capacity is mediated by mirror neurons, a class of premotor and parietal visuomotor neurons in the monkey that activate both during action execution and during action observation. Thus, these neurons constitute a matching system, enabling individuals to automatically understand others' actions. Here the main features of mirror neurons in monkeys and the evidence of the presence of a similar mirror system in humans is described. Then, the way in which the mirror system is involved in intention understanding is shown in both monkeys and humans. Finally, the issue of the plasticity of the mirror system is addressed, suggesting its possible use in rehabilitation in humans.

Introduction

Classical behavioural and psychophysical studies (Jeannerod, 1988; Rosenbaum *et al.*, 2007) and more recent neurophysiological experiments (see Fogassi, 2009) have shown that the motor system is organized at different levels. At the top level we can put *action*. Action has an ultimate goal (*e.g.*, eating a piece of apple) and is formed by a series of motor acts. *Motor acts*, which constitute the second level, are movements aimed towards a goal (*e.g.*, grasping a piece of apple or bringing it to the mouth). The *movement* is the third level and can be defined as the displacement of single joints. In order to attain the intended goal of an action, single motor acts must be organized into structured sequences and fluently linked with each other. Each motor act is accomplished by combining two or more movements in a synergic way. All the described levels are represented in different sectors of the motor system. Actions and motor acts are coded by higher-order cortical areas, and movements are coded by primary motor cortex or even by subcortical areas. Finally, movements are implemented through commands of spinal motor neurons to muscles. This premise constitutes a background for understanding that cognitive properties, contrary to what was previously thought, can emerge from motor organization.

A traditional view of the brain's information processing emphasized the role of the posterior part of cortex in elaborating uni-modal or poly-modal sensory input in order to achieve perception. In this view, the role of the frontal part of the cortex and, in particular, of the motor cortex, was that of producing behavioural responses appropriate to the objects of perception. Thanks to the work of the past three decades, this clear-cut distinction between action and perception was challenged, and the concept of the cortical flow of information changed. In fact, many neurophysiological experiments in the macaque monkey demonstrated that the motor cortex (*i.e.*, the posterior half of the frontal lobe) stores motor representations that can be directly addressed by sensory inputs, through the reciprocal anatomic connections between parietal and frontal motor cortices (Rizzolatti *et al.*, 1998). Thus, it became clear that action and perception are strictly linked and, in some sense, represent two different aspects of our means of achieving a knowledge of the world.

A first important finding that changed the concept of the motor cortex was that neurons of this cortical sector discharge during goal-related motor acts, such as reaching for an object, pushing it, grasping it, *etc.*, rather than during simple movements, such as joint dislocations. In particular, single neurons of ventral premotor area F5 activate when a monkey executes motor acts such as grasping, manipulating, holding, or tearing objects (Rizzolatti *et al.*, 1988). Some of them show a high level of goal abstraction, discharging when the monkey grasps food with the left hand, with the right hand, or with the mouth and, as has been recently reported, when the goal is achieved not only with the natural effector (*i.e.*, the hand or the mouth), but also with a tool, after a period of motor training in the use of it (Umiltà *et al.*, 2008). In this study, monkeys had to learn to grasp a piece of food with normal or inverted pliers, so that the finger movements that allowed the animal to take possession of food were opposite in the two cases. It has been found that the same neuron discharged when the monkey closed the fingers to achieve the food (normal pliers) or when it extended them (inverted pliers), thus coding the goal of the act independent of the type of movement employed to achieve it.

Altogether, these findings suggest that neurons of area F5 represent an 'internal motor knowledge' or a 'storage' of motor representations. This storage can be addressed by sensory inputs through the anatomic connections between parietal and motor cortex (see Rizzolatti *et al.*, 1998), thus allowing two main functions: (*a*) the transformation of an external input (*e.g.*, an object) into a motor format (*e.g.*, grasping); and (*b*) a sensorimotor matching mechanism, providing an automatic attribution of motor meaning to the sensory input addressing motor representations. Because of their joint action in the realization of these processes, the parietal and motor cortex can be included in the same 'motor system'. As a matter of fact, many neurons of the motor cortex respond to several types of sensory inputs, and many neurons of parietal cortex show motor properties beyond the sensory ones.

An example of a sensorimotor process that allows the individual to achieve a specific understanding of the external world is the mirror matching mechanism. In the next section the basic properties of mirror neurons in the monkey and of the mirror system in humans will be described.

Review of the topic

Mirror neurons in the monkey

Mirror neurons (MNs), as first described in area F5 of the monkey ventral premotor cortex, are visuomotor neurons that activate when the monkey *performs* a hand or mouth goal-directed motor act (*e.g.*, grasping, biting, tearing, or manipulating an object) and when it *observes* the same, or a similar, act performed by the experimenter or by a conspecific (Di Pellegrino *et al.*, 1992; Gallese *et al.*, 1996; Ferrari *et al.*, 2003; Rizzolati *et al.*, 1996a). The response of most MNs is invariant with respect to many visual aspects, such as distance, type of object, or hand. Recently, however, two studies have demonstrated some interesting details of the response of MNs. In fact, when we understand motor acts done by others, this cognitive process includes both the understanding of the goal of the observed motor act and the details of it. For example, I recognize that another individual is tearing a piece of paper and that he is performing this act at a certain distance from me, in a frontal perspective. In accord with this behavioural observation, a recent study showed that mirror neurons can be modulated by the visual perspective from which a motor act is seen by an observer (Caggiano *et al.*, 2011). In this study, the responses of MNs of monkey premotor area F5 to movies showing grasping motor acts seen from different perspectives (frontal, lateral, egocentric) were recorded. The first finding of this work was that mirror neurons are activated also by actions observed in movies, although a comparison with the response to natural actions showed that this latter response was normally higher. The second result was that only 25 per cent of the recorded mirror neurons responded to the visual presentation of motor acts in movies, independent of the visual perspective from which they were presented. The other neurons showed significant view-tuning, with different view preferences. These findings suggest that there are mirror neurons whose function is that of encoding the goal of motor acts, while other mirror neurons also contribute by providing details on specific aspects of the observed act. It is likely that this second function occurs through the feedback connections that the motor cortex sends to the posterior, high-order visual areas.

In another investigation (Caggiano *et al.*, 2009) MNs have been analyzed according to the space sector in which the observed agent performed the action. Under one condition the experimenter grasped a piece of food within the monkey's reaching space (peripersonal space); under the other he performed the same motor act far from the monkey (extrapersonal space). Some mirror neurons discharged more strongly when the experimenter grasped a piece of food within the monkey's peripersonal space, whereas other neurons behaved in the opposite way, coding others' actions performed in the extrapersonal space. Interestingly, when the monkey's working space was shortened by the presence of a barrier, extrapersonal neurons that responded less in the peripersonal space, started discharging strongly also within it, as if this space, because of the barrier, had become far. These data suggest that mirror neurons could code other's actions within different spaces. Possibly, this differential response could be linked to the possibility of social interactions with others. Peripersonal neuronal discharge would trigger in the observer immediate cooperative or competitive behaviour, while extrapersonal ones would trigger a more complex behaviour, for example, an approach of the observer to the action agent in order to interact.

The idea that mirror neurons crucially contribute to our understanding of motor events has been supported by further neurophysiological investigations, one of which demonstrated that MNs discharged both when the monkey could fully observe a grasping act and when it could see only part of it because the hand–target interaction was hidden behind a screen (Umiltà *et al.*, 2001). It is worth noting that the discharge was absent when the monkey knew that no object was present behind the screen (mimicked hidden motor act), suggesting that mirror neurons have access to prior contextual information (memory of the object presence, vision of the reaching component of the act) in order to retrieve the motor representation corresponding to the observed motor act, despite the absence of its full visual description.

In another study, the sensory information regarding the motor act was presented to the monkey in an acoustic and/or a visual format. Kohler and colleagues (2002) showed that a subclass of mirror neurons, called 'audio-visual mirror neurons', discharge not only when a monkey executes and observe a noisy act (*i.e.*, breaking a peanut), but also when it simply listens to the sound produced by that act, suggesting that its meaning can be accessed through different sensory modalities.

The two latter studies clearly show that mirror neuron discharge can be elicited in partial or complete absence of vision of the motor act and that other modalities carrying information about biological actions can address the internal motor representation of those actions, allowing the observer/listener to retrieve action meaning.

The most important property of MNs is the congruence they show between the effective observed and the effective executed motor act. This aspect is crucial for a theory based on matching observation with execution. In fact, the output of mirror neurons, as all the other neurons in the premotor cortex, is motor. Every presynaptic input capable of activating mirror neurons above threshold determines their activation, which is a motor output. Thus, it is important to verify the congruence between visual and motor response. Ninety per cent of mirror neurons are congruent in terms of goal (Gallese *et al.*, 1996). However, this congruence may be stricter or broader, depending on whether the motor act eliciting the visual response is the same as that eliciting the motor response or whether it differs, for example, regarding the higher or lower specificity of one of the two responses. Whatever the type of congruence, the matching mechanism allows the visual/acoustic input to retrieve the goal of the corresponding motor representation.

Where does the main source of visual information for mirror neurons come from? The anterior region of the superior temporal sulcus (STSa) contains visual neurons responding to the observation of head orientation, faces, locomotion, and arm movements, (Perrett *et al.*, 1989). Among them there are also neurons responding to the observation of goal-directed movements performed with the forelimb, even though no motor-related discharge has been described. This region has strong anatomic connections with the inferior parietal lobule (IPL) (Rozzi *et al.*, 2006), but not with F5. Thus, one could postulate that IPL could be the first node of an IPL–F5 circuit processing biologically meaningful movements. In support of this, MNs have been found also in IPL, and in particular in area PFG[1] (Gregoriou *et al.*, 2006; Rozzi *et al.*, 2008). The properties of these MNs are similar to those of F5, but there are also some differences (Rozzi *et al.*, 2008). For example, there are more visual responses to dyadic hand interaction and fewer to mouth motor acts with respect to F5 mirror neurons. In addition, very often, in order to have an effective visual response, the monkey must look at the scene. This constraint is normally not required for F5 MNs.

[1] The IPL has been subdivided by Pandya and Seltzer (1982), into three cytoarchitectonic areas, from rostral to caudal: PF, PG and Opt. They also introduced PFG as a transition between PF and PFG. This was considered a distinct area in the more recent classification of Gregoriou *et al.* (2006).

The anatomic link between F5 and PFG sectors containing mirror neurons has been recently directly documented (Bonini *et al.*, 2010). This link, together with that of PFG with the superior temporal gyrus makes these areas work as a functional circuit, in which the STS node provides the main source of biological visual information, while PFG and F5 have the major role of matching the visual description of a motor act with its motor representation.

The mirror system in humans

A system matching observation and execution of action is hardly lost in human evolution. In fact, the existence of a mirror system (MS) in humans has been demonstrated with electrophysiologic (TMS, EEG, MEG) and neuroimaging (PET, fMRI) techniques. For example, Fadiga and colleagues (1995) stimulated the hand representation of the motor cortex of subjects observing an experimenter grasping an object. The stimulation showed a specific enhancement, during grasping observation with respect to control conditions, of the electromyographic activity (motor-evoked potentials [MEPs]) of those muscles that subjects normally use to execute the observed motor act.

Transcranial magnetic stimulation (TMS), however, gives only an approximate location of the activated anatomic areas. Several PET and fMRI studies demonstrated that observation of actions activate three main areas, mainly in the left hemisphere: one around the STS, a second one in the supramarginal gyrus (part of IPL), and a third in the ventral premotor cortex plus the posterior sector of the inferior frontal gyrus (IFG), this latter corresponding to areas 44 and 45, that together form the so-called Broca's area (the 'speech' area) (Buccino *et al.*, 2001; Frey & Gerry, 2006; Grèzes *et al.*, 2003; Iacoboni *et al.*, 1999; Koski *et al.*, 2003; Rizzolatti *et al.*, 1996b; see also Rizzolatti *et al.*, 2009). The areas activated in IFG and IPL correspond anatomically to the areas where MNs have been found in monkeys (F5 and PFG, respectively). The area activated inside the STS is the likely homologue of the monkey area described by Perrett and colleagues, containing neurons responding during observation of biological actions, but devoid of motor properties (Perrett *et al.*, 1989).

More recent fMRI studies confirmed that action observation activates the above-described parieto-frontal circuit that, in many cases, includes also the anterior intraparietal area (AIP) (Shmuelof & Zohari, 2008). Finally, electroencephalographic (EEG) and magnetoencephalographic (MEG) investigations, beyond confirming the activation of the frontal cortex during action observation (Cochin *et al.*, 1999; Nishitani & Hari, 2000), showed also that, in temporal terms, activation of the IFG precedes that of precentral cortex.

While the first PET and some fMRI studies mainly showed the activation, during observation, of a "grasping" circuit, it has been recently demonstrated (Filimon *et al.*, 2007) that the observation of pure reaching movements directed towards an object activate a more dorsal circuit, namely the dorsal premotor cortex (PMd) and the superior parietal lobule (SPL), together with the inferior parietal sulcus (IPS), indicating that the sector of activation depends on the observed effector (hand, arm). A study by Buccino and colleagues (2001) well clarifies this concept, demonstrating a somatotopic activation, with some degree of overlap, of frontal and parietal cortices during subjects' observation of goal-related motor acts performed with different effectors (*i.e.*, mouth, hand and leg). This nicely corresponds to the somatotopic arrangement found in these cortices during the execution of these same motor acts (Penfield & Rasmussen, 1950; Rozzi *et al.*, 2008).

As described above, some mirror neurons can be activated by observation of motor acts performed with tools (Ferrari *et al.*, 2005; Rochat *et al.*, 2010). Do the areas of the human mirror system also activate during observation of actions performed with a non-biological effector?

Gazzola and colleagues (2007a) instructed volunteers to observe video-clips in which either a human or a robot arm grasped objects. In spite of differences in shape and kinematics between the human and robot arms, the parieto-frontal mirror circuit was activated in both conditions. This result was further extended by Peeters and colleagues (2009), who performed an fMRI experiment in which both monkeys and humans had to observe motor acts performed by a human hand, a robot hand, and different types of tools. The results showed that, regardless of the type of effector used, the ventral premotor–inferior parietal circuit was always active in both humans and monkeys. However, only in humans, during tool action observation, was there a specific activation of a rostral sector of the left anterior supramarginal gyrus (aSMG). This activation was not present in monkeys, even after training to use the tools that they would then observe during fMRI scanning. Since it is known that monkeys only rarely use tools without training, these data suggest that during evolution the achievement of the capacity to use tools and to understand their meaning corresponded to the formation of an extracortical region.

Intention understanding

A motor act (*e.g.*, grasping) can be included in several actions having different ultimate goals. A series of experiments in monkeys was aimed at assessing whether mirror neurons in the parietal and premotor cortex coding grasping motor acts are influenced by the action goal in which this act is embedded (Fogassi *et al.*, 2005; Bonini *et al.*, 2010). Grasping neurons were recorded while the monkey executed a motor task and observed the same task, performed by an experimenter, in which the same motor act (grasping) was embedded into two different actions (eating or placing). The results showed that a number of both parietal and premotor purely motor and mirror neurons discharged differently during both execution and observation of the grasping act, depending on the goal of the action in which the act was embedded. Thus, the modulation of grasping neurons reflects the action goal during action execution. During observation, the recruitment of the same mechanism enables the observing individual to *predict* the final goal (intention) of the observed agent. In other words, the mirror matching mechanism provides an automatic understanding not only of others' motor acts, but also of others' intentions.

A recent study in which the monkey had to perform more complex actions (Bonini *et al.*, 2011) revealed that the action goal modulates the activity of grasping neurons right from the time of the early phases of the action, suggesting the presence of a mechanism, probably located in the prefrontal cortex, selecting actions on the basis of context.

As in monkeys, there is evidence that the mirror mechanism might play a role in understanding others' intentions also in humans. An fMRI study by Iacoboni and colleagues (2005) showed that when the context indicated to observing subjects the intention underlying an observed action, there was a differential activation of the right IFG (Iacoboni *et al.*, 2005) when the 'intention' condition was compared with control conditions in which only the context or only the action were shown. A similar result was obtained by Hamilton and Grafton in a repetition-suppression fMRI experiment (2008). Volunteers were presented with movies showing actions (*e.g.*, pushing or pulling a lid) that could lead to the same or to a different outcome (*e.g.*, opening or closing a box). The results showed that the responses in the right inferior parietal lobule and right inferior frontal cortex decreased (*e.g.*, adapted) when participants saw movies of actions that had the same outcome, regardless of the individual movements involved.

The studies reviewed above indicate that the parieto-frontal mirror network subserves the understanding of motor intentions underlying the actions of others. This does not mean that the parieto-frontal mirror mechanism covers all types of intention understanding. While motor intention can be automatically understood through a process of retrieval of action representations, the interpretation of others' behaviour can require propositional attitudes that imply a more time-consuming mechanism, probably involving other cortical areas, considered to be part of the 'mentalistic network' (see Brass *et al.*, 2007; de Lange *et al.*, 2008; Liepelt *et al.*, 2008).

Plasticity of the mirror system

A very important issue that requires a deeper investigation is whether mirror neuron activity can be modified by experience and learning. A hint in this direction comes from two above-mentioned studies reporting the presence of F5 mirror neurons responding to the observation of grasping motor acts performed by an experimenter with a tool. The study of Rochat and colleagues (2010) indicates that when a novel motor act is incorporated in the one's motor repertoire, the new motor representation is integrated in the mirror neuron system, thus allowing a motor resonance during the observation of this act. In the study of Ferrari and colleagues (2005), the recorded neurons responded when the monkey observed motor acts performed by an experimenter with a tool (a stick or a pair of pliers). On the motor side, these neurons responded when the monkey executed hand and mouth motor acts. Since in this experiment monkeys were not trained to use the observed tools, the presence of this particular type of mirror neuron can be due to a relatively long visual exposure to tool actions, so that the tool became a kind of prolongation of the hand. However, also in the case of these neurons, there was a congruence between the visual and the motor response in terms of the goal of the coded motor act.

Two fMRI studies in humans showed that experience or training in dance can influence the mirror system. In the first (Calvo-Merino *et al.*, 2005), participants, who included classical dancers, dancers of *capoeira* (a Brazilian martial-arts dance), and persons naïve in professional dance and *capoeira* observed video-clips showing steps of either classical dance or *capoeira*. All groups had an activation of the mirror system, as would be expected because of action observation. More interestingly, the observation of *capoeira* relative to classical dance caused a greater activation in precentral and parietal cortex of *capoeira* dancers, while the opposite was observed in classical dancers during observation of classic ballet. Naïve subjects did not show any differential activation between the two conditions.

In the second study, Cross and colleagues (2006) asked expert dancers to learn and rehearse novel, complex whole-body sequences of modern dance for five weeks. Functional MRI was performed every week while the dancers observed and imagined performing movement sequences, half of which were rehearsed and half unpracticed. The results showed that the activation of the mirror system was modulated by the dancers' motor experience, with an increase of activity in PMv and IPL during observation of the rehearsed sequences.

The mirror system reveals plasticity in some pathologic situations as well. For example, Gazzola *et al.* (2007b) performed an fMRI study in which participants, two aplasic individuals born without arms or hands, and typically developing (TD) individuals had to observe goal-related hand motor acts and to execute mouth, hand (only TDs), and foot motor acts. This study demonstrated that during observation aplasic subjects presented an activation of the mirror system similar to that of controls. Second, during hand motor-act observation, these subjects had an activation that included the mouth and foot representation of the motor cortex. This second finding has been explained by a recruitment, during observation, of cortical representations involved in the execution of motor acts that achieve similar goals (*e.g.*, taking possession of an object) using different effectors. Thus, it appears that the mirror system can undergo plastic changes similar to those already demonstrated in sensory systems after deprivation of afferent input.

A second example of this concept comes from an investigation by Ricciardi and colleagues (2009), who showed that when congenitally blind patients listen to the sound of actions there is an activation of a fronto-parieto-temporal system corresponding to the regions activated in the normally sighted control subjects during observation of and listening to the same actions. This means that the mirror system is activated by action sounds. Furthermore, the sound of familiar actions caused a greater activation of this system in both blind and normally sighted subjects.

Taken together, these examples demonstrate that there is a plasticity of the mirror system, and that this relies on a reorganization of the motor representations. These findings allow us to also hypothesize that the intrinsic plasticity of the observation/execution system can be exploited for rehabilitative purposes. Only recently has action observation therapy been employed for systematic investigation on its effect related to brain modification. Ertelt and colleagues (2007) employed action observation therapy on stroke patients with mild paresis of the hand. These patients were subdivided into two groups: one (the experimental group) had to observe and reproduce motor acts of increasing complexity, whereas the other (the control group) had to observe videos showing geometric symbols and letters and then perform the same motor acts as the first group, as instructed by the therapist. After the end of this 18-day therapy, only the experimental group showed an improvement of the functional scales used to evaluate motor performance. Moreover, an fMRI study performed on patients of both groups, before and after rehabilitation, showed that during execution of an object manipulation task there was an increased activation in the experimental group as compared to the control group in some areas of both hemispheres, such as the ventral premotor cortex (PMv), supplementary motor area (SMA), SMG, and superior temporal sulcus. Most of these areas belong to the classical observation/execution mirror system.

Conclusions

In this article, the properties of the mirror system in both monkeys and humans have been described. It has also been shown that this system possesses a plasticity that can be also revealed in pathologic situations. In the last decade it has been proposed that an impairment of the mirror mechanism could account for the core deficit of autistic spectrum disorders, which are characterized by difficulty in intersubjective relations. In support of this notion, electrophysiologic and fMRI studies showed a decrease in the functioning of the mirror circuit in patients with autism-spectrum disorders (Dapretto *et al.*, 2006; Oberman *et al.*, 2005). However, because autistic children often present with motor impairments, it has been proposed that a deficit in motor organization could also explain part of their problems in understanding others' intentions and emotions. A series of studies showed indeed that autistic children, with respect to TD children, lack the typical fluidity that characterizes the organization of intentional actions (Cattaneo *et al.*, 2007; Fabbri-Destro *et al.*, 2009). This deficiency, interpreted in the light of the above-described intentional circuits, would explain why they are not able to understand intentions when they can rely only on pragmatic information (Boria *et al.*, 2009). These observations open the way to further investigations of the autistic motor system and of the relation between action execution and action perception. Furthermore, such further studies could represent a crucial step for devising rehabilitation therapies based on neurophysiological models.

References

Bonini, L., Rozzi, S., Ugolotti Serventi, F., Simone, L., Ferrari, P.F. & Fogassi, L. (2010): Ventral premotor and inferior parietal cortices make distinct contribution to action organization and intention understanding. *Cerebr. Cortex* **20,** 1372–1385. doi:10.1093/cercor/bhp200.

Bonini, L., Ugolotti Serventi, F., Simone, L., Rozzi, S., Ferrari, P.F. & Fogassi, L. (2011): Grasping neurons of monkey parietal and premotor cortices encode action goals at distinct levels of abstraction during complex action sequences. *J. Neurosci.* **31,** 5876 –5887.

Boria, S., Fabbri-Destro, M., Cattaneo, L., Sparaci, L., Sinigaglia, C., Santelli, E., *et al.* (2009): Intention understanding in autism. *PloS One* **4,** e5596.

Brass, M., Schmitt, R.M., Spengler, S. & Gergely, G. (2007): Investigating action understanding: inferential processes versus action simulation. *Curr. Biol.* **17,** 2117–2121.

Buccino, G., Binkofski, F., Fink, G.R., Fadiga, L., Fogassi, L., Gallese, V., *et al.* (2001): Action observation activates premotor and parietal areas in a somatotopic manner: an fMRI study. *Eur. J. Neurosci.* **13,** 400–404.

Caggiano, V., Fogassi, L., Rizzolatti, G., Thier, P. & Casile, A. (2009): Mirror neurons differentially encode the peripersonal and extrapersonal space of monkeys. *Science* **324,** 403–406.

Caggiano, V., Fogassi, L., Rizzolatti, G., Pomper, J.K., Thier, P., Giese, M.A. & Casile, A. (2011): View-based encoding of actions in mirror neurons of area f5 in macaque premotor cortex. *Curr. Biol.* **21,** 144–148. E-pub 2011 Jan 13.

Calvo-Merino, B., Glaser, D.E., Grezes, J., Passingham, R.E. & Haggard, P. (2005): Action observation and acquired motor skills: an FMRI study with expert dancers. *Cereb. Cortex* **15,** 1243–1249.

Cattaneo, L. Fabbri-Destro, M., Boria, S., Pieraccini, C., Monti, A., Cossu, G. & Rizzolatti, G. (2007): Impairment of actions chains in autism and its possible role in intention understanding. *Proc. Natl. Acad. Sci. USA* **104,** 17825–17830.

Cochin, S., Barthelemy, C., Roux, S. & Martineau, J. (1999): Observation and execution of movement: similarities demonstrated by quantified electroencephalograpy. *Eur. J. Neurosci.* **11,** 1839–1842.

Cross, E.S., de Hamilton, A.F. & Grafton, S.T. (2006): Building a motor simulation de novo: observation of dance by dancers. *NeuroImage* **31,** 1257–1267.

Dapretto, M., Davies, M.S., Pfeifer, J.H., Scott, A.A., Sigman, M., Bookheimer, S.Y. & Iacoboni, M. (2006): Understanding emotions in others: mirror neuron dysfunction in children with autism spectrum disorders. *Nat. Neurosci.* **9,** 28–30.

de Lange, F.P., Spronk, M., Willems, R.M., Toni, I. & Bekkering, H. (2008): Complementary systems for understanding action intentions. *Curr. Biol.* **18,** 454–457.

Di Pellegrino, G., Fadiga, L., Fogassi, L., Gallese, V. & Rizzolatti, G. (1992): Understanding motor events: a neurophysiological study. *Exp. Brain Res.* **91,** 176–180.

Ertelt, D., Small, S., Solodkin, A., Dettmers, C., McNamara, A., Binkofski, F. & Buccino, G. (2007): Action observation has a positive impact on rehabilitation of motor deficits after stroke. *NeuroImage* **36** (Suppl. 2), T164–173.

Fabbri-Destro, M., Cattaneo, L., Boria, S. & Rizzolatti, G. (2009): Planning actions in autism. *Exp. Brain Res.* **192,** 521–525. E-pub 2008 Oct 7.

Fadiga, L., Fogassi, L., Pavesi, G. & Rizzolatti, G. (1995): Motor facilitation during action observation: a magnetic stimulation study. *J. Neurophysiol.* **73,** 2608–2611.

Ferrari, P.F., Gallese, V., Rizzolatti, G. & Fogassi, L. (2003): Mirror neurons responding to the observation of ingestive and communicative mouth actions in the monkey ventral premotor cortex. *Eur. J. Neurosci.* **17,** 1703–1714.

Ferrari, P.F., Rozzi, S. & Fogassi, L. (2005): Mirror neurons responding to observation of actions made with tools in monkey ventral premotor cortex. *J. Cogn. Neurosci.* **17,** 212–226.

Filimon, F., Nelson, J.D., Hagler, D.J. & Sereno, M.I. (2007): Human cortical representations for reaching: mirror neurons for execution, observation, and imagery. *NeuroImage* **37,** 1315–1328.

Fogassi, L., Ferrari, P.F., Gesierich, B., Rozzi, S., Chersi, F. & Rizzolatti G. (2005): Parietal lobe: from action organization to intention understanding. *Science* **308,** 662–667.

Fogassi, L. (2009): Codifica dello scopo degli atti motori e delle azioni: un approccio neurofisiologico. *Teorie e Modelli* **XIV (1),** 25–40.

Frey, S.H. & Gerry, V.E. (2006): Modulation of neural activity during observational learning of actions and their sequential orders. *J. Neurosci.* **26,** 13194–13201.

Gallese, V., Fadiga, L., Fogassi, L. & Rizzolatti, G. (1996): Action recognition in the premotor cortex. *Brain* **119,** 593–609.

Gazzola, V., Rizzolatti, G., Wicker, B. & Keysers, C. (2007a): The anthropomorphic brain: the mirror neuron system responds to human and robotic actions. *NeuroImage* **35,** 1674–1684.

Gazzola, V., van der Worp, H., Mulder, T., Wicker, B., Rizzolatti, G. & Keysers, C. (2007b): Aplasics born without hands mirror the goal of hand actions with their feet. *Curr. Biol.* **17,** 1235–1240.

Gregoriou, G.G., Borra, E., Matelli, M., Luppino, G. 2006. Architectonic organization of the inferior parietal convexity of the macaque monkey. *J. Comp. Neurol.* **496,** 422-451.

Grèzes, J., Armony, J.L., Rowe, J. & Passingham, R.E. (2003): Activations related to "mirror" and "canonical" neurons in the human brain: an fMRI study. *NeuroImage* **18,** 928–937.

Hamilton, A.F. & Grafton, S.T. (2008): Action outcomes are represented in human inferior frontoparietal cortex. *Cereb. Cortex* **18,** 1160-1168. E-pub 2007 Aug 28.

Iacoboni, M., Woods, R.P., Brass, M., Bekkering, H., Mazziotta, J.C. & Rizzolatti, G. (1999): Cortical mechanisms of human imitation. *Science* **286,** 2526–2528.

Iacoboni, M., Molnar-Szakacs, I., Gallese, V., Buccino, G., Mazziotta, J.C. & Rizzolatti, G. (2005): Grasping the intentions of others with one's own mirror neuron system. *PLoS Biol.* **3,** e79.

Jeannerod, M. (1988): *The Neural and Behavioural Organization of Goal-Directed Movements.* Oxford: Clarendon Press.

Kohler, E., Keysers, C., Umiltà, M.A., Fogassi, L., Gallese, V. & Rizzolatti, G. (2002): Hearing sounds, understanding actions: action representation in mirror neurons. *Science* **297,** 846–848.

Koski, L., Iacoboni, M., Dubeau, M.C., Woods, R.P. & Mazziotta, J.C. (2003): Modulation of cortical activity during different imitative behaviors. *J. Neurophysiol.* **89,** 460–471.

Liepelt, R., Von Cramon, D.Y. & Brass, M. (2008): How do we infer other's goals from non stereotypic actions? The outcome of context-sensitive inferential processing in right inferior parietal and posterior temporal cortex. *NeuroImage* **43,** 784–792.

Nishitani, N. & Hari, R. (2000): Temporal dynamics of cortical representation for action. *Proc. Natl. Acad. Sci. USA* **97,** 913–918.

Oberman, L.M., Hubbard, E.M., McCleery, J.P., Altschuler, E.L., Ramachandran, V.S. & Pineda, J.A. (2005): EEG evidence for mirror neuron dysfunction in autism spectrum disorders. *Brain Res. Cogn. Brain Res.* **24,** 190–198.

Peeters, R., Simone, L., Nelissen, K., Fabbri-Destro, M., Vanduffel, W., Rizzolatti, G. & Orban, G.A. (2009): The representation of tool use in humans and monkeys: common and unique human features. *J. Neurosci.* **29,** 11523–11539.

Penfield, W. & Rasmussen, T. (1950): *The Cerebral Cortex of Man: A Clinical Study of Localization and Function.* New York: Macmillan.

Perrett, D.I., Harries, M.H., Bevan, R., Thomas, S., Benson, P.J., Mistlin, A.J., *et al.* (1989): Frameworks of analysis for the neural representation of animate objects and actions. *J. Exp. Biol.* **146,** 87–113.

Ricciardi, E., Bonino, D., Sani, L., Vecchi, T., Guazzelli, M., Haxby, J.V., *et al.* (2009): Do we really need vision? How blind people "see" the actions of others. *J. Neurosci.* **29,** 9719–9724.

Rizzolatti, G., Camarda, R., Fogassi, L., Gentilucci, M., Luppino, G. & Matelli, M. (1988): Functional organization of inferior area 6 in the macaque monkey: II. Area F5 and the control of distal movements. *Exp. Brain Res.* **71,** 491–507.

Rizzolatti, G., Fadiga, L., Gallese, V. & Fogassi, L. (1996a) Premotor cortex and the recognition of motor actions. *Brain Res. Cogn. Brain Res.* **3,** 131–141.

Rizzolatti, G., Fadiga, L., Matelli, M., Bettinardi, V., Paulesu, E., Perani, D. & Fazio, F. (1996b): Localization of grasp representations in humans by PET: 1. Observation versus execution. *Exp. Brain Res.* **111,** 246–252.

Rizzolatti, G., Luppino, G. & Matelli, M. (1998): The organization of the cortical motor system: new concepts. *Electroencephalogr. Clin. Neurophysiol.* **106,** 283–296.

Rizzolatti, G., Fogassi, L. & Gallese, V. (2009): The mirror neuron system: a motor-based mechanism for action and intention understanding. In: *The Cognitive Neuroscience IV,* ed. M. Gazzaniga, pp. 625–640. Cambridge, MA: The MIT Press.

Rochat, M.J., Caruana, F., Jezzini, A., Escola, L., Intskirveli, I., Grammont, F., *et al.* (2010): Responses of mirror neurons in area F5 to hand and tool grasping observation. *Exp. Brain Res.* **204,** 605–616.

Rosenbaum, D.A., Cohen, R.G., Jax, S.A., Weiss, D.J. & van der Wel, R. (2007): The problem of serial order in behavior: Lashley's legacy. *Hum. Mov. Sci.* **26,** 525–554.

Rozzi, S., Calzavara, R., Belmalih, A., Borra, E., Gregoriou, G.G., Matelli, M. & Luppino, G. (2006): Cortical connections of the inferior parietal cortical convexity of the macaque monkey. *Cereb. Cortex* **16,** 1389–1417.

Rozzi, S., Ferrari, P.F., Bonini, L., Rizzolatti, G. & Fogassi, L. (2008): Functional organization of inferior parietal lobule convexity in the macaque monkey: electrophysiological characterization of motor, sensory and mirror responses and their correlation with cytoarchitectonic areas. *Eur. J. Neurosci.* **28,** 1569–1588.

Shmuelof, L. & Zohary, E. (2008): A mirror representation of others' actions in the human anterior parietal cortex. *Nat. Neurosci.* **11,** 1267–1269.

Umiltà, M.A., Kohler, E., Gallese, V., Fogassi, L., Fadiga, L., Keysers, C. & Rizzolatti, G. (2001): I know what you are doing: a neurophysiological study. *Neuron* **31,** 155–165.

Umiltà, M.A., Escola, L., Intskirveli, I., Grammont, F., Rochat, M., Caruana, F., *et al.* (2008): How pliers become fingers in the monkey motor system. *Proc. Natl. Acad. Sci. USA* **105,** 2209–2213.

Brain Lesion Localization and Developmental Functions, D. Riva, C. Njiokiktjien and S. Bulgheroni (eds.)

Chapter 4

Memory and frontal lobe in typical and atypical development

Stefano Vicari, Floriana Costanzo, Pamela Varvara and Deny Menghini

Child and Adolescence Neuropsychiatry Unit, Department of Neurosciences, Children's Hospital Bambino Gesù, piazza Sant'Onofrio 4, 00165 Rome, Italy
stefano.vicari@opbg.net

Summary

Human memory is a multi-componential function with distinct brain regions serving specific memory functions. The frontal lobe, with its specialized subregions, is one of the primary structures implicated in several memory processes such as working memory, episodic memory, and procedural and implicit learning. Studies on typical and atypical developmental populations have contributed to clarify the role of the frontal lobe in memory. Several data on individuals with intellectual disabilities documented deficits in working memory's central executive system related to frontal lobe abnormalities. In typically developed populations, a higher use of strategic mechanisms in episodic memory (*e.g.*, recall) has been related to increased prefrontal cortex activity; however, in persons with Down syndrome reduced use of strategic mechanisms in verbal recall has been associated with an abnormal neuroanatomic reorganization of the right orbitofrontal cortex. Moreover, the recollection component of episodic memory has been found to be impaired in individuals with Williams syndrome and associated with their abnormalities in frontal lobe regions. Similarly, the implicit learning deficits found in Williams syndrome and in dyslexic individuals have been associated with frontal cortex abnormalities. In this chapter, the role of the frontal lobe in developmental disorders and its significant implications for rehabilitation of memory are discussed.

Introduction

According to structural approaches to memory, various regions of neuroarchitecture serve specific functions. In agreement with Atkinson and Shiffrin (1971), Squire (1987) distinguished between short-term memory (STM) and long-term memory (LTM). These two systems are characterized by their differences: retention capacity (which is limited to only a few items for STM and is practically unlimited for LTM); information coding (which is mainly phonological coding in the STM and is based on semantic processing of stimuli for LTM); and mnesic trace deterioration rate (which lasts for a few seconds without reiteration for STM and is variable but relatively slow for LTM).

Concerning STM, the working memory (WM) model has been developed by Baddeley and his colleagues (Baddeley, 1986; Baddeley & Hitch, 1974). WM is defined as a limited capacity system for the temporary storage of information held for further manipulation and is not subserved by a unitary store but by the cooperation of two major systems. The first is a central executive system, a limited-capacity central processor able to temporarily store and process information from many modalities. The second major system of the WM model actually consists of a number of peripheral slave systems, or limited-capacity systems, which temporarily store and rehearse information belonging to a single modality when the flow of data surpasses the capacity of the central executive system.

In the LTM domain, explicit or declarative memory and implicit or procedural memory have to be distinguished. Explicit memory is involved in intentional and/or conscious recall and recognition of experiences and information. A further distinction within explicit memory should be made between episodic and semantic memory (Tulving, 1992). Episodic memory concerns memory for past events of our life and its relation with space and temporal information, while semantic memory concerns factual and concept knowledge and is organized in an associative manner without chronological order information (Squire, 1987). Two components of episodic memory storage can also be distinguished: *recollection*, which involves remembering specific contextual details about a prior learned episode, and *familiarity*, which involves simply knowing an item that was presented before (Yonelinas, 2002). Conversely, implicit memory facilitates performance of perceptual, cognitive, and motor tasks without any conscious reference to previous experiences (for a review, see Tulving and Schacter, 1990). Explicit and implicit memory systems are not completely independent, but cooperate with each other.

Because of frontal lobe connections with numerous brain regions (*e.g.*, basal ganglia, medial temporal lobe, parietal lobe, and cerebellum), there is evidence of its crucial role in memory processes such as WM, episodic LTM, and implicit and procedural learning. The frontal lobe structures are vulnerable to the effects of increasing age and continue to mature well into the adolescent years and through early adulthood (*e.g.*, Finn *et al.*, 2010, Sowell *et al.*, 2001) and differential performance on these memory processes can be expected during development.

Review of the topic

Working memory

WM comprises a set of cognitive processes required for many, if not all, forms of learning. A critical neural substrate for WM, the prefrontal cortex, continues to mature through early adulthood. Using a longitudinal design, Finn *et al.* (2010) showed that the recruitment of prefrontal cortex during a WM task is correlated with performance only in late adolescence. Thus, the neural circuitry underlying WM changes during adolescent development.

Accordingly, studies on the development of WM capacity in a typically developed (TD) population showed that verbal span increases with age. Hulme and Mackenzie (1992) described a verbal span of three at 4 years, of six at 10–12 years and of seven to eight at 16 years. The main increment is more evident between 4 and 10 years of age, while afterwards it seems minimal. In addition, Italian studies confirmed the main increment of both verbal and visual span between 4 and 10 years of age (Cornoldi, 1992; Orsini *et al.*, 1987). However, such an increment has been associated with increasing specialization and efficiency in the elaboration of memorandums (Gathercole & Hitch, 1993; Hulme & Mackenzie, 1992) rather than with the growth of the STM store.

As concerns neurodevelopmental disorders, results on WM's ability are controversial. Some studies demonstrated that individuals with Williams syndrome (WS) have a global impairment of WM (Sampaio *et al.*, 2008), whereas others studies documented the greater strength in a dual WM task for WS individuals in comparison to that of a group with Down syndrome (DS) and one with intellectual disability (ID) of mixed aetiology. Furthermore, WS individuals have shown a general superiority for the verbal WM, with a rather compromised spatial ability compared to visual ability (Vicari & Carlesimo, 2006; Vicari *et al.*, 2003a; 2006). These results are not confirmed by other studies that found no impairment for spatial WM as opposed to visual memory in individuals with WS (Jarrold *et al.*, 2007). A better understanding of the findings on WM in WS was provided by the study by O'Hearn *et al.* (2009), who documented how the WM impairment could be overcome under some conditions – for example, by using a delayed recognition paradigm. In a recent study (Menghini *et al.*, 2010) a group of persons with WS were compared to a group of mentally age-matched TD children in verbal and visuo-spatial STM and WM tasks. The results confirmed data in the literature describing preserved verbal STM in individuals with WS, in contrast with deficient visuospatial STM abilities (Jarrold *et al.*, 1999, 2007; Vicari *et al.*, 1996a). However, dissociation was not found between verbal and visuospatial WM, which were equally compromised. This result was interpreted in light of Baddeley's model (Baddeley, 2001) as the expression of deficient functioning of the central executive system component of the WM.

WM has also been investigated in people with DS, and it has been found to be generally compromised (Vicari *et al.*, 1995) on account of the reduced resources of the executive system. The documented deficit in the central executive system for individuals with DS and with WS can be to some extent explained by a numbers of anomalies found in the frontal lobe anatomy of these individuals. Volumetric MRI studies have reported reduced volume of frontal cortices in nondemented adults with DS compared to controls (Jernigan *et al.*, 1993; Kesslak *et al.*, 1994), as well as reduced volume of the left medial frontal lobe (White *et al.*, 2003). Abnormalities in gray matter of frontal areas (bilateral superior and inferior frontal gyri) have been recently confirmed (Menghini *et al.*, 2011a).

Episodic long-term memory

Behavioural and functional neuroimaging findings suggest that different regions within the frontal lobes contribute to LTM functioning, offering an explanation for the variability on memory dysfunction observed in patients with frontal lobe damage and frontal lobe epilepsy (Centeno *et al.*, 2010). A number of studies have stressed the importance of the prefrontal cortex in performing explicit memory-retrieval tasks (*e.g.*, Dobbins *et al.*, 2004; Ranganath, 2004). It is generally assumed that control processes mediated by the prefrontal cortex are responsible for guiding the efficient search for relevant items (*e.g.*, Dobbins *et al.*, 2002), for setting up retrieval strategies, and for adapting retrieval to the current task demands (Czernochowski *et al.*, 2005). In everyday life, we often must remember the past in the absence of helpful cues in the environment. In these cases, the brain directs retrieval by relying on internally maintained cues and strategies. Free recall is a widely used behavioural paradigm for studying retrieval with minimal cue support. During free recall, individuals often recall semantically related items consecutively – an effect termed *semantic clustering* – and previous studies have sought to understand clustering to gain leverage on the basic mechanisms supporting strategic recall. Successful recall and semantic clustering depend on the prefrontal cortex. The question remains open as to whether one or several frontal control mechanisms operate during encoding and recall. Applying a recently developed method (Oztekin *et al.*, 2010) to assess event-related fMRI signal changes during free recall, Long *et al.* (2010) found that during encoding dorsolateral prefrontal cortex activation was predictive of subsequent semantic clustering. In contrast, subregions of ventrolateral prefrontal cortex were predictive of subsequent recall, whether clustered or nonclustered, and were inversely associated with clustering during recall. These results suggested that the dorsolateral prefrontal cortex supports relational processes at encoding that are sufficient to produce category clustering effects during recall. Conversely, controlled retrieval mechanisms supported by the ventrolateral prefrontal cortex sustain item-specific search during recall (Long *et al.*, 2010).

Free-recall impairment has been largely documented in developmental disorders, showing inconsistent findings. Early studies (Ellis & Allison, 1988) reported that individuals with intellectual disability (ID)[1] performed significantly worse than a TD group in a free recall of lists of words and pictures, but were as accurate as the controls in a frequency judgment of words. In a free-recall test of a word list, TD children scored higher than individuals with familial ID, who, in turn, scored higher than individuals with organic ID. In 1963, Rossi reported a reduced use of semantic strategies by people with ID in a task involving free recall of related word lists, whereas subsequent studies reported opposite results (Winters & Semchuk, 1986). Inconsistencies between studies in memory profile of persons with ID could be due to the different aetiology of ID. Indeed, in a study of individuals with Down syndrome, ID of unspecified aetiology, and mentally age-matched TD controls, Carlesimo *et al.* (1997) found that the DS group scored significantly lower than the other groups in verbal-recall tasks (*e.g.*, recalling a list of words and a short story) and visuospatial recall tasks (*e.g.*, reproducing Rey's figure), concluding that individuals with DS have a severe impairment of explicit LTM. Converging evidence (*e.g.*, Nadel, 1999; Nichols *et al.*, 2004; Pennington *et al.*, 2003; Vicari *et al.*, 2000, 2006) reported individuals with DS recalling fewer words than mental-age-matched TD controls. In the case of individuals with WS, Vicari *et al.* (1996b) documented lower performance of children with WS than mental-age-matched TD children in verbal LTM (*i.e.*, in word-list delayed free recall and recognition).

In summary, individuals with DS show diffuse and general impairment in free recall relative to mental-age-matched TD controls, whereas those with WS usually exhibited a less severe pattern, with some aspects of verbal recall preserved relative to TD children. This difference could be due to a documented deficit in individuals with DS in the use of strategic mechanisms for free recall (Carlesimo *et al.* 1997; Vicari, 2004; Vicari *et al.*, 2000, 2002).

Frontal lobe abnormalities have been documented in individuals with DS (Menghini *et al.*, 2011a; White *et al.*, 2003). However, the relationship between brain anatomy and neuropsychological profile is poorly understood. In a recent voxel-based morphometry study (Menghini *et al.*, 2011a), the direct association between structural brain measures and behavioural data has been investigated. The different neuropsychological measures derived from cognitive tasks, including memory, were correlated to grey matter density measures in DS individuals. Results documented a direct correlation between grey matter density in the right orbitofrontal cortex and verbal memory. Functionally, the orbitofrontal cortex is activated for emotionally salient items during verbal memory tasks (Johnson *et al.*, 2004), whereas anatomically the left orbitofrontal cortex volume is related to the semantic organization of verbal memory tasks in schizophrenic patients (Matsui *et al.*, 2008). This finding indicates in DS an abnormal anatomic contribution of the right orbitofrontal cortex on tasks specifically requiring participation of the left hemisphere, suggesting atypical neuroanatomic reorganization related to verbal LTM abilities; this could explain these subjects' particular difficulty on tasks requiring the organization of verbal material according to its categorical structure (Carlesimo *et al.*, 1997).

[1] http://www.britishpathe.com/category.php?id=10&o=0

The role of the frontal lobe in explicit LTM has been also recognized in the componential analysis of performance on explicit memory tasks including recognition memory tasks. Two different kinds of access to stored memories can be distinguished: recollection and familiarity (Mandler, 1980; Tulving, 1985; Yonelinas, 2002). Recollection involves mentally reliving the specific episode during which an item was encountered; it permits remembering the spatial–temporal context in which the event occurred and other information associated with it. Conversely, familiarity entails the feeling of having previously encountered the stimulus target without the retrieval of other details, that is, contextual or associated information.

Distinct cortical areas in the frontal lobes likely play a differential role in recollection and familiarity; even if data reported in the literature are controversial (Davidson *et al.*, 2006; MacPherson *et al.*, 2008). It is generally assumed that control processes mediated by the prefrontal cortex are responsible for guiding the efficient search for relevant item attributes or item–context attribute conjunctions (*e.g.*, see Dobbins *et al.*, 2002). In a source memory study, Kirwan *et al.* (2008) demonstrated that brain activity in the medial temporal lobe is predictive of subsequent memory strength, whereas activity in the prefrontal cortex is predictive of subsequent recollection. Both recollection- and familiarity-based responses are associated with right dorsolateral prefrontal cortex activity, but recollection involves additional prefrontal activity (Skinner & Fernandes, 2007). An earlier study also found frontal lobe activity during learning that was related to subsequent source memory success. Cansino *et al.* (2002) compared source-correct to source-incorrect trials when item memory strength was high, and found two regions in the frontal lobe (left superior and inferior frontal gyri) where activity was greater for source-correct than source-incorrect trials.

Frontal control mechanisms are essential for the monitoring and verification of the products of memory retrieval as documented by clinical studies examining patients with frontal lobe damage. Indeed, Mayes *et al.* (2002) demonstrated that frontal lobe–damaged patients were able to perform at close to normal levels in an item-recognition test, but were at floor levels when source information was asked for. In a similar vein, elderly people have been demonstrated to suffer from less-effective control functioning and to have larger problems with source memory requirements than would be expected from their item memory performance (*e.g.*, Dywan *et al.*, 1998; Friedman & Miyake, 2000; Trott *et al.*, 1999). Since the frontal lobe structures not only are vulnerable to the effects of increasing age, but also have a very protracted development and continue to mature well into the adolescent years (*e.g.*, Sowell *et al.*, 2001), it can be assumed that cognitive control processes continue to develop along with frontal lobe maturation.

Few studies have investigated the contribution of recollection and familiarity to the memory performance of individuals with developmental disorders. Most of the evidence in this regard comes from studies that provided indirect estimates of recollection and familiarity by contrasting performance on tests of recognition (which involve both recollection and familiarity processes) with those of free recall (which involves recollection processes only). Jarrold *et al.* (2007) reported a more severe deficit on tests of free recall than recognition in individuals with WS or DS compared to chronological-age-matched controls. However, Vicari (2001) reported preserved free recall and recognition (verbal and visual) in individuals with WS, and Carlesimo *et al.* (1997) documented reduced free recall and recognition in individuals with DS. Finally, Ornstein *et al.* (2008) described preserved free recall but impaired recognition memory in individuals with Fragile-X syndrome compared to mental-age-matched controls. Recollection and familiarity were also recently studied in individuals with autism by Bigham *et al.* (2010).

Impaired performance in participants with high-functioning autism in recollection, but not in familiarity, was found. In the same study, these authors also reported evidence of reduced recollection processes in a group of low-functioning individuals with autism.

In a recent study, Costanzo *et al.* (2011) demonstrated reduced recollection and spared familiarity in the explicit memory performances of individuals with WS. These results provide direct evidence of dissociation between recollection and familiarity in a neurodevelopmental disorder.

Procedural and implicit learning

Procedural and implicit learning (IL) play a central role in a number of cognitive functions, such as acquisition of motor sequences, stimulus–response associations, priming effect, and classical conditioning (Clark & Squire, 1998; Richter *et al.*, 2004). A complete definition of the neural network involved in IL is still a matter of investigation. Empirical evidence based on studies including patients with brain damage supports a primary role of the frontal cortex, especially premotor areas, together with the basal ganglia and the cerebellum in the implicit acquisition of motor sequences (Doyon *et al.*, 1997; Knopman & Nissen, 1991; Pascual-Leone *et al.*, 1993).

Recent neurologic and physiologic data suggest that IL is impaired in individuals with dyslexia (Vicari *et al.*, 2003b, 2005). The brain areas involved in the IL deficit exhibited by dyslexics have been studied during a motor sequence learning task (Nicolson *et al.*, 1999; Menghini *et al.*, 2006). In particular, fMRI results (Menghini *et al.*, 2006) showed an abnormal activation in dyslexics in the parietal cortex, the supplementary motor area, and the cerebellum.

Menghini *et al.* (2008) have been also conducted an anatomic investigation on the brain regions involved in the IL of dyslexics. Consistently with functional data, dyslexics showed reduced grey matter volumes in the parietal lobe and precuneus and in the supplementary motor area.

The performances of dyslexics have been compared with those of a chronological-age- and gender-matched group of TD children in a task measuring learning by observation (Menghini *et al.*, 2011b). Learning by observation is a very efficient form of knowledge acquisition that occurs as a function of observing, retaining, and replicating novel behaviour executed by others. In the study by Menghini *et al.* (2011b) participants were assigned to three different experimental conditions. The authors found that dyslexic children were severely impaired in learning a sequence by observation. By contrast, they were able to detect a sequence by trial and error, and became as efficient as normal readers in reproducing an observed sequence after a session of learning by doing. Thus, the authors concluded that the impaired ability to learn by observation could be reversed by agentive experience with a powerful learning mechanism. More generally, the beneficial effect of practice on the ability to learn by observation could provide dyslexic children with a useful chance to acquire new cognitive abilities through a more fine-tuned teaching approach. Furthermore, a significant occurrence of perseverative errors in dyslexics has been found and it may account for the prefrontal dysfunctions documented in the presence of dyslexia (Hauser, 1999).

Fewer studies have been devoted to investigating IL in individuals with ID, documenting differences in IL abilities of distinct groups of individuals with ID. Even if WS individuals exhibited deficits in IL, persons with DS showed a similar IL pattern of their TD controls, thus confirming the presence of different patterns of procedural learning in the two syndromes (Vicari *et al.*, 2007).

Conclusion

The frontal lobe is one of the cortical regions to undergo the greatest expansion in the course of both evolution and individual maturation. The protracted, relatively large, development correlates with the development of cognitive functions, in particular memory, which neuropsychological studies in animals and humans have ascribed to this cortex.

Since memory is a multi-componential function, with distinct brain regions serving specific memory functions, the specialized subregions of the frontal lobe are differently involved in each memory process.

The relationship between frontal lobe maturation and children's memory may be reflective of the development towards the more adult-like frontal lobe function; however, in the case of atypical development, it may become manifest in a series of memory deficits.

Data from genetic syndromes with anomalies of the frontal lobe, as DS and WS, documented a deficit of WM and LTM (recall and recollection) at different levels. Moreover, developmental disorders, such as dyslexia, show IL and observational learning impairment, in part associated with frontal lobe activity.

Findings derived from both typical and atypical child populations have proven to be essential to clarify memory processes. Future studies will need to better characterize the complex and dynamic relationship between the frontal cortex and neuropsychological mechanisms underlying human memory. In particular, early investigations and interventions on memory competencies that might be impaired in children with developmental disabilities are crucial to avoid negative outcomes and to support memory development in children.

References

Atkinson, R.C. & Shiffrin, R.M. (1971): The control of short-term memory. *Sci. Am.* **225,** 82–90.

Baddeley, A.D. (1986): *Working Memory,* p. 289. Oxford, UK: Oxford University Press.

Baddeley, A.D. (2001): Is working memory still working? *Am. Psychol.* **56,** 851–864.

Baddeley, A.D. & Hitch, G. (1974): Working memory. *Psychol. Learn. Motiv.* **8,** 47–90.

Bigham, S., Boucher, J., Mayes, A. & Anns, S. (2010): Assessing recollection and familiarity in autistic spectrum disorders: methods and findings. *J. Autism Dev. Disord.* **40,** 878–889.

Cansino, S., Maquet, P., Dolan, R.J. & Rugg, M.D. (2002): Brain activity underlying encoding and retrieval of source memory. *Cereb. Cortex* **12,** 1048–1056.

Carlesimo, G.A., Marotta, L. & Vicari, S. (1997): Long-term memory in mental retardation: evidence for a specific impairment in subjects with Down's syndrome. *Neuropsychologia* **35,** 71–79.

Centeno, M., Thompson, P.J., Koepp, M.J., Helmstaedter, C. & Duncan, J.S. (2010): Memory in frontal lobe epilepsy. *Epilepsy Res.* **91,** 123–132.

Clark, R.E. & Squire, L.R. (1998): Classical conditioning and brain systems: the role of awareness. *Science* **280,** 77–81.

Cornoldi, C. (1992): Lo sviluppo della memoria. In: *Il Pensiero in Erba*, ed. A. Dentici, pp. 99–126. Milano: Franco Angeli.

Costanzo, F., Vicari, S. & Carlesimo, G.A. (2011): Familiarity and recollection in Williams syndrome. *Cortex* doi:10.1016/j.cortex.2011.06.007.

Czernochowski, D., Mecklinger, A., Johansson, M. & Brinkmann, M. (2005): Age-related differences in familiarity and recollection: ERP evidence from a recognition memory study in children and young adults. *Cogn. Affect. Behav. Neurosci.* **5,** 417–433.

Davidson, P.S., Troyer, A.K. & Moscovitch, M. (2006): Frontal lobe contributions to recognition and recall: linking basic research with clinical evaluation and remediation. *J. Int. Neuropsychol. Soc.* **12,** 210–223.

Dobbins, I.G., Foley, H., Schacter, D.L. & Wagner, A.D. (2002): Executive control during episodic retrieval: multiple prefrontal processes subserve source memory. *Neuron* **35,** 989–996.

Dobbins, I.G., Simons, J.S. & Schacter, D.L. (2004): fMRI evidence for separable and lateralized prefrontal memory monitoring processes. *J. Cogn. Neurosci.* **16,** 908–920.

Doyon, J., Gaudreau, D., Laforce, R.,Jr., Castonguay, M., Bédard, P.J., Bédard, F. & Bouchard, J.P. (1997): Role of the striatum, cerebellum, and frontal lobes in the learning of a visuomotor sequence. *Brain Cognit.* **34,** 218–245.

Dywan, J., Segalowitz, S.J. & Webster, L. (1998): Source monitoring: ERP evidence for greater reactivity to nontarget information in older adults. *Brain Cognit.* **36,** 390–430.

Ellis, N. & Allison, P. (1988): Memory for frequency of occurrence in retarded and nonretarded persons. *Intelligence* **12,** 61–76.

Finn, A.S., Sheridan, M.A., Kam, C.L., Hinshaw, S. & D'Esposito, M. (2010): Longitudinal evidence for functional specialization of the neural circuit supporting working memory in the human brain. *J. Neurosci.* **30,** 11062–11067.

Friedman, N.P. & Miyake, A. (2000): Differential roles for visuospatial and verbal working memory in situation model construction. *J. Exp. Psychol. Gen.* **129,** 61–83.

Gathercole, S.E. & Hitch, G.J. (1993): Developmental changes in short-term memory: a revised working memory perspective. In: *Theories of Memory*, eds. A.F. Collins, S.E. Gathercole, M.A. Conway & P.E. Morris, pp. 189–209. Hove, U.K.: Lawrence Erlbaum Associates.

Hauser, M.D. (1999): Perseveration, inhibition and the prefrontal cortex: a new look. *Curr. Opin. Neurobiol.* **9,** 214–222.

Hulme, C. & MacKenzie, S. (1992): *Working Memory and Severe Learning Difficulties*, p.141. Hove, U.K.: Lawrence Erlbaum Associates.

Jarrold, C., Baddeley, A.D. & Hewes, A.K. (1999): Genetically dissociated components of working memory: evidence from Down's and Williams syndrome. *Neuropsychologia* **37,** 637–651.

Jarrold, C., Phillips, C. & Baddeley, A.D. (2007): Binding of visual and spatial short-term memory in Williams syndrome and moderate learning disability. *Dev. Med. Child Neurol.* **49,** 270–273.

Jernigan, L., Bellugi, U., Sowell, E., Doherty, S. & Hesselink, J.R. (1993): Cerebral morphologic distinctions between Williams and Down syndromes. *Arch. Neurol.* **50,** 186–191.

Johnson, M.K., Mitchell, K.J., Raye, C.L. & Greene, E.J. (2004): An age-related deficit in prefrontal cortical function associated with refreshing information. *Psychol. Sci.* **15,** 127–132.

Kesslak, J.P., Nagata, S.F., Lott, I. & Nalcioglu, O. (1994): Magnetic resonance imaging analysis of age-related changes in the brains of individuals with Down's syndrome. *Neurology* **44,** 1039–1045.

Kirwan, C.B., Wixted, J.T. & Squire, L.R. (2008): Activity in the medial temporal lobe predicts memory strength, whereas activity in the prefrontal cortex predicts recollection. *J. Neurosci.* **15,** 1541–1548.

Knopman, D. & Nissen, M.J. (1991): Procedural learning is impaired in Huntington's disease: evidence from the serial reaction time task. *Neuropsychologia* **29,** 245–354.

Long, N.M., Oztekin, I. & Badre, D. (2010): Separable prefrontal cortex contributions to free recall. *J. Neurosci.* **30,** 10967–10976.

MacPherson, S.E., Bozzali, M., Cipolotti, L., Dolan, R.J., Rees, J.H. & Shallice, T. (2008): Effect of frontal lobe lesions on the recollection and familiarity components of recognition memory. *Neuropsychologia* **46,** 3124–3132.

Mandler, G. (1980): Recognizing: the judgment of previous occurrence. *Psychol. Rev.* **87,** 252–271.

Matsui, M., Suzuki, M, Zhou, S.Y., Takahashi, T., Kawasaki, Y., Yuuki, H., *et al.* (2008): The relationship between prefrontal brain volume and characteristics of memory strategy in schizophrenia spectrum disorders. *Prog. Neuropsychopharmacol. Biol. Psychiatry* **32,** 1854–1862.

Mayes, A.R., Holdstock, J.S., Isaac, C.L., Hunkin, N.M. & Roberts, N. (2002): Relative sparing of item recognition memory in a patient with adult-onset damage limited to the hippocampus. *Hippocampus* **12,** 325–340.

Menghini, D., Hagberg, G.E., Caltagirone, C., Petrosini, L. & Vicari, S. (2006): Implicit learning deficits in dyslexic adults: an fMRI study. *Neuroimage* **33,** 1218–12126.

Menghini, D., Hagberg, G.E., Petrosini, L., Bozzali, M., Macaluso, E., Caltagirone, C. & Vicari, S. (2008): Structural correlates of implicit learning deficits in subjects with developmental dyslexia. *Ann. N. Y. Acad. Sci.* **1145,** 212–221.

Menghini, D., Addona, F., Costanzo, F. & Vicari, S. (2010): Executive functions in individuals with Williams syndrome. *J. Intellect. Disabil. Res.* **54,** 418–432.

Menghini, D., Costanzo, F. & Vicari, S. (2011a): Relationship between brain and cognitive processes in Down syndrome. *Behav. Genet.* **41,** 381–393.

Menghini, D., Vicari, S., Mandolesi, L. & Petrosini, L. (2011b): Is learning by observation impaired in children with dyslexia? *Neuropsychologia* **49,** 1996–2003.

Nadel, L. (1999): Down syndrome in cognitive perspective. In: *Neurodevelopmental Disorders*, ed. H. Tager-Flusberg, pp. 197–221. Cambridge: MIT Press.

Nichols, S., Jones, W., Roman, M.J., Wulfeck, B., Delis, D.C., Reilly, J. & Bellugi, U. (2004): Mechanisms of verbal memory impairment in four neurodevelopmental disorders. *Brain Lang.* **88,** 180–189.

Nicolson, R.I., Fawcett, A.J., Berry, E.L., Jenkins, I.H., Dean, P. & Brooks, D.J. (1999): Association of abnormal cerebellar activation with motor learning difficulties in dyslexic adults. *Lancet* **353,** 1662–1667.

O'Hearn, K., Courtney, S., Street, W. & Landau, B. (2009): Working memory impairment in people with Williams syndrome: effects of delay, task and stimuli. *Brain Cognit.* **69,** 495–503.

Ornstein, P.A., Schaaf, J.M., Hooper, S.R., Hatton, D.D., Mirrett, P. & Bailey, D.B., Jr (2008): Memory skills of boys with fragile X syndrome. *Am. J. Ment. Retard.* **113,** 453–465.

Orsini, A., Grossi, D., Capitani, E., Laiacona, M., Papagno, C. & Vallar, G. (1987): Verbal and spatial immediate memory span: normative data from 1,355 adults and 1,112 children. *Ital. J. Neurol. Sci.* **6,** 539–548.

Oztekin, I., Long, N.M. & Badre, D. (2010): Optimizing design efficiency of free recall events for FMRI. *J. Cogn. Neurosci.* **22,** 2238–2250.

Pascual-Leone, A., Grafman, J., Clark, K., Stewart, M., Massaquoi, S., Lou, J.S. & Hallett, M. (1993): Procedural learning in Parkinson's disease and cerebellar degeneration. *Ann. Neurol.* **34,** 594–602.

Pennington, B.F., Moon, J., Edgin, J., Stedron, J. & Nadel, L. (2003): The neuropsychology of Down syndrome: evidence for hippocampal dysfunction. *Child Dev.* **74,** 75–93.

Ranganath, C. (2004): The 3-D prefrontal cortex: hemispheric asymmetries in prefrontal activity and their relation to memory retrieval processes. *J. Cogn. Neurosci.* **16,** 903–907.

Richter, S., Matthies, K., Ohde, T., Dimitrova, A., Gizewski, E., Beck, A., *et al.* (2004): Stimulus-response versus stimulus-stimulus-response learning in cerebellar patients. *Exp. Brain. Res.* **158,** 438–449.

Rossi, E.L. (1963): Associative clustering in normal and retarded children. *Am. J. Ment. Defic.* **67,** 691–699.

Sampaio, A., Sousa, N., Férnandez, M., Henriques, M. & Gonçalves, O.F. (2008): Memory abilities in Williams syndrome: dissociation or developmental delay hypothesis? *Brain Cognit.* **66,** 290–297.

Skinner, E.I. & Fernandes, M.A. (2007): Neural correlates of recollection and familiarity: a review of neuroimaging and patient data. *Neuropsychologia* **45,** 2163–2179.

Sowell, E.R., Delis, D., Stiles, J. & Jernigan, T.L. (2001): Improved memory functioning and frontal lobe maturation between childhood and adolescence: a structural MRI study. *J. Int. Neuropsychol. Soc.* **7,** 312–322.

Squire, L.R. (1987): *Memory and Brain*, p. 336. Oxford, UK: Oxford University Press.

Trott, C.T., Friedman, D., Ritter, W., Fabiani, M. & Snodgrass, J.G. (1999): Episodic priming and memory for temporal source: event-related potentials reveal age-related differences in prefrontal functioning. *Psychol. Aging* **14,** 390–413.

Tulving, E. (1985): Memory and consciousness. *Can. Psychol.* **26,** 1–12.

Tulving, E. (1992): Memory systems and the brain. *Clin. Neuropharmacol.* **15,** 327A–328A.

Tulving, E. & Schacter, D.L. (1990): Priming and human memory systems. *Science* **247,** 301–306.

Vicari, S. (2001): Implicit versus explicit memory function in children with Down and Williams syndrome. *Down Syndr. Res. Pract.* **7,** 35–40.

Vicari, S. (2004): Memory development and intellectual disabilities. *Acta Paediatr. Suppl.* **445,** 1–6.

Vicari, S. & Carlesimo, G.A. (2006): Short-term memory deficits are not uniform in Down and Williams syndromes. *Neuropsychol. Rev.* **16,** 87–94.

Vicari, S., Carlesimo, A. & Caltagirone, C. (1995): Short-term memory in persons with intellectual disabilities and Down's syndrome. *J. Intellect. Disabil. Res.* **39,** 532–537.

Vicari, S., Carlesimo, G., Brizzolara, D. & Pezzini, G. (1996a): Short-term memory in children with Williams syndrome: a reduced contribution of lexical – semantic knowledge to word span. *Neuropsychologia* **34,** 919–925.

Vicari, S., Brizzolara, D., Carlesimo, G.A., Pezzini, G. & Volterra, V. (1996b): Memory abilities in children with Williams syndrome. *Cortex* **32,** 503–514.

Vicari, S., Bellucci, S. & Carlesimo, G.A. (2000): Implicit and explicit memory: a functional dissociation in persons with Down syndrome. *Neuropsychologia* **38,** 240–251.

Vicari, S., Caselli, M.C., Gagliardi, C., Tonucci, F. & Volterra, V. (2002): Language acquisition in special population: a comparison between Down and Williams syndromes. *Neuropsychologia* **40,** 2461–2470.

Vicari, S., Bellucci, S. & Carlesimo, G.A. (2003a): Visual and spatial working memory dissociation: evidence from Williams syndrome. *Dev. Med. Child Neurol.* **45,** 269–273.

Vicari, S., Marotta, L., Menghini, D., Molinari, M. & Petrosini, L. (2003b): Implicit learning deficit in children with developmental dyslexia. *Neuropsychologia* **41,** 108–114.

Vicari, S., Finzi, A., Menghini, D., Marotta, L., Baldi, S. & Petrosini L. (2005): Do children with developmental dyslexia have an implicit learning deficit? *J. Neurol. Neurosurg. Psychiatry* **76,** 1392–1397.

Vicari, S., Bellucci, S. & Carlesimo, G.A. (2006): Evidence from two genetic syndromes for the independence of spatial and visual working memory. *Dev. Med. Child Neurol.* **48,** 126–131.

Vicari, S., Verucci, L., Carlesimo, G.A. (2007): Implicit memory is independent from IQ and age but not from etiology: evidence from Down and Williams syndromes. *J. Intellect. Disabil. Res.* **51,** 932–941.

White, N.S., Alkire, M.T. & Haier, R.J. (2003): A voxel-based morphometric study of nondemented adults with Down syndrome. *NeuroImage* **20,** 393–403.

Winters, J.J., Jr. & Semchuk, M.T. (1986): Retrieval from long-term store as a function of mental age and intelligence. *Am. J. Ment. Defic.* **90,** 440–448.

Yonelinas, A.P. (2002): The nature of recollection and familiarity: a review of 30 years of research. *J. Mem. Lang.* **46,** 441–517.

Brain Lesion Localization and Developmental Functions, D. Riva, C. Njiokiktjien and S. Bulgheroni (eds.)

Chapter 5

Development of executive function

Giovanni Valeri

Child Neuropsychiatry Unit, Department of Neurosciences, IRCCS Children Hospital Bambino Gesù, piazza Sant'Onofrio 4, 00165 Rome, Italy
giovanni.valeri@opbg.net

Summary

During the last two decades, great progress has been made in our understanding of the development of the executive function (EF) in childhood. It is now known that: (*1*) EF is a *unitary* construct with partially dissociable components (Garon *et al.*, 2008; Miyake *et al.*, 2000); this model shows *continuity* in the structure of EF from preschool to adulthood. (*2*) EF begins to emerge in the first few years of life (*e.g.*, Diamond, 1990) and continues to develop through the preschool period (Garon *et al.*, 2008; Hughes *et al.*, 2010; Wiebe *et al.*, 2008), the school-age period (Lehto *et al.*, 2003), adolescence (Blakemore & Choudhury, 2006; Sommerville & Casey, 2010), and as far as adulthood (Huizinga *et al.*, 2006). (*3*) EF shows robust *associations* with cognitive characteristics, such as language ability and understanding of false-beliefs (*e.g.*, Hughes, 1998), and associations with family factors, such as socioeconomic status (Hughes & Ensor, 2005; Mezzacappa, 2004). (*4*) EF *predicts* school readiness (Blair & Peters, 2003) and success in numeracy and literacy (Blair & Razza, 2007). (*5*) EF can be improved in at-risk children through *preschool intervention* programs (Diamond *et al.*, 2007).

Introduction

During the last two decades interest has been increasing in the broad construct of *executive function* (EF) in childhood. This construct, which has long been linked to the prefrontal cortical network (*e.g.*, see Luria, 1966), includes a number of cognitive processes that are integral to the emerging self-regulation of behavior and developing social and cognitive competence in children. These cognitive processes include: the *inhibition* of prepotent responding, the maintenance of information in *working memory*, and the appropriate *shifting* and sustaining attention for the purpose of goal-directed action.

Over the past decades, great strides have been made in our understanding of the development of EF in childhood. In particular, recent years have seen a massive growth in the number of developmentally appropriate tasks available for assessing EF in children (*e.g.*, see Carlson, 2005; Espy *et al.*, 1999; Zelazo & Muller, 2002). Carlson (2005), for example, studied the performance of 602 typically developing children, aged 2 to 6 years, on several EF tasks. She analyzed and reported: (*i*) age trends in performance, and (*ii*) task difficulty scales at 2, 3, 4, and 5 to 6 years. The analysis of Carlson informs theories of EF development and offers researchers (and clinicians) an evidence-based guide to task selection and design.

These child-friendly tasks have led to dramatic improvements in our understanding of the development of EF. However, as Garon *et al.* (2008) noted in their review, simplifying adult tasks to make them age-appropriate for young children, carries the danger of losing the critical EF component. Thus the first step to take is to establish the *construct validity* of EF tasks for children.

Studies of adults (*e.g.*, Friedman & Miyake, 2004; Miyake *et al.*, 2000) have demonstrated advantages in the use of confirmatory factor analysis (CFA), a structural equation modeling technique, to assess the validity of different theoretical models. One of the strengths of the CFA is that it is theory driven, and thus researchers can explicitly test their model against competing models. An additional advantage is that CFA extracts common variance from measures. In recent years, this CFA approach has been extended to studies of preschool children (Hughes *et al.*, 2010; Wiebe *et al.*, 2008), school-aged children (*e.g.*, Brookshire *et al.*, 2004; Gathercole *et al.*, 2004; Lehto *et al.*, 2003), and young adults (Huizinga *et al.*, 2006).

Taken together, the findings from these studies suggest a *remarkable continuity* in the structure of EF from preschool to adulthood.

Review of the topic

Definition of the executive function

Historically, there have been two broad approaches to the development of EF frameworks.

– The first considers EF as a *unitary construct* with constituent subprocesses (*e.g.*, Baddeley, 1986; Shallice, 1988). In the theories of both investigators a *central attention system* is thought to regulate various subprocesses. Developmentally, Posner and Rothbart have also argued that a *central attention system* underlies the important changes taking place in EF control from 2 to 6 years of age (Posner & Rothbart, 1998, 2007; Rothbart & Posner, 2001). In contrast to a 'central attention system', Dempster (1992) has suggested that a general *inhibitory process* is responsible for developmental changes in EF. Some evidence supports the *unitary* EF view. Different measures of EF are intercorrelated for both children and adults, suggesting a common process (Carlson *et al.*, 2004; Friedman & Miyake, 2004; Hughes & Ensor, 2005; Lehto *et al.*, 2003; Miyake *et al.*, 2000). Evidence indicates further that performance on a variety of EF tasks is highly correlated with a central attention process (Kane & Engle, 2003). Finally, there seems to be a general developmental spurt in the performance of many EF tasks at certain ages, notably between 3 to 6 years of age (Carlson, 2005; Diamond, 2002; Rothbart & Posner, 2001).

– The second broad theoretical approach emphasizes *dissociable EF processes*; those most frequently cited in the developmental literature are *working memory* and *inhibition* (*e.g.*, Carlson & Moses, 2001; Diamond, 1990; Pennington, 1997). Diamond (2002) argues that working memory and inhibition are dissociable components that have different developmental trajectories. In support of this view, variation exists in the developmental timing of various EF abilities (Carlson, 2005; Luciana & Nelson, 2002; Murray & Kochanska, 2002; Rosso *et al.*, 2004).

Many proponents of the componential view have used *factor analysis* to delineate components in EF (*e.g.*, Hughes, 1998; Pennington, 1997). Findings from this work indicate that performance on different EF tasks clusters into distinct functional domains (Carlson & Moses, 2001; Friedman & Miyake, 2004; Hughes, 1998; Lehto *et al.*, 2003; Miyake *et al.*, 2000; Murray & Kochanska, 2002; Pennington, 1997).

Other researchers have separated out EF components on the basis of *prefrontal networks* (Casey *et al.*, 2001). Evidence from neuropsychological studies of patients with lesions of the prefrontal cortex indicates that different EF processes have differential associations with areas of the prefrontal cortex (Brookshire *et al.*, 2004; Stuss *et al.*, 2002).

– Over the last decade, evidence has been accumulating to support *both unitary* and *componential views* of EF, and so the literature has shifted toward the integration of these perspectives (Baddeley, 2002; Friedman & Miyake, 2004; Lehto *et al.*, 2003; Miyake *et al.*, 2000; Shallice, 2002). This is well represented by the integrative EF model proposed for adults by Miyake *et al.* (2000), who have argued for a *common EF mechanism*, similar to either 'executive attention' or a 'central inhibitory system', as well as *partially dissociable EF components*.

Although there is evidence for both unitary and componential views of EF, only recently have the two views been compared systematically. Miyake *et al.* (2000) used CFA, a structural equation modeling technique, to assess the validity of their model. In reviewing the literature on EF, Miyake *et al.* found that the three most common EF components were mental set shifting, information updating, and monitoring (which has been interpreted by most authors as working memory), and inhibition of prepotent responses. For each of these components, they used three common EF measures. The best model was one in which the three latent EF variables were partially independent but still correlated with one another. Further, this model was a better fit than a model in which the three EF variables were completely independent or one in which all measures formed a single central EF component.

Different researchers have applied this integrated model to children: Lehto *et al.* (2003) studied EF in 8- to 13-year-olds, in whom EF measures were found to cluster into three factors: working memory, set shifting, and inhibition. Again, CFA indicated that the best fit was a model with three partially dissociable but moderately intercorrelated latent variables.

In another study that used CFA on data from a sample of 7-to-21 year-olds, Huizinga *et al.* (2006) found partial support for Miyake's model. Like Lehto *et al.*, they found evidence of dissociation between the measures underlying the three EF components. An advantage of this study was that Huizinga *et al.* conducted a multiple-group CFA in order to compare latent factors across development. However, whereas two latent variables could be extracted from the working memory and set-shifting measures, this was not the case for the three inhibition measures, which did not load onto a common factor. It is possible that the wide age range used in this study (7- to 21-year-olds) may have complicated the results, as variance in task performance would be due to development in addition to components in EF. Huizinga *et al.* found that the same common underlying factors were evident over separate age groups, providing support for the stability of executive components through middle childhood, adolescence, and adulthood.

Some studies applied this integrative model to preschool children: Wiebe *et al.* (2008) used CFA to understand EF in preschool children, studying a sample of 243 normally developing children between 2.3 and 6 years of age. CFA was used to compare multiple models of executive control empirically. A single-factor was sufficient to account for the data.

Hughes *et al.* (2010) used a CFA of data from a socially diverse sample of 191children, aged 4 to 6 years for a longitudinal study of EF in children. This study showed the validity of EF as a latent construct underpinning performance at ages 4 and 6 years on tests of planning, inhibitory control, and working memory, supporting, in this way, the validity of a single EF construct at both time-points.

Summing up, these studies show that EF is a unitary construct with partially dissociable components, through infancy to adulthood.

Development of executive function

Executive function begins to emerge very early – for example Diamond (1990) shows that infants of 8 months begin to have EF, which continues to develop through preschool (Garon *et al.* 2008), school age (Letho *et al.*, 2003), adolescence (Blakemore & Choudhury, 2006), and as far as adulthood (Huizinga *et al.*, 2006).

Preschool

Factor analytic techniques (such as exploratory factor analysis or principal components analysis) have, until recently, rarely been used to examine EF in preschool children. Here, exceptions include: Hughes's (1998) study that included tasks designed to be developmentally appropriate for preschool; Espy's *et al.* (1999) study of very young children's performance on delayed-response tasks (such as the A-not-B task) and Kochanska's *et al.* (2001) study of self-regulation, a construct that is closely akin to EF but that also includes socioemotional dimensions. Kochanska *et al.* studied longitudinally 'the development of self-regulation in the first four years of life', when the children were 14, 22, 33, and 45 months of age. Wiebe *et al.* (2008) used CFA to study EF in preschool children. A sample of 243 normally developing children between 2.3 and 6 years of age completed a battery of age-appropriate executive control tasks.

CFA was used to compare, empirically, multiple models of executive control. A single-factor was sufficient to account for the data. Furthermore, the fit of the unitary model was invariant across subgroups of children divided by socioeconomic status or sex. Girls displayed a higher level of latent executive control than boys, and children of higher and lower socioeconomic status did not differ in level. In typically developing preschool children, tasks conceptualized as indexes of working memory and inhibitory control in fact measured a single cognitive ability despite surface differences between task characteristics. Interestingly, although the latent EF variable applied equally to boys and girls, and to children from different socioeconomic backgrounds, it explained more variance in performance for younger than for older children, suggesting that EF may drive task performance somewhat differently with development.

Hughes's *et al.* (2010) longitudinal study of EF in children aged 4 to 6 years yielded three main findings. First, CFA supported the application of a single EF latent construct to describe variation in children's scores on three distinct tasks (tapping inhibitory control, working memory, and planning). This model was supported both at age 4 and at age 6 and applied equally to girls and boys. Second, there was sufficient evidence of measurement invariance to conduct a latent growth model (LGM). Together, the models suggest that age-related improvements in children's task performance across these time-points may reflect a genuine increase in EF ability, rather than an artifact of non-executive task demands. Third, while verbal mental age and family income both predicted baseline individual differences, only verbal mental age independently predicted variation in the rate at which EF improved across time-points. However, this predictive effect was in the opposite direction to that hypothesized: across the transition to school, verbally-less-able children (but not children from low income families) showed greater gains in EF than their peers.

Garon *et al.* (2008) have adopted, following Miyake *et al.* (2000), an integrative model for their review of the literature on EF development during the preschool period. They have focused on the three EF components specified by Miyake *et al.*: updating/working memory, response inhibition, and set shifting. Given that attention has been widely viewed as pivotal to the construct of a central executive (Baddeley, 2002; Kane & Engle, 2003), they have also provided an overview of the development of attention. Garon's review illustrates how EF components are built upon simpler cognitive skills, and can be said to be the result of a coordination of simpler skills. Garon *et al.* suggest that by the end of the preschool period, EF organization is characterized by partially dissociable components. For instance, factor analysis of data from children 2 to 5 years of age indicates that measures of EF cluster into distinct factors (Carlson, 2005). However, the data also suggest that the development of this hierarchical structure is not a linear process. Garon *et al.* have focused on skills that they consider critical for EF development, such as the ability to 'hold in mind' and delay responses. The 'combination skills' are the ones that have been more closely linked with actual components of EF, as well as the central executive.

Selective attention is a prerequisite skill in any EF task; it allows children to focus on relevant aspects of the task and to disengage attention when warranted. The development in attention set the stage for EF components to develop:

– The first EF component to develop is working memory. There is evidence that children can hold simple representations in mind during the first 6 months of life. More complex skills, such as updating and manipulating information, which require coordination with the attention system, become apparent by 15 months.

– Simple forms of response inhibition develop within the latter half of the 1st year, reflecting the infant's growing ability to impose cognitive control over behavior. Once infants are able to delay responses, the ability to reduce conflict between dominant and subdominant responses develops. Dealing with simple conflict, such as controlling a direct reach, develops at approximately 12 months of age. Coordination of working memory and response inhibition develop around 2 years of age, when children are able to use a rule held in mind to inhibit a prepotent response and execute a subdominant response.

– Set shifting is the most complex EF component. Because of its nature, there is no pure set-shifting task, as shifting naturally builds upon the first two EF components (response inhibition and working memory). Shifting tasks require children to shift from a mental set that has been formed.

Garon *et al.* suggest that there are two main stages in EF development during the preschool period:

– Before a child has reached 3 years of age, many of the basic skills needed to perform EF tasks are emerging. During this period, there is a developmental surge in which the infant gains more voluntary control over attention. Critical concomitant achievements that become possible include the capacities to hold and manipulate representations in the mind, to inhibit a response using a rule held in mind, and to respond and allocate attention flexibly.

– The period between 3 and 5 years is very important for EF development. The literature indicates that there are significant age-related improvements in all three EF components during this period. These are well represented in Carlson's (2005) findings for a wide variety of EF tasks.

It is interesting to note that Hughes's (1998) longitudinal data provide support for the idea of a progressive integration and coordination: correlations between EF tasks increased from 3 years to 4 years, which she interpreted as evidence for increasing coherence of EF.

Summing up, the work of Garon *et al.* (2008) has revealed an interesting pattern of developments from infancy to 5 years, with individual EF components emerging before 3 years of age. Most researchers agree that the years from 3 to 5 constitute an important period in the development of EF. Garon *et al.* suggest that the resolution of a high degree of conflict is common to tasks that are challenging for 3-year-olds. They propose that improved performance from 3 to 5 years reflects development of the attention system and its connectivity with other brain areas underlying component EFs. This is consistent with the view of Rothbart and Posner (2001) and others (*e.g.*, Eigsti *et al.*, 2006), who have argued that changes in the attention system are particularly critical in allowing the developing child to resolve various forms of conflict.

As we have already seen in recent years, the CFA approach has been extended to studies of school-aged children (*e.g.*, Brookshire *et al.*, 2004; Gathercole *et al.*, 2004; Lehto *et al.*, 2003).

Adolescence

Adolescence is a time of considerable development at the levels of behaviour, cognition, and brain. Histologic and brain imaging studies have demonstrated specific changes in neural architecture during puberty and adolescence, outlining trajectories of grey and white matter development (Casey *et al.*, 2008). The brain development is associated with specific changes in EF and social cognition during puberty and adolescence (Blakemore & Choudhury, 2006).

Changes at the level of the brain and cognition may map onto behaviours commonly associated with adolescence: a developmental period characterized by suboptimal decisions and actions that give rise to an increased incidence of unintentional injuries and violence, alcohol and drug abuse, unintended pregnancy, and sexually transmitted diseases.

Because MRI studies have demonstrated changes in frontal cortex during adolescence, EF abilities might be expected to improve during this time. For example, selective attention, decision-making, and response-inhibition skills, along with the ability to carry out multiple tasks at once, might improve during adolescence.

Behavioural studies show that performance of adolescents on tasks including inhibitory control (Leon-Carrion *et al.*, 2004; Luna *et al.*, 2004), processing speed (Luna *et al.*, 2004), working memory, and decision-making (Hooper *et al.*, 2004; Luciana *et al.*, 2005) continues to develop during adolescence. Luna *et al.* (2004), for example, showed that performance on an oculomotor task undergoes a large improvement from childhood to adolescence, followed by a plateau between adolescence and early adulthood.

Another study investigating performance on a variety of executive function tasks between the ages of 11 and 17 demonstrated a linear improvement in performance on some tasks but not others (Anderson *et al.*, 2001). Improvement during adolescence was observed on tasks of selective attention, working memory, and problem solving. Different aspects of executive function, therefore, may have different developmental trajectories.

Prospective memory is the ability to hold in mind an intention to carry out an action at a future time, such as remembering to make a phone call at a specific time in the future. Prospective memory is associated with frontal lobe activity, and has been shown to develop through childhood as we develop our future-oriented thought and action (Ellis & Kvavilashvili, 2000). *Multitasking* is believed to be a test of prospective memory as it requires participants to remember to perform a number of different tasks, mirroring the requirements of everyday life. In a study of the development of prospective memory from childhood to adulthood, a multitask paradigm was used to test children (aged between 6 and 14) and adults (Mackinlay *et al.*, 2003).

Participants were scored for both efficiency and the strategies used to carry out the task effectively. A significant improvement in both the efficiency and quality of strategies was found between the ages of 6 and 10. However, between the ages of 10 and 14, there was no significant change in performance. The adult group (mean age 25), on the other hand, significantly outperformed the children. The authors therefore suggested that prospective memory continues to develop during adolescence, in line with the notion of frontal maturation in the brain. It is possible that the lack of improvement in performance between the 10- and 14-year-olds was related to their pubertal status.

A nonlinear pattern of development was found in a behavioural study that used a match-to-sample task (McGivern *et al.*, 2002). In this task, volunteers were shown pictures of faces showing particular emotional expressions (happy, sad, angry), or words describing those emotions ('happy', 'sad', 'angry'), and were asked to specify, as quickly as possible, the emotion presented in the face or word. In a third condition, volunteers were shown both a face and a word, and had to decide whether the facial expression matched the emotional word. The rationale behind the design of the task was that the face/word condition places high demands on frontal lobe circuitry since it requires working memory and decision-making. The task was given to a large group of children aged 10 to 17 years and a group of young adults aged 18 to 22 years. The results revealed that at the age of onset of puberty, at 11–12 years, there was a decline in performance in the matching face and word condition.

Traditional neurobiologic and cognitive explanations for adolescent behaviour have failed to account for the *nonlinear* changes in behavior observed during adolescence, relative to childhood and adulthood. Casey *et al.* (2008) posits 'the adolescent brain' as a biologically plausible conceptualization of the neural mechanisms underlying these nonlinear changes in behaviour characterized by a heightened responsiveness to incentives, while impulse control is still relatively immature during this period. Recent human imaging and animal studies provide a biological basis for this view, suggesting differential development of limbic reward systems relative to top-down control systems (prefrontal cortex) during adolescence relative to childhood and adulthood. This developmental pattern may be exacerbated in those adolescents with a predisposition toward risk-taking, increasing the risk for poor outcomes.

Association between EF and other factors

Executive function shows strong associations with cognitive characteristics, such as language ability and understanding of false beliefs (*e.g.*, Hughes, 1998); EF equally shows associations with family factors, such as socioeconomic status (SES) (Hughes & Ensor, 2005; Mezzacappa, 2004). Studies have shown cross-sectional associations between individual differences in EF and both the characteristics of the child (gender, verbal ability, theory of mind) and family socioeconomic status. Good performance on EF tasks is more common among girls than boys (Hughes & Ensor, 2005; Hughes *et al.*, 2010; Wiebe *et al.*, 2008), in children with high verbal ability (*e.g.*, Hughes, 1998; Hughes & Ensor, 2005), and in children from high SES families (*e.g.*, Noble *et al.*, 2007).

However, it is hard to judge from existing evidence whether these associations are similar or distinct for different age groups (in part because the EF tasks used typically vary across studies). As a result, it is not clear whether gender, verbal ability, and SES also predict *developmental change* in executive function.

As noted in a recent review (Hackman & Farah, 2009), a lack of longitudinal data is a significant constraint on theoretical models of the processes underpinning the robust association between poverty (low SES) and poor EF. As these authors report, this association cannot be fully explained in terms of SES-related differences in the quantity and quality of education, as it is also evident in studies of very young children (*e.g.*, Farah *et al.*, 2006; Hughes & Ensor, 2005; Noble *et al.*, 2007). We know that the environmental effects of poverty are strongest for children from families exposed to multiple stressors. The effects of the family environment on children's developing EF are mediated by different factors.

Consistent with direct effects of the social environment on EF, findings from a recent longitudinal study (Hughes & Ensor, 2009) indicate that several aspects of family life predict improvements in EF in children between the ages of 2 and 4. These include maternal scaffolding, opportunities for indirect observational learning, and low levels of family chaos or inconsistent parenting.

Predictions

Executive function predicts school readiness (Blair & Peters, 2003) and success in numeracy and literacy. EF is more strongly associated with school readiness than are intelligence quotient (IQ) or entry-level reading or math skills (Blair & Razza, 2007). Kindergarten teachers rank skills like self-discipline and attentional control as more critical for school readiness than content knowledge. EF is important for academic achievement throughout the school years. Working memory and inhibition independently predict math and reading scores in preschool through high school (Bull & Scerif, 2001; Gathercole *et al.*, 2005).

Intervention and prevention

Empirically, two sets of findings suggest that environmental factors can promote EF development: First, a previous longitudinal study demonstrated that high maternal scaffolding and low family chaos each independently predicted improvements in EF between the ages of 2 and 4 (Hughes & Ensor, 2009). Second, a recent intervention for children attending Head Start programs has been shown to yield significant gains in EF (Diamond *et al.*, 2007).

Many children begin school lacking in EF skills. Teachers receive little instruction in how to improve EF and, in the USA, preschoolers are removed from class for poor self-control at alarming rates. Previous attempts to improve children's EF have often been costly and of limited success (Dowsett & Livesey, 2000; Rueda *et al.*, 2005). Poor EF is associated with such problems as ADHD, teacher burnout, student dropout, drug use, and crime. Young lower-income children have disproportionately poor EF (Noble *et al.*, 2007), and they fall progressively farther behind in school each year.

The work of Diamond *et al.* (2007) shows that EF can be improved in 4- to 5-year-olds in regular public school classes with regular teachers. The curriculum outlined in *Tools of the Mind* ('Tools') (Bodrova & Leong, 1996) successfully moves children with poor EF to a more optimal state. It is not known how much it would help children who begin with better EF. Most interventions for at-risk children target *consequences* of poor EFs rather than seeking means of *prevention*, as does Tools. Diamond *et al.* hypothesize that improving EF early may have increasing benefits over time and may reduce the need for costly special education, societal costs from unregulated antisocial behavior, and the number of diagnoses of EF disorders (*e.g.*,

ADHD and conduct disorder). Finally, Diamond (2011) shows modulation of EF by biology (genes and neurochemistry) and the environment (including school programs) with implications for clinical disorders and for education.

As we have already seen, EF is critical for success in school and in life. Many children begin school lacking needed EF skills. Disturbances in EF occur in many mental health disorders, such as ADHD and depression. Unusual properties of the prefrontal dopamine system contribute to the PFC's vulnerability to environmental and genetic variations that have little effect elsewhere. EF depends on a late-maturing brain region (PFC), yet it can be improved even in infants and preschoolers without specialists or fancy equipment. Recent research shows that activities often budgetarily squeezed out of school curricula (such as play, physical education, and the arts), rather than detracting from academic achievement, help improve EF and enhance academic outcomes. Such additions to the curriculum may also head off problems before they lead to diagnoses of EF impairments, including ADHD. Many issues are not simply education issues or health issues; rather, they are both.

Conclusions

During the last two decades, great progress has been made in our understanding of the development of executive function in childhood (Diamond, 2006). It is now known that EF, in children and in adults, is a unitary construct with partially dissociable components (working memory, inhibition and set shifting) through infancy to adulthood (Garon *et al.*, 2008; Miyake *et al.*, 2000).

Executive function begins to emerge in the first few years of life (Diamond, 1990), continues to develop, in a nonlinear process through preschool (Garon *et al*, 2008; Huizinga *et al.*, 2010; Wiebe *et al.*, 2008), school age (Letho *et al.*, 2003), adolescence (Blakemore & Choudhury, 2006; Sommerville & Casey, 2010), extending as far as adulthood (Huizinga *et al.*, 2006).

Development of EF during adolescence shows some specificity. An article by Casey *et al.* (2008) on 'the adolescent brain' lays out the theoretical rationale supporting the relationship between specific dynamic frontostriatal interaction and risky behaviour in adolescence.

EF shows robust associations with cognitive characteristics, such as *verbal ability* and *social cognition* (*e.g.*, Hughes, 1998). The associations with family factors, such as *socioeconomic status* (Hughes & Ensor, 2005; Mezzacappa, 2004) seem mediated by maternal scaffolding and family chaos: each independently predicts improvements in EF between the ages of 2 and 4 (Hughes & Ensor, 2009).

EF *predicts* school readiness (Blair & Peters, 2003) and ability in numeracy and literacy: EF is more strongly associated with school success than is intelligence quotient (IQ) or entry-level reading or math skills (Blair & Razza, 2007).

Finally, EF can be improved in at-risk children through preschool intervention programs (Diamond *et al.*, 2007).

References

Anderson, V., Anderson, P., Northam, E., Jacobs, R & Catroppa, C. (2001): Development of executive functions through late childhood and adolescence in an Australian sample. *Dev. Neuropsychol.* **20,** 385–406.

Baddeley, A. (1986): *Working Memory.* Oxford, UK: Oxford University Press.

Baddeley, A. (2002): Fractionating the central executive. In: *Principles of Frontal Lobe Function*, eds. D. Stuss & R. Knight, pp. 246–260. New York: Oxford University Press.

Blair, C. & Peters, R. (2003): Physiological and neurocognitive correlates of adaptive behavior in preschool among children in Head Start. *Dev. Neuropsychol.* **24,** 479–497.

Blair, C. & Razza, R. (2007): Relating effortful control, executive function, and false belief understanding to emerging math and literacy ability in kindergarten. *Child Dev.* **78,** 647–663.

Blakemore, S.J. & Choudhury, S. (2006): Development of the adolescent brain: implications for executive function and social cognition. *J. Child Psychol. Psychiatry* **47,** 296–312.

Bodrova, E. & Leong, D. (1996): *Tools of the Mind: The Vygotskian Approach to Early Childhood Education.* Englewood Cliffs, NJ: Merrill/Prentice Hall.

Brookshire, B., Levin, H., Song, J. & Zhang, L. (2004): Components of executive function in typically developing and head-injured children. *Dev. Neuropsychol.* **25,** 61–83.

Bull, R. & Scerif, G. (2001): Executive functioning as a predictor of children's mathematics ability: inhibition, switching, and working memory. *Dev. Neuropsychol.* **19,** 273–293.

Carlson, S. (2005): Developmentally sensitive measures of executive function in preschool children. *Dev. Neuropsychol.* **28,** 595–616.

Carlson, S. & Moses, L. (2001): Individual differences in inhibitory control and children's theory of mind. *Child Dev.* **72,** 1032–1053.

Carlson, S., Mandell, D. & Williams, L. (2004): Executive function and theory of mind: stability and prediction from ages 2 to 3. *Dev. Psychol.* **40,** 1105–1122.

Casey, B., Durston, S. & Fossella, J. (2001): Evidence for a mechanistic model of cognitive control. *Clin. J. Neurosci. Res.* **1,** 267–282.

Casey, B., Getz, S. & Galvan, A. (2008): The adolescent brain. *Dev. Rev.* **28,** 62–77.

Dempster, F. (1992): The rise and fall of the inhibitory mechanism: toward a unified theory of cognitive development and aging. *Dev. Rev.* **12,** 45–75.

Diamond, A. (1990): Developmental time course in human infants and infant monkeys, and the neural bases of inhibitory control in reaching. *Ann. N.Y. Acad. Sci.* **608,** 637–704.

Diamond, A. (2002): Normal development of prefrontal cortex from birth to young adulthood: cognitive functions, anatomy, and biochemistry. In: *Principles of Frontal Lobe Function*, eds. D. Stuss & R. Knight, pp. 466–503. New York: Oxford University Press.

Diamond, A. (2006): The early development of executive functions. In: *Lifespan Cognition: Mechanisms of Change*, eds. E. Bialystok & F. Craik, pp.70–95. New York: Oxford University Press.

Diamond, A. (2011): Biological and social influences on cognitive control processes dependent on prefrontal cortex. *Prog. Brain Res.***189,** 19–39.

Diamond, A., Barnett, W., Thomas, J. & Munro, S. (2007): Preschool program improves cognitive control. *Science* **318,** 1387–1388.

Dowsett, S. & Livesey, D. (2000): The development of inhibitory control in preschool children: effects of executive skills training. *Dev. Psychobiol.* **36,** 161–174.

Eigsti, I.M, Zayas, V., Mischel, W., Shoda, Y, Ayduk, O, Dadlani M.B., *et al.* (2006) Predicting cognitive control from preschool to late adolescence and young adulthood. *Psychol. Sci.* **17,** 478–484.

Ellis, J. & Kvavilashvili, L. (2000): Prospective memory in 2000: past, present and future directions. *Appl. Cogn. Psychol.* **14,** S1–S9.

Espy, K., Kaufmann, P., McDiarmid, M. & Glisky, M. (1999): Executive functioning in preschool children: performance on A-not-B and other delayed response format tasks. *Brain Cognit.* **41,** 178–199.

Farah, M., Shera, D., Savage, J., Betancourt, L., Giannetta, J., Brodsky, N., *et al.* (2006). Childhood poverty: specific associations with neurocognitive development. *Brain Res.* **1110,** 166–174.

Friedman, N. & Miyake, A. (2004): The relations among inhibition and interference control functions: a latent-variable analysis. *J. Exp. Psychol. Genl.* **133,** 101–135.

Garon, N., Bryson, S. & Smith, I. (2008): Executive function in preschoolers: a review using an integrative framework. *Psychol. Bull.* **134,** 31–60.

Gathercole, S., Pickering, S., Ambridge, B. & Wearing, H. (2004): The structure of working memory from 4 to 15 years of age. *Dev. Psychol.* **40,** 177–190.

Gathercole, S., Tiffany, C., Briscoe, J., Thorn, A. & ALSPAC Team (2005): Developmental consequences of poor phonological short-term memory function in childhood: a longitudinal study. *J. Child Psychol. Psychiatry* **46,** 598–611.

Hackman, D. & Farah, M. (2009). Socioeconomic status and the developing brain. *Trends Cogn. Sci.* **13,** 65–73.

Hooper, C.J., Luciana, M., Conklin, H.M. & Yarger, R.S. (2004): Adolescents' performance on the development of decision making and ventromedial prefrontal cortex. *Dev. Psychol.* **40,** 1148–1158.

Hughes, C. (1998). Executive function in preschoolers: Links with theory of mind and verbal ability. *Br. J. Dev. Psychol.* **16,** 233–253.

Hughes, C. & Ensor, R. (2005): Theory of mind and executive function in 2-year-olds: a family affair? *Dev Neuropsychol.* **28,** 645–668.

Hughes, C. & Ensor, R. (2009). How do families help or hinder the emergence of early executive function. *New Direct. Child Adolesc. Dev.* **123,** 35–50.

Hughes, C., Ensor, R, Wilson, A. & Graham, A. (2010): Tracking executive function across the transition to school: a latent variable approach. *Dev. Neuropsychol.* **35,** 20–36.

Huizinga, M., Dolan, C. & van der Molen, M. (2006): Age-related change in executive function: developmental trends and a latent variable analysis. *Neuropsychologia* **44,** 2017–2036.

Kane, M. & Engle, R. (2003): Working-memory capacity and the control of attention: the contributions of goal neglect, response competition, and task set to Stroop interference. *J. Exp. Psychol. Genl.* **132,** 47–70.

Kochanska, G., Coy, K.C. & Murray, K.T., (2001): The development of self-regulation in the first four years of life. *Child. Dev.* **72,** 1091–1101.

Lehto, J., Juujärvi, P., Kooistra, L. & Pulkkinen, L. (2003): Dimensions of executive functioning: Evidence from children. *Br. J. Dev. Psychol.* **21,** 59–80.

Leon-Carrion, J., Garcia-Orza, J. & Perez-Santamaria, F.J. (2004): The development of the inhibitory component of the executive functions in children and adolescents. *Int. J. Neurosci.* **114,** 1291–1311.

Luciana, M. & Nelson, C. (2002): Assessment of neuropsychological function through use of the Cambridge Neuropsychological Testing Automated Battery: performance in 4- to 12-year-old children. *Dev. Neuropsychol.* **22,** 595–624.

Luciana, M., Conklin, H.M., Cooper, C.J. & Yarger, R.S. (2005): The development of nonverbal working memory and executive control processes in adolescents. *Child Dev.* **76,** 697–712.

Luna, B., Garver, K.E., Urban, T.A., Lazar, N.A. & Sweeney, J.A. (2004): Maturation of cognitive processes from late childhood to adulthood. *Child Dev.* **75,** 1357–1372.

Luria, A.R. (1966). *Higher Cortical Functions in Man.* New York: Basic Books.

Mackinlay, R., Charman, T. & Karmiloff-Smith, A. (2003): Remembering to remember: a developmental study of prospective memory in a multitasking paradigm. Poster presented at biennial meeting of the Society for Research in Child Development, 24–27 April, Tampa, Florida.

McGivern, R.F., Andersen, J., Byrd, D., Mutter, K.L. & Reilly, J. (2002): Cognitive efficiency on a match to sample task decreases at the onset of puberty in children. *Brain Cognit.* **50,** 73–89.

Mezzacappa, E. (2004): Alerting, orienting, and executive attention: developmental properties and sociodemographic correlates in an epidemiological sample of young, urban children. *Child Dev.* **75,** 1373–1386.

Miyake, A., Friedman, N., Emerson, M., Witzki, A., Howerter, A. & Wager, T. (2000): The unity and diversity of executive functions and their contributions to complex "frontal lobe" tasks: a latent variable analysis. *Cogn. Psychol.* **41,** 49–100.

Murray, K. & Kochanska, K. (2002): Effortful control: factor structure and relation to externalizing and internalizing behaviors. *J. Abnorm. Child Psychol.* **30,** 503–514.

Noble, K., McCandliss, B. & Farah, M. (2007): Socioeconomic gradients predict individual differences in neurocognitive abilities. *Dev. Sci.* **10,** 464–480.

Pennington, B. (1997): Dimensions of executive functions in normal and abnormal development. In: *Development of the Prefrontal Cortex: Evolution, Neurobiology, and Behavior,* eds. N. Krasnegor, G. Lyon & P. Goldman-Rakic, pp. 265–282. Baltimore, MD: Brookes Publishing.

Posner, M. & Rothbart, M. (1998): Attention, self-regulation and consciousness. *Phil. Trans. Royal Soc. London, Ser. B* **353,** 1915–1927.

Posner, M.I. & Rothbart, M.K. (2007): Research on attention networks as a model for the integration of psychological science. *Annu. Rev. Psychol.* **58,** 1–23.

Rothbart, M. & Posner, M. (2001): Mechanism and variation in the development of attentional networks. In: *Handbook of Developmental Cognitive Neuroscience*, eds. C. Nelson & M. Luciana, pp. 353–363. Cambridge, MA: MIT Press.

Rosso, I., Young, A., Femia, L. & Yurgelun-Todd, D. (2004): Cognitive and emotional components of frontal lobe functioning in childhood and adolescence. *Ann. N.Y. Acad. Sci.* **1021,** 355–362.

Rueda, M.R., Rothbart, M.K., McCandliss, B.D., Saccomanno, L., Posner, M.I. (2005): Training, maturation, and genetic influences on the development of executive attention. *Proc. Natl. Acad. Sci. USA* **102,** 14931–14947.

Shallice, T. (1988): *From Neuropsychology to Mental Structure.* Cambridge, UK: Cambridge University Press.

Shallice, T. (2002): Fractionation of the supervisory system. In: *Principles of Frontal Lobe Function,* eds. D. Stuss & R. Knight, pp. 261–277. New York: Oxford University Press.

Sommerville, L.H. & Casey, B.J. (2010): Developmental neurobiology of cognitive control and motivational systems. *Curr. Opin. Neurobiol.* **20,** 236–241.

Stuss, D., Alexander, M., Floden, D., Binns, M., Levine, B., McIntosh, A., *et al.* (2002): Fractionation and localization of distinct frontal lobe processes: evidence from focal lesions in humans. In: *Principles of Frontal Lobe Function,* eds. D. Stuss & R. Knight, pp. 392–407. New York: Oxford University Press.

Wiebe, S., Espy, K. & Charak, D. (2008): Using confirmatory factor analysis to understand executive control in preschool children: I. Latent structure. *Dev. Psychol.* **44,** 575–587.

Zelazo, P. & Muller, U. (2002): Executive function in typical and atypical development. In: *Handbook of Childhood Cognitive Development,* ed. U. Goswami, pp. 445–469. Oxford, UK: Blackwell.

Brain Lesion Localization and Developmental Functions, D. Riva, C. Njiokiktjien and S. Bulgheroni (eds.)
© 2011 John Libbey Eurotext, pp. 53–62.

Chapter 6

Neuropsychology of epilepsies involving the frontal lobe in children

Chiara Vago, Sara Bulgheroni and Daria Riva

Developmental Neurology Division, Fondazione IRCCS Istituto Neurologico 'C. Besta', via Celoria 11, 20133 Milan, Italy
neuropsicologia@istituto-besta.it

Summary

Focal or partial epilepsies are often associated with cognitive, behavioural, and emotional problems that also interfere with a patient's adaptive functioning. From a neuropsychological standpoint, the frontal location of the epileptic focus is crucial, since this area of the brain is involved in processing executive functions and metacognitive skills, in motor planning, and in impulse control. There are reports in the literature of impaired executive functions in children with frontal epileptic disorders, but no uniform neuropsychological and behavioural profile has been established as yet for such cases. Specific neuropsychological problems depend on the site and side of the epileptogenic focus, the frequency and severity of the seizures, and age-related factors. This chapter discusses epilepsies involving the frontal lobe in children, reviewing the recent literature. First, we briefly describe the characteristics of the EEG discharges and then concentrating on the neuropsychological and behavioral consequences in the light of the complexity of the frontal regions; finally, we consider the interactions between EEG characteristics, demographic variables, and neuropsychological outcome.

Introduction

The frontal lobes of the brain are characterized by a complex organization in terms of its neuroanatomy and connections, which support the higher-level integration circuits. This complexity determines a marked variability in the epileptic manifestations with a rapid and both inter- and intra-hemispheric propagation (Patrikelis *et al.*, 2009).

Specific neuropsychological and behavioural problems vary according to the site and side of the epileptogenic focus, the frequency and severity of the seizures, and age-related factors. The involvement of the frontal lobe is crucial because this area of the brain is involved in processing executive functions, which can be seen as a multiple of inter-related, interdependent process-related systems that function together as an integrated supervisory or control system (Lezak *et al.*, 2004). Anderson (2002) proposed a model of executive functions comprising four discrete but inter-related executive domains working together to enable 'executive control'. These domains are: (*i*) attention control, that is, the capacity to selectively attend to specific stimuli and inhibit prepotent responses, and to focus attention for a prolonged period of time, and the regulation and monitoring of actions; (*ii*) information processing, which includes fluency, efficiency, and speed of output; (*iii*) cognitive flexibility, or the ability to shift between response sets, learn from mistakes and devise alternative strategies, as well as working memory and divided attention; and (*iv*) the goal-setting domains, or the ability to develop new initiatives and concepts, plan actions in advance, and take an efficient, strategic approach to a task.

Frontal lobe epilepsy

Frontal lobe epilepsy (FLE) accounts for 20–30 per cent of cases of childhood focal epilepsy. The EEG shows partial frontal anomalies, frequently with a secondary generalization and a rapid and diffuse propagation of the epileptic activity to the contralateral hemisphere. The seizures caused by this type of anomaly are usually short-lived and rich in motor signs, and they often occur at night. Their particular features depend on the side and the precise site affected by the epileptic focus (Patrikelis *et al.*, 2009).

The number of studies on adults with FLE has increased in recent years: these patients generally have an impaired response inhibition and impulse control, and deficits in attention, motor programming, and speed (for a review, see Patrikelis *et al.*, 2009). Fewer studies have been conducted on patients during the age of development. Children with FLE share many of the features of frontal lobe dysfunctions with those in adult patients, but the different neuropsychological test methods used and, more importantly, the late development of the frontal lobe and the functions it serves make it impossible to extend findings in adults to patients of developmental age.

Most studies are consistent in reporting globally normal cognitive skills (Culhane-Shelburne *et al.*, 2002; Hernandez *et al.*, 2002, 2003; Luton *et al.*, 2010; Riva *et al.*, 2002, 2005), irrespective of the features of the seizure; however, a retrospective study of 21 children with FLE conducted by Prevost *et al.* (2006) found that only 52 per cent of them had a normal IQ when tested with the Wechsler scales. Most studies on FLE children investigate the efficiency of their executive functions by comparing them with children who have temporal lobe epilepsy (TLE) or generalized epilepsy with absences (GEA), as well as with typically developing children and assessing school-aged subjects.

FLE children have disorganized behaviour in the goal-setting domain, with impaired problem-solving skills, a limited capacity to rely on previously-learned strategies and in developing new strategies, and designing an efficient action plan in advance. In the London Tower Test, which assesses the ability to make plans and to anticipate his/her own actions, children with FLE have shorter planning times initially, but are subsequently slow to complete the task, which leads to longer total execution times. These findings suggest an impaired capacity to plan behaviour as a function of their goal, which is associated with a tendency towards impulsiveness, factors that give rise to a slower and less accurate global performance in completing a task (Hernandez *et al.*, 2002).

In information processing, FLE children have a reduced output, with slow responses and continuous hesitations in verbal fluency tasks, with both phonemic (Hernandez *et al.*, 2002; Riva *et al.*, 2005) and semantic cues (Luton *et al.*, 2010), as well as in graphic fluency tasks (Riva *et al.*, 2002, 2005).

As for FLE children's cognitive flexibility, there are clinical reports of rigid and inflexible patterns of behaviour, problems in switching from one activity or procedure to another, and failure to adapt to new or unusual demands. Neuropsychological tools have not proved sensitive enough to detect these problems, however. To the best of our knowledge, it was only in the study conducted by Igarashi *et al.* (2002) that the Wisconsin Card Sorting Test was able to identify such impairments, with a higher number of perseverative errors in FLE children. Riva *et al.* (2002) also reported an impaired performance, with a larger number of perseverative responses and numerous non-perseverative errors, but these data were not confirmed in a subsequent study conducted on a larger sample (Riva *et al*, 2005).

In terms of attention skills, Culhane-Shelburne *et al.* (2002) found that school-aged FLE children made more mistakes in the Stroop Color Word Test. Using the Continuous Performance Test, Hernandez *et al.* (2003) also found that FLE children make more mistakes, particularly in terms of false positives. These findings suggest an impulsive response mode and a more limited capacity to inhibit irrelevant but highly activated response patterns.

Auclair *et al.* (2005) reported a deficient preparatory attention, which was investigated by a task in which children had to react to a target presented in the middle of a display, while ignoring a distracter appearing to the right or left of the target before the target appeared, with a frequency that varied within a set of tests (0 per cent, 33 per cent, 67 per cent). Children with FLE had slower reaction times in responding to the target stimulus as a function of the percentage rate of appearance of the distracter during the course of the test. This gives the impression that children with FLE have an abnormal sensitivity to the possible onset of a distracter and a consequently weaker capacity to resist interference.

Memory skills are also affected in FLE children. Rather than in encoding, they reportedly have difficulty in using appropriate memory strategies for organizing material and thereby improving its learning and subsequent recall (Culhane-Shelburne *et al.*, 2002; Hernandez *et al.*, 2003; Riva *et al.*, 2002). In addition, they apparently have difficulty in inhibiting irrelevant responses, experiencing a stronger influence of retroactive and proactive interferences, and a larger number of intrusions (Hernandez *et al.*, 2003). In copy and recall tasks using visual material, they show a poor visuoperceptual organization and a greater impulsiveness in making their copy, which determines a lower accuracy when it comes to recalling the figure (Hernandez *et al.*, 2003).

As for the fine manual and bimanual coordination skills, there are reports of delays and a limited manual dexterity, with slow and stiff or quick, impulsive movements (Hernandez *et al.*, 2002; Riva *et al.*, 2002, 2005). A difficulty in planning and maintaining a fluid sequence of movements has also been described, with a tendency for the children to use spatial or verbal strategies to guide their movements, particularly in tasks requiring reciprocal, non-symmetrical gestures involving both hands (Hernandez *et al.*, 2002). The impairment seems to be worse for the non-dominant arm and in inter-manual tests; this would seem to indicate that frontal epilepsy interferes with the more complex aspects of motor activity.

FLE has effects not only on higher cognitive functioning, but also on the behavioural and emotional spheres. Recent studies have mentioned irritability, hyperactivity, impulsiveness, and mood changes, with a high comorbidity with ADHD (Parisi *et al.*, 2010). Using the Child Behavior Checklist, Hernandez *et al.* (2003) found high scores on both the Attention problems scale (confirming problems relating to lack of attention, distractibility, impulsiveness) and on the Thought problems scale (on which parents reported recurrent ideas and repetitive behaviour patterns). In their normal daily environment, FLE children have a limited capacity for self-regulation and ability to work unassisted; they are easily distracted and have difficulty in completing the task assigned to them, as well as in assessing their actions as they proceed (Luton *et al.*, 2010).

Adaptive and social functioning are also affected. Culhane-Shelburne *et al.* (2002) reported slightly lower than normal scores in all the areas investigated by the Vineland Adaptive Behaviour Scales, *i.e.*, communication, daily abilities, and socialization. It is also significant that parents reported having lower expectations concerning the academic performance of their children with frontal epilepsy and of their ability to become independent and successful in life (Hernandez *et al.*, 2003).

On the correlation between neuropsychological findings and clinical variables, it is important first to comment generally on the fact that most studies only provide descriptive data, without using statistical analyses. There is a general consensus in the literature that neuropsychological function impairments are worse, the earlier the age of onset of the epileptic seizures (Hernandez *et al.*, 2002, 2003; Prevost *et al.*, 2006; Riva *et al.*, 2002, 2005). The frequency of the seizures has only been correlated with the neuropsychological findings by our own group, which found a significant link in a first study (Riva *el al.*, 2002) that was not confirmed in a subsequent study group (Riva *et al.*, 2005). The side of the epileptic focus is usually classified as right, left, unilateral or bilateral, and no studies have found any significant correlation between this aspect and the neuropsychological data. This is presumably because of the tendency for the frontal epileptic focus to propagate to the contralateral hemisphere; it may also be that cerebral functions are redistributed following a very early onset of epilepsy (Riva *et al.*, 2002, 2005).

Benign epilepsy of childhood with centrotemporal spikes

Benign epilepsy with centrotemporal spikes (BECTS) or rolandic epilepsy accounts for 15 per cent of all cases of childhood epilepsy. The location of the interictal epileptic activity may vary: it prominently involves the temporal or rolandic areas but other regions may be involved, such as frontal regions. Spikes are often multifocal, moreover, presenting bilaterally and asynchronously, and they may even be located ipsilaterally to the side of the body affected by the ictal phenomena. Seizures usually occur at night, with focal paresthesias and tonic or clonic facial contractions, and they may subsequently become generalized. They occur when the child is between 3 and 13 years of age. The EEG spikes fade away spontaneously during puberty at the latest, irrespective of any use of antiepileptic medication (Stephani & Carlsson, 2006).

Studies on the neuropsychological outcome in children with BECTS are now numerous; most of them report globally normal cognitive skills (Northcott *et al.*, 2005; Riva *et al.*, 2007; Völkl-Kernstock *et al.*, 2006) and a broad array of neuropsychological impairments with a far from uniform profile. It is generally agreed, however, that the related impairments are mild and do not seem to interfere with daily functioning. Deficiencies have emerged in language skills, in terms of expressive vocabulary (Baglietto *et al.*, 2001; Völkl-Kernstock *et al.*, 2009), comprehension (Danielsson & Petermann, 2009; Riva *et al.*, 2007, Völkl-Kernstock *et al.*, 2009), and meta-phonological awareness (Northcott *et al.*, 2005), as well as learning difficulties (Piccinelli *et al.*, 2008), affecting reading (Ay *et al.*, 2009; Fonseca *et al.*, 2009; Papavasiliou *et al.*, 2005; Staden *et al.*, 1998), and spelling (Monjauze *et al.*, 2005; Papavasiliou *et al.*, 2005; Staden *et al.*, 1998). Another interesting research topic concerns the effects of rolandic spikes on functional language lateralization: Bulgheroni *et al.* (2008) suggested that the superiority of the left hemisphere in processing phonological stimuli is functionally disturbed by interictal spikes, leading to a bi-hemispheric representation of the phonological processing of verbal auditory stimuli. fMRI analyses recently showed that language-related activation was less lateralized to the left hemisphere in the anterior brain regions in BECTS children than in controls (Lillywhite *et al.*, 2009).

As for memory, there are reports of difficulties in short (Danielsson & Petermann, 2009; Northcott *et al.*, 2005; Weglage *et al.*, 1997) and long-term verbal memory (Northcott *et al.*, 2005) in the learning of verbal information (Croona *et al.*, 1999; Staden *et al.*, 1998) and also in visual and spatial memory (Baglietto *et al.* 2001; Danielsson & Petermann, 2009; Völkl-Kernstock *et al.*, 2009). Our group assessed verbal learning and retrieval, and the related use of learning strategies. Children under 10 years of age with BECTS had significant learning difficulties and were less efficient in using semantic clustering strategies with respect to age-matched controls, while no such difference emerged for the over-10-year-olds. This suggests that the ability to use more efficient strategies spontaneously matures later in BECTS children (Vago *et al.*, 2008).

Studies on attention and executive abilities in BECTS children have shown mild impairments in auditory attention (Ay *et al.*, 2009), information processing (Baglietto *et al.*, 2001; D'Alessandro *et al.*, 1990), inhibitory processes (Deltour *et al.*, 2007, 2008), problem solving (Croona *et al.*, 1999), and cognitive flexibility (Croona *et al.*, 1999; Deltour *et al.*, 2007).

As regards behaviour, there are reports of impulsiveness (Massa *et al.*, 2001; Metz-Lutz *et al.*, 1999) and hyperactivity (Giordani *et al.*, 2006; Holtmann *et al.*, 2006; Völkl-Kernstock *et al.*, 2009).

When neuropsychological data are correlated with clinical variables, an early age of onset of the epileptic seizures coincides with a worse impairment of neuropsychological functioning (Deltour *et al.*, 2007; Piccinelli *et al.*, 2008). Some works reported a link between spike frequency and neuropsychological data (Nicolai *et al.*, 2007; Piccinelli *et al.*, 2008; Riva *et al.*, 2007; Weglage *et al.*, 1997), but this was not confirmed in other studies (Massa *et al.*, 2001; Pinton *et al.*, 2006; Riva *et al.*, 2007). Several studies also considered the site of the epileptic focus, usually classified as right, left, or bilateral (Bedoin *et al.*, 2006; Deltour *et al.*, 2007; Northcott *et al.*, 2005; Riva *et al.* 2007; Staden *et al.*, 1998), and some of them identified a side-related effect. For instance in the study by Bedoin *et al.* (2006) BECTS children with right focus were impaired in the visual-spatial task relative to those with left focus, and the typical left-hemisphere advantage was not reported in the verbal task in children with left focus. Riva *et al.* (2007) found that children with a right focus had worse results in the Vocabulary subtest of the WISC-R and in the lexical comprehension test, by comparison with a healthy control group, whereas children with a left focus fared less well in phonemic fluency tasks. The discordance of the data may be because BECTS is a form of epilepsy with signs of cortical hyperexcitability that vary with time in terms of rate, side, and site, so the pattern of neuropsychological deficiencies may have changed (to some degree at least) based on the EEG variables considered by the time the test was administered.

The literature is generally consistent in saying that neuropsychological functioning improves when the EEG trace returns to normal (Baglietto *et al.*, 2001; D'Alessandro *et al.*, 1995; Deonna *et al.*, 2000; Northcott *et al.*, 2007; Völkl-Kernstock *et al.*, 2009).

The difficulties identified in dealing with executive tasks (Ay *et al.*, 2009; Baglietto *et al.*, 2001; Croona *et al.*, 1999; D'Alessandro *et al.*, 1990; Riva *et al.*, 2007; Vago *et al.*, 2008) are suggestive of a frontal lobe dysfunction, which leads us to surmise that, although the epileptic focus typical of BECTS is concentrated mainly in the central region, its variable propagation may interfere with the activity of other regions too (such as the frontal area), disrupting functions not directly processed by the centrotemporal regions and giving rise to malfunctions apparently not strictly related to the primary site of the typical BECTS focus.

In addition to the behavioural findings emerging from neuropsychological tests, neuroimaging studies have confirmed that children with BECTS and neuropsychological impairments have disturbed prefrontal and frontal lobe growth by comparison with controls, particularly during the active phase of the epileptic anomalies (Kanemura *et al.*, 2011).

Continuous spike and waves during slow sleep syndrome

Continuous spike and wave in slow sleep (CSWS) is a term used to describe a clinical epileptic syndrome associated with electrical status epilepticus in sleep (ESES). The EEG trace shows a dramatic activation of epileptiform discharges during sleep, while it frequently shows anomalies in wakefulness that are focal, multifocal, or diffuse, often with a frontotemporal, frontocentral, or centrotemporal predominance (Nickels & Wirrell, 2008). In the past it has been considered that the diffuse and generalized anomalies with continuous spike and wave complexes had to occupy at least 85 per cent of the total period of slow sleep and persist on three or more readings over a period of at least a month (De Negri, 1997; Patry *et al.*, 1971). This definition has been judged excessively strict in the more recent literature, and it has been suggested instead that ESES-related syndromes derive from a combination of clinical and electrographic features (Galanopoulou *et al.*, 2000; Nickels & Wirrell, 2008).

CSWS syndrome is considered rare, with an incidence of less than 1 per cent of all childhood epilepsies (Nickels & Wirrel, 2008). The age of onset varies for CSWS, which can develop any time between 1 and 14 years of age, peaking in children between 4 and 8 years old (Tassinari & Rubboli, 2006). It can last from months to years. The picture of ESES usually disappears spontaneously during the second decade of life. Epilepsy persists after puberty in one in three patients, however, despite the disappearance of the ESES (Scholtes *et al.*, 2005).

It is hard to establish the exact incidence of neuropsychological impairment because most reports describe only single cases or numerically limited series, and the related data analyses are often not very accurate (Galonopoulou *et al.*, 2000). Although most patients reportedly have a normal neuropsychological and motor development prior to the onset of their symptoms (Morikawa *et al.*, 1995; Tassinari *et al.*, 1992), previous neurological deficits are reported in approximately one in three patients (MacAllister & Schaffer, 2007). Whatever the patients' prior cognitive status and development, the onset of CSWS is associated with a new, progressive regression in global skills (Tassinari *et al.*, 2000). Only a few studies of the past reported on cases of CSWS with no correlated cognitive impairments (Aicardi & Chevrie, 1982; Gökyiğit *et al.*, 1986). To be specific, during periods of ESES there are reports of a markedly impaired IQ and deteriorations in language skills, with a tendency for expressive aphasia, and lexical and syntactic difficulties, while comprehension is usually preserved (Debiais *et al.*, 2007; MacAllister & Schaffer, 2007). Learning difficulties at school are described too, as is poor reasoning (Roulet-Perez *et al.*, 1993) and short-term memory deficits (De Negri *et al.*, 1997; Roulet-Perez *et al.*, 1993; Tassinari *et al.*, 1992, 2000). Motor impairments develop too, such as ataxia, dystonia, and dyspraxia (Maquet *et al.*, 1995; Tassinari *et al.*, 2000).

Children with CSWS often develop behavioural issues, and there are reports of a reduced attention span and hyperkinesia, aggressiveness, and disinhibition (Scholtes *et al.*, 2005; Tassinari *et al.*, 1992; Veggiotti *et al.*, 1998), as well as bizarre behaviour (Kyllerman *et al.*, 1996;

Morikawa *et al.*, 1995; Roulet-Perez *et al.*, 1993), emotional lability, anxiety, and phobias (Morikawa *et al.*, 1995; Roulet-Perez *et al.*, 1993), and autistic-like behaviour (Bulteau *et al.*, 1995; Kyllerman *et al.*, 1996). For a review of the spectrum of neuropsychological and behavioural abnormalities associated with CSWS, see Galanopoulou *et al.* (2000).

As concerns the correlation with clinical variables, the prognosis is better for patients with a shorter-lived CSWS (Rousselle & Revol, 1995). The related cognitive deterioration is less severe when the patients' age at the onset of CSWS is at least 8–9 years old, while there is no proof of any direct link between the severity of cognitive impairment and the severity of the epilepsy (Scholtes *et al.*, 2005). As for the site of the interictal foci, this seems to play a major part in influencing the degree and type of cognitive dysfunction in CSWS patients (Tassinari & Rubboli, 2006): CSWS patients with mainly cognitive and behavioural dysfunctions tended to have a frontal focus, while those with dysfunctions mainly relating to language skills had a temporal focus. There was a considerable overlap between the study groups, however, which makes it difficult to draw clear distinctions between them (Rousselle & Revol, 1995). When the EEG picture improves, there are also reportedly significant, but still only partial, improvements in the cognitive, motor, and behavioural sphere (Paquier *et al.*, 2009; Tassinari & Rubboli, 2006).

Conclusions

Epileptic anomalies involving the frontal lobe have a negative effect on executive abilities (abilities primarily processed by the frontal lobe). The recent literature has not drawn a uniform neuropsychological profile of the various types of frontal lobe epilepsy, since the reported deficits vary in severity and in the specific skills affected. A reduced capacity for the inhibitory control of previously learned, strongly activated responses is the dysfunction most frequently described, irrespective of the type of task involved. The selective impairment of certain executive skills, while others are spared, provides further evidence of the fact that dysexecutive syndrome is by no means a unitary disorder (Lezak *et al.*, 2004, Stuss & Alexander, 2000).

As for the clinical variables, we can generally say that the extent of neuropsychological impairments correlates with both the severity of the epileptic anomalies and the patient's age at onset of the condition: a diffuse epileptic activity and an earlier age of onset interfere more heavily with a patient's performance in neuropsychological tests. The onset of epilepsy can therefore interfere with the frontal lobe's maturation and the development of the skills that it processes. In future studies, it would consequently be interesting to lower the age for the children's neuropsychological assessment, investigating cases occurring in preschool-aged children to establish their functioning profile, as well as with a view to focusing their rehabilitation therapy on the skills most severely affected and following them up during their years at school.

The fact that we have no clear neuropsychological profile for reference makes it necessary to conduct in-depth neuropsychological assessments to investigate a given individual's functioning profile. This assessment should also consider how the child functions in daily life because neuropsychological tests involve completing a single task within a limited time and after receiving more or less clear indications on when the test would start and end. Such conditions differ considerably from those of real life, when scarcely structured settings demand decision-making and strategic processes of far greater complexity.

Executive functions are also activated when several processes have to be coordinated, or when the complexity of a task makes it necessary to process new types of information. Most cognitive tasks implicate variable degrees of executive skills, so it is important to observe *how* a proposed task is completed, *e.g.*, by observing how children approach the task, how they plan and organize their actions to achieve the required result, and whether or not they assess what they have done.

References

Aicardi, J. & Chevrie, J.J. (1982): Atypical benign partial epilepsy of childhood. *Dev. Med. Child Neurol.* **24,** 281–292.

Anderson, P. (2002): Assessment and development of executive function (EF) during childhood. *Child Neuropsychol.* **8,** 71–82.

Auclair, L., Jambaqué, I., Dulac, O., LaBerge, D. & Sieroff, E. (2005): Deficit of preparatory attention in children with frontal lobe epilepsy. *Neuropsychologia* **43,** 1701–1712.

Ay, Y., Gokben, S., Serdaroglu, G., Polat, M., Tosun, A., Tekgul, H., *et al.* (2009): Neuropsychologic impairment in children with rolandic epilepsy. *Pediatr. Neurol.* **41,** 359–363.

Baglietto, M.G., Battaglia, F.M., Nobili, L., Tortorelli, S., De Negri, E., Calevo, M.G., *et al.* (2001): Neuropsychological disorders related to interictal epileptic discharges during sleep in benign epilepsy of childhood with centrotemporal or Rolandic spikes. *Dev. Med. Child Neurol.* **43,** 407–412.

Bedoin, N., Herbillon, V., Lamoury, I., Arthaud-Garde, P., Ostrowsky, K., De Bellescize, J., *et al.* (2006): Hemispheric lateralization of cognitive functions in children with centrotemporal spikes. *Epilepsy Behav.* **9,** 268–274.

Bulgheroni, S., Franceschetti, S., Vago, C., Usilla, A., Pantaleoni, C., D'Arrigo, S. & Riva, D. (2008): Verbal dichotic listening performance and its relationship with EEG features in benign childhood epilepsy with centrotemporal spikes. *Epilepsy Res.* **79,** 31–38.

Bulteau, C., Plouin, P., Jambaqué, J., Renaux, V., Quillerou, D. & Boidein, F. (1995): Case reports. In: *Continuous Spikes and Waves during Slow Sleep, Electrical Status Epilepticus during Slow Wave Sleep: Acquired Epileptic Aphasia and Related Conditions,* eds. A. Beaumanoir, M. Bureau, T. Deonna, *et al.*, pp. 175–182. London: John Libbey.

Croona, C., Kihlgren, M., Lundberg, S., Eeg-Olofsson, O. & Eeg-Olofsson, K.E. (1999): Neuropsychological findings in children with benign childhood epilepsy with centrotemporal spikes. *Dev. Med. Child Neurol.* **41,** 813–818.

Culhane-Shelburne, K., Chapieski, L., Hiscock, M. & Glaze, D. (2002): Executive functions in children with frontal and temporal lobe epilepsy. *J. Int. Neuropsychol. Soc.* **8,** 623–632.

D'Alessandro, P., Piccirilli, M., Tiacci, C., Ibba, A., Maiotti, M., Sciarma, T. & Testa, A. (1990): Neuropsychological features of benign partial epilepsy in children. *Ital. J. Neurol. Sci.* **11,** 265–269.

Danielsson, J. & Petermann, F. (2009): Cognitive deficits in children with benign rolandic epilepsy of childhood or rolandic discharges: a study of children between 4 and 7 years of age with and without seizures compared with healthy controls. *Epilepsy Behav.* **16,** 646–651.

Debiais, S., Tuller, L., Barthez, M.A., Monjauze, C., Khomsi, A., Praline, J., *et al.* (2007): Epilepsy and language development: the continuous spike-waves during slow sleep syndrome. *Epilepsia* **48,** 1104–1110.

Deltour, L., Quaglino, V., Barathon, M., De Broca, A. & Berquin, P. (2007): Clinical evaluation of attentional processes in children with benign childhood epilepsy with centrotemporal spikes (BCECTS). *Epileptic Disord.* **9,** 424–431.

Deltour, L., Querné, L., Vernier-Hauvette, M.P. & Berquin, P. (2008): Deficit of endogenous spatial orienting of attention in children with benign epilepsy with centrotemporal spikes (BECTS). *Epilepsy Res.* **79,** 112–119.

De Negri, M. (1997): Electrical status epilepticus during sleep (ESES). Different clinical syndromes: towards a unifying view? *Brain Dev.* **19,** 447–451.

Deonna, T., Zesiger, P., Davidoff, V., Maeder, M., Mayor, C. & Roulet, E. (2000): Benign partial epilepsy of childhood: a longitudinal neuropsychological and EEG study of cognitive function. *Dev. Med. Child Neurol.* **42,** 595–603.

Fonseca, L.C., Tedrus, G.M., de Oliveira, E.D. & Ximenes, V.L. (2009): Benign childhood epilepsy with centrotemporal spikes: word and pseudoword discrimination. *Arq. Neuropsiquiatr.* **67,** 450–456.

Galanopoulou, A.S., Bojko, A., Lado, F. & Moshé, S.L. (2000): The spectrum of neuropsychiatric abnormalities associated with electrical status epilepticus in sleep. *Brain Dev.* **22,** 279–295.

Giordani, B., Caveney, A.F., Laughrin, D., Huffman, J.L., Berent, S., Sharma, U., *et al.* (2006): Cognition and behavior in children with benign epilepsy with centrotemporal spikes (BECTS). *Epilepsy Res.* **70,** 89–94.

Gökyiğit, A., Apak, S. & Calişkan, A. (1986): Electrical status epilepticus lasting for 17 months without behavioural changes. *Electroencephalogr. Clin. Neurophysiol.* **63,** 32–34.

Hernandez, M.T., Sauerwein, H.C., Jambaqué, I., De Guise, E., Lussier, F., Lortie, A., *et al.* (2002): Deficits in executive functions and motor coordination in children with frontal lobe epilepsy. *Neuropsychologia* **40,** 384–400.

Hernandez, M.T., Sauerwein, H.C., Jambaqué, I., de Guise, E., Lussier, F., Lortie, A., *et al.* (2003): Attention, memory, and behavioral adjustment in children with frontal lobe epilepsy. *Epilepsy Behav.* **4,** 522–536.

Holtmann, M., Matei, A., Hellmann, U., Becker, K., Poustka, F. & Schmidt, M.H. (2006): Rolandic spikes increase impulsivity in ADHD: a neuropsychological pilot study. *Brain Dev.* **28,** 633–640.

Igarashi, K., Oguni, H., Osawa, M., Awaya, Y., Kato, M., Mimura, M. & Kashima, H. (2002): Wisconsin card sorting test in children with temporal lobe epilepsy. *Brain Dev.* **24,** 174–178.

Kanemura, H., Hata, S., Aoyagi, K., Sugita, K. & Aihara, M. (2011): Serial changes of prefrontal lobe growth in the patients with benign childhood epilepsy with centrotemporal spikes presenting with cognitive impairments/behavioral problems. *Brain Dev.* **33,** 106–113.

Kyllerman, M., Nydén, A., Praquin, N., Rasmussen, P., Wetterquist, A.K. & Hedström, A. (1996): Transient psychosis in a girl with epilepsy and continuous spikes and waves during slow sleep (CSWS). *Eur. Child Adolesc. Psychiatry* **5,** 216–221.

Lezak, M.D., Howieson, D.B. & Loring, D.W. (2004): *Neuropsychological Assessment* (4th ed.). New York: Oxford University Press.

Lillywhite, L.M., Saling, M.M., Harvey, A.S., Abbott, D.F., Archer, J.S., Vears, D.F., *et al.* (2009): Neuropsychological and functional MRI studies provide converging evidence of anterior language dysfunction in BECTS. *Epilepsia* **50,** 2276–2284.

Luton, L.M., Burns, T.G. & DeFilippis, N. (2010): Frontal lobe epilepsy in children and adolescents: a preliminary neuropsychological assessment of executive function. *Arch. Clin. Neuropsychol.* **25,** 762–770.

MacAllister, W.S. & Schaffer, S.G. (2007): Neuropsychological deficits in childhood epilepsy syndromes. *Neuropsychol. Rev.* **17,** 427–444.

Maquet, P., Hirsch, E., Metz-Lutz, M.N., Motte, J., Dive, D., Marescaux, C. & Franck, G. (1995): Regional cerebral glucose metabolism in children with deterioration of one or more cognitive functions and continuous spike-and-wave discharges during sleep. *Brain* **118,** 1497–1520.

Massa, R., de Saint-Martin, A., Carcangiu, R., Rudolf, G., Seegmuller, C., Kleitz, C., *et al.* (2001): EEG criteria predictive of complicated evolution in idiopathic rolandic epilepsy. *Neurology* **57,** 1071–1079.

Metz-Lutz, M.N., Kleitz, C., de Saint Martin, A., Massa, R., Hirsch, E. & Marescaux, C. (1999): Cognitive development in benign focal epilepsies of childhood. *Dev. Neurosci.* **21,** 182–190.

Monjauze, C., Tuller, L., Hommet, C., Barthez, M.A. & Khomsi, A. (2005): Language in benign childhood epilepsy with centro-temporal spikes abbreviated form: rolandic epilepsy and language. *Brain Lang.* **92,** 300–308.

Morikawa, T., Seino, M. & Watanabe, M. (1995): Long-term outcome of CSWS syndrome. In: *Continuous Spikes and Waves during Slow Sleep – Electrical Status Epilepticus during Slow Sleep*, eds. A. Beaumanoir, M. Bureau, T. Deonna, L. *et al.*, pp. 175–182. London: John Libbey.

Nickels, K. & Wirrell, E. (2008): Electrical status epilepticus in sleep. *Semin. Pediatr. Neurol.* **15,** 50–60.

Nicolai, J., van der Linden, I., Arends, J.B., van Mil, S.G., Weber, J.W., Vles, J.S. & Aldenkamp, A.P. (2007): EEG characteristics related to educational impairments in children with benign childhood epilepsy with centrotemporal spikes. *Epilepsia* **48,** 2093–2100.

Northcott, E., Connolly, A.M., Berroya, A., Sabaz, M., McIntyre, J., Christie, J., *et al.* (2005): The neuropsychological and language profile of children with benign rolandic epilepsy. *Epilepsia* **46,** 924–930.

Northcott, E., Connolly, A.M., Berroya, A., McIntyre, J., Christie, J., Taylor, A., *et al.* (2007): Memory and phonological awareness in children with benign rolandic epilepsy compared to a matched control group. *Epilepsy Res.* **75,** 57–62.

Papavasiliou, A., Mattheou, D., Bazigou, H., Kotsalis, C. & Paraskevoulakos, E. (2005): Written language skills in children with benign childhood epilepsy with centrotemporal spikes. *Epilepsy Behav.* **6,** 50–58.

Paquier, P.F., Verheulpen, D., De Tiège, X. & Van Bogaert, P. (2009): Acquired cognitive dysfunction with focal sleep spiking activity. *Epilepsia* **50,** 29–32.

Parisi, P., Moavero, R., Verrotti, A. & Curatolo, P. (2010): Attention deficit hyperactivity disorder in children with epilepsy. *Brain Dev.* **32,** 10–16.

Patrikelis, P., Angelakis, E. & Gatzonis, S. (2009): Neurocognitive and behavioral functioning in frontal lobe epilepsy: a review. *Epilepsy Behav.* **14,** 19–26.

Patry, G., Lyagoubi, S. & Tassinari, C.A. (1971): Subclinical 'electrical status epilepticus' induced by sleep in children: a clinical and electroencephalographic study of six cases. *Arch. Neurol.* **24,** 242–252.

Piccinelli, P., Borgatti, R., Aldini, A., Bindelli, D., Ferri, M., Perna, S., *et al.* (2008): Academic performance in children with rolandic epilepsy. *Dev. Med. Child Neurol.* **50,** 353–356.

Pinton, F., Ducot, B., Motte, J., Arbuès, A.S., Barondiot, C., Barthez, M.A., *et al.* (2006): Cognitive functions in children with benign childhood epilepsy with centrotemporal spikes (BECTS). *Epileptic Disord.* **8,** 11–23.

Prévost, J., Lortie, A., Nguyen, D., Lassonde, M. & Carmant, L. (2006): Nonlesional frontal lobe epilepsy (FLE) of childhood: clinical presentation, response to treatment and comorbidity. *Epilepsia* **47,** 2198–2201.

Riva, D., Saletti, V., Nichelli, F. & Bulgheroni, S. (2002): Neuropsychologic effects of frontal lobe epilepsy in children. *J. Child Neurol.* **17,** 661–667.

Riva, D., Avanzini, G., Franceschetti, S., Nichelli, F., Saletti, V., Vago, C., *et al.* (2005): Unilateral frontal lobe epilepsy affects executive functions in children. *Neurol. Sci.* **26,** 263–270.

Riva, D., Vago, C., Franceschetti, S., Pantaleoni, C., D'Arrigo, S., Granata, T. & Bulgheroni, S. (2007): Intellectual and language findings and their relationship to EEG characteristics in benign childhood epilepsy with centrotemporal spikes. *Epilepsy Behav.* **10,** 278–285.

Roulet Perez, E., Davidoff, V., Despland, P.A. & Deonna, T. (1993): Mental and behavioural deterioration of children with epilepsy and CSWS: acquired epileptic frontal syndrome. *Dev. Med. Child. Neurol.* **35,** 661–674.

Rousselle, C. & Revol, M. (1995): Relations between cognitive functions and continuous spikes and waves during slow sleep. In: *Continuous Spikes and Waves during Slow Sleep – Electrical Status Epilepticus during Slow Sleep*, eds. A. Beaumanoir, M. Bureau, T. Deonna, *et al.*, pp. 175–182. Mariani Foundation Paediatric Neurology Series – III. London: John Libbey.

Scholtes, F.B., Hendriks, M.P. & Renier, W.O. (2005): Cognitive deterioration and electrical status epilepticus during slow sleep. *Epilepsy Behav.* **6,** 167–173.

Staden, U., Isaacs, E., Boyd, S.G., Brandl, U., Neville, B.G. (1998): Language dysfunction in children with Rolandic epilepsy. *Neuropediatrics* **29,** 242–248.

Stephani, U. & Carlsson, G. (2006): The spectrum from BCECTS to LKS: the Rolandic EEG trait-impact on cognition. *Epilepsia* **47,** 67–70.

Stuss, D.T. & Alexander, M.P. (2000): Executive functions and the frontal lobes: a conceptual view. *Psychol. Res.* **63,** 289–298.

Tassinari, C.A., Michelucci, R., Forti, A., Salvi, F., Plasmati, R., Rubboli, G., *et al.* (1992): The electrical status epilepticus syndrome. *Epilepsy Res. Suppl.* **6,** 111–115.

Tassinari, C.A., Rubboli, G., Volpi, L., Meletti, S., d'Orsi, G., Franca, M., *et al.* (2000): Encephalopathy with electrical status epilepticus during slow sleep or ESES syndrome including the acquired aphasia. *Clin. Neurophysiol.* **111,** 94–102.

Tassinari, C.A. & Rubboli, G. (2006): Cognition and paroxysmal EEG activities: from a single spike to electrical status epilepticus during sleep. *Epilepsia* **47,** 40–43.

Vago, C., Bulgheroni, S., Franceschetti, S., Usilla, A. & Riva, D. (2008): Memory performance on the California Verbal Learning Test of children with benign childhood epilepsy with centrotemporal spikes. *Epilepsy Behav.* **13,** 600–606.

Veggiotti, P., Beccaria, F., Papalia, G., Termine, C., Piazza, F. & Lanzi, G. (1998): Continuous spikes and waves during sleep in children with shunted hydrocephalus. *Childs Nerv. Syst.* **14,** 188–194.

Völkl-Kernstock, S., Willinger, U. & Feucht, M. (2006): Spacial perception and spatial memory in children with benign childhood epilepsy with centro-temporal spikes (BCECTS). *Epilepsy Res.* **72,** 39–48.

Völkl-Kernstock, S., Bauch-Prater, S., Ponocny-Seliger, E. & Feucht, M. (2009): Speech and school performance in children with benign partial epilepsy with centro-temporal spikes (BCECTS). *Seizure* **18,** 320–326.

Weglage, J., Demsky, A., Pietsch, M. & Kurlemann, G. (1997): Neuropsychological, intellectual, and behavioral findings in patients with centrotemporal spikes with and without seizures. *Dev. Med. Child. Neurol.* **39,** 646–651.

Brain Lesion Localization and Developmental Functions, D. Riva, C. Njiokiktjien and S. Bulgheroni (eds.)

Chapter 7

Social problem-solving after traumatic brain injury in children

Gerri Hanten*, Elisabeth A. Wilde*,o,#, and Harvey S. Levin*,o,§

Cognitive Neuroscience Laboratory, Departments of Physical Medicine and Rehabilitation, Neurology^o, Neurosurgery and Paediatrics§, and Radiology#, Baylor College of Medicine, 1709 Dryden Road, Suite 1200, Houston, Texas 77030, USA*
ghanten@bcm.edu
hlevin@bcm.edu
ewilde@bcm.edu

Summary

Clinicians and investigators have long recognized that peer relations and psychosocial development in general are impaired after severe traumatic brain injury in children and adolescents. These observations have been confirmed by controlled studies of social problem-solving by children with TBI, which affects brain regions identified with social cognition, including orbitofrontal and mesial prefrontal cortex and white matter tracts that connect these regions to posterior brain regions. These studies employ narratives along with virtual reality environments, as well as fMRI and DTI imaging to illuminate correlates of the social problem-solving deficits that persist in these children. Both focal lesions and shearing of white matter tracts ostensibly contribute to this impairment of social problem-solving, which does not appear to resolve over time.

Introduction

Clinicians and investigators have documented that social development is often adversely affected by traumatic brain injury (TBI) in children and adolescents. For example, reports of social development following prefrontal injury in children have noted intractable psychosocial impairment even in the presence of relatively normal intellectual development. However, these early reports were based on observations of individual children or series of patients. This paper addresses the vulnerability of social brain networks to TBI and the consequences for social problem-solving in children and adolescents. We report controlled studies showing that children and adolescents exhibit impaired social problem-solving following moderate to severe TBI. These studies, which have presented social narratives and more recently used virtual environments to more realistically depict social dilemmas among youths, have found that impaired social problem-solving persists after moderate to severe TBI without evidence for 'closing the gap' relative to performance by youth without TBI. In addition, we show that TBI has an impact on brain regions identified with social cognition, including the orbitofrontal and mesial prefrontal cortex and white matter tracts that connect these regions to posterior brain regions. Finally our findings using functional magnetic resonance imaging implicate cortical reorganization of social functions as a result of TBI in the pediatric age range.

Review of the topic

Pathophysiology of traumatic brain injury

Traumatic brain injury (TBI) is the most frequent cause of acquired brain injury in children. Closed head trauma resulting from motor vehicle crashes, falls, and sports-related injuries is by far the most common mechanism of TBI in children. This type of injury imparts acceleration–deceleration and/or blunt trauma to the brain. Brain swelling is a complication of TBI, which is especially common in children and can result in elevated intracranial pressure and ischaemia if uncontrolled. The pathophysiology of TBI due to closed head trauma includes both focal lesions, such as contusions and hematomas, and diffuse brain injury. In contrast to focal vascular lesions, which have been the focus of studies on development of language and visuospatial ability, TBI associated with closed head trauma generally produces axonal injury, which occurs in a continuum of severity depending on the traumatic forces and may be either focal or diffuse (Adelson & Kochanek, 1998). The shearing and stretching of white matter tracts may have a profound effect on myelination and growth of connections among prefrontal subregions and with connections to posterior cerebral cortex and subcortical regions. In summary, there is considerable heterogeneity in the pattern of focal and diffuse brain injury resulting from closed head trauma in children.

Advanced imaging techniques for understanding TBI-related injury and impact on development

Advanced methods of brain imaging have generated new tools for gaining understanding of the complexities of function in social cognition and other domains after brain injury. More automated and detailed analysis of regional brain volume and cortical thickness on high-resolution structural magnetic resonance imaging (MRI) has proven useful in furthering our understanding of TBI-related change and how this relates to social-cognitive abilities in the developing brain. Diffusion tensor imaging (DTI) is a relatively recent type of advanced MRI, which assesses the integrity of white matter microstructure by measuring the diffusion of water parallel to and perpendicular to the longitudinal axis of white matter tracts. Diffusion is particularly affected by characteristics of myelin surrounding the axons, such as myelin thickness. To the extent that white matter tracts have matured (*e.g.*, myelinated) and their integrity is preserved, water preferentially diffuses parallel to their long axis (*i.e.*, anisotropic diffusion. DTI-derived metrics have yielded additional information about brain-behaviour relations following TBI). Finally, recent studies examining aspects of social cognition after TBI have utilized functional MRI (fMRI).

In a recent fMRI study, Newsome and colleagues (2008) examined brain activation in adolescents with moderate to severe TBI and age- and socioeconomic-matched typically developing controls when they performed a task in which they judged personality traits from different perspectives in themselves (self) and a well-known other person (other) whom they nominated. The two independent variables were Target, that is, the person in whom the trait was evaluated (self or other), and Perspective, the viewpoint person from which the trait was evaluated (self or other). For example, the subject might see the following stimuli, corresponding to the experimental conditions: (1) *You think you are cheerful*: Target = self; perspective = self; (2) *You think Sammy is cheerful:* Target = other; perspective = self: (3) *Sammy thinks he is cheerful*: Target = other; perspective = other: (4) *Sammy thinks you are cheerful*: Target = self; perspective = other. It was hypothesized that disruption of circuitry involving mesial prefrontal cortex, medial parietal cortex, and temporal regions would result in more extensive activation in adolescents with moderate to severe TBI to compensate for reduced neural resources (Newsome *et al.*, 2008).

The analysis confirmed the expectation that frontal-temporal regions would be activated in trait attribution task performance. Although there were no regions in which activation pattern for the Target × Perspective interaction was greater in the control group of children, activation was greater for the TBI group (relative to controls) in left hemispheric regions corresponding to the posterior cingulate, the cuneus, lingual gyrus, parahippocampal gyrus, inferior parietal white matter, supramarginal gyrus white matter, and bilaterally, the thalamus.

Social cognitive development after prefrontal lesions

In children with TBI, ventral medial prefrontal and orbitofrontal lesions have been associated with disorders of comportment, *e.g.*, a lack of empathy, difficulty acquiring social rules of conduct, and behavioural dysregulation (Tranel & Eslinger, 2000). Additionally, some studies of children with ventral medial prefrontal lesions have demonstrated insensitivity to the future consequences of their behaviour (Anderson *et al.*, 1999). These observations have been corroborated by administering a test of moral reasoning, which reveals in the children with ventral medial prefrontal lesions an egocentric approach rather than the capacity to appreciate the perspective of others.

Adults with childhood-onset of injury with ventral medial prefrontal lesions have demonstrated poor performance on a gambling task that involves selecting cards from a deck that provides more consistent, albeit modest rewards over trials rather than alternative, disadvantageous decks which are associated initially with large rewards followed by large penalties (Anderson *et al.*, 1999; Anderson *et al.*, 1999). The lack of learning demonstrated in discovering the advantageous deck has been interpreted as evidence of a disconnection between the emotional response to loss by selecting cards from the disadvantageous deck and the cognitive operations guided by prefrontal cortex to shift to a different deck of cards. In our own lab, we found that children with ventral medial prefrontal lesions did not show impairment on the gambling task, but age-matched children with amygdala lesions did (Hanten *et al.*, 2006), which is not inconsistent with the above hypothesis.

Neural correlates of social problem-solving after TBI

Advanced methods of brain imaging have generated new tools for gaining understanding of the complexities of function after brain injury. Recent studies have revealed that specialized regions of the brain interconnect to form distributed networks that may support multiple cognitive and social-cognitive functions (Fig. 1). For example, as can be seen in Figure 2, the circuitry that subserves executive functioning and social cognition partially overlap, but there are regions that are selectively activated by executive function and others that primarily support social cognition. Further, these functional networks change with development, both in the physical structures and the relationships between behaviour and the brain (Adolphs *et al.*, 2001; Johnson *et al.*, 2005). Many studies have linked broad regions (*e.g.*, the frontal lobes) to equally broad cognitive processes (executive functioning), and some theorists suggest that the specific

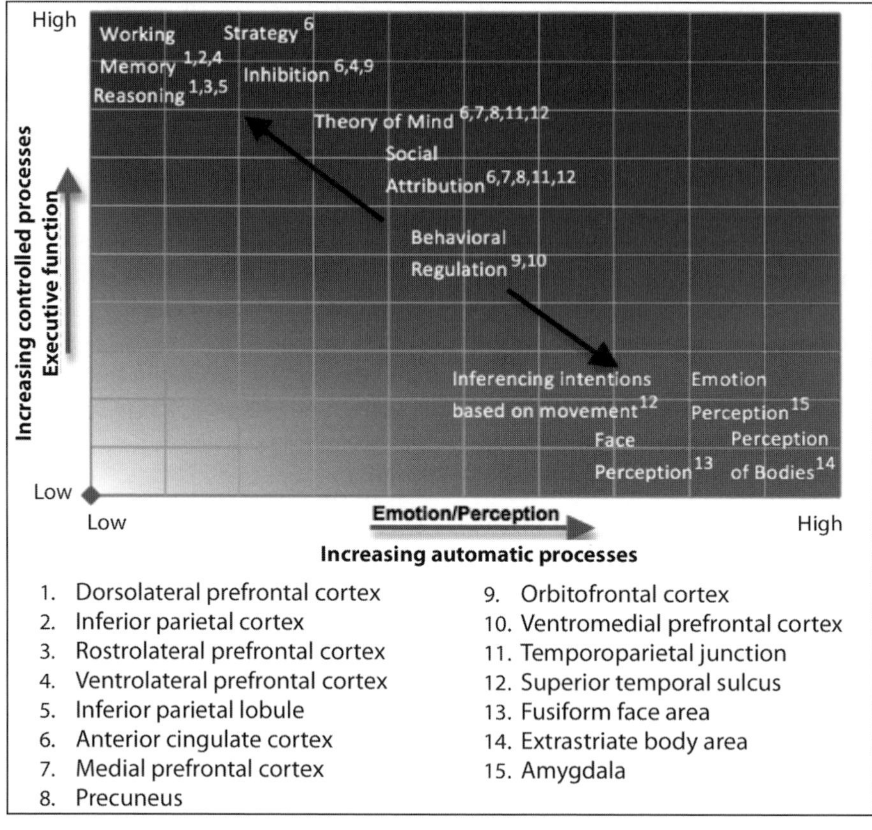

Fig. 1. Relation among functional domains of executive function, social cognition, emotional processing, and their underlying circuitry.

pattern of regions involved may be an emergent property of individual tasks (D'Esposito, 2007, 2008). Nonetheless, links have been drawn between defined behaviours and specific brain structures (Bechara *et al.*, 1994; Stewart *et al.*, 2001).

TBI frequently gives rise to both focal lesions and diffuse axonal injury, especially in the frontal, temporal, and parietal regions (Kim *et al.*, 2008; Levine *et al.*, 2008; Oni *et al.*, 2010; Wilde *et al.*, 2005). Damage to these regions, and in particular the ventral medial areas, has been associated with deficits in social cognition (Yeates *et al.*, 2007). Further, abnormal cortical thinning in these regions has been reported in children with TBI (McCauley *et al.*, 2010; Merkeley *et al.*, 2008), which differs from the pattern of cortical thinning associated with typical development in this age range (Giedd *et al.*, 1999).

Given the probability of damage to neural circuitry supporting social and emotional skills, it is perhaps not surprising that social functioning is commonly impaired after childhood TBI (Hanten *et al.*, 2008; Turkstra *et al.*, 2001; Yeates *et al.*, 2004). After TBI, children and adolescents are reported to be lonely and socially dissatisfied, have fewer friends, and tend to rely on family for social needs more than do uninjured peers (Yeates *et al.*, 2007). Several studies have sought to identify mechanisms underlying negative social outcome, and studies of children in adolescence, a stage of development in which social interaction increases dramatically in typically developing youth, have revealed specific aspects of social processing that are impaired

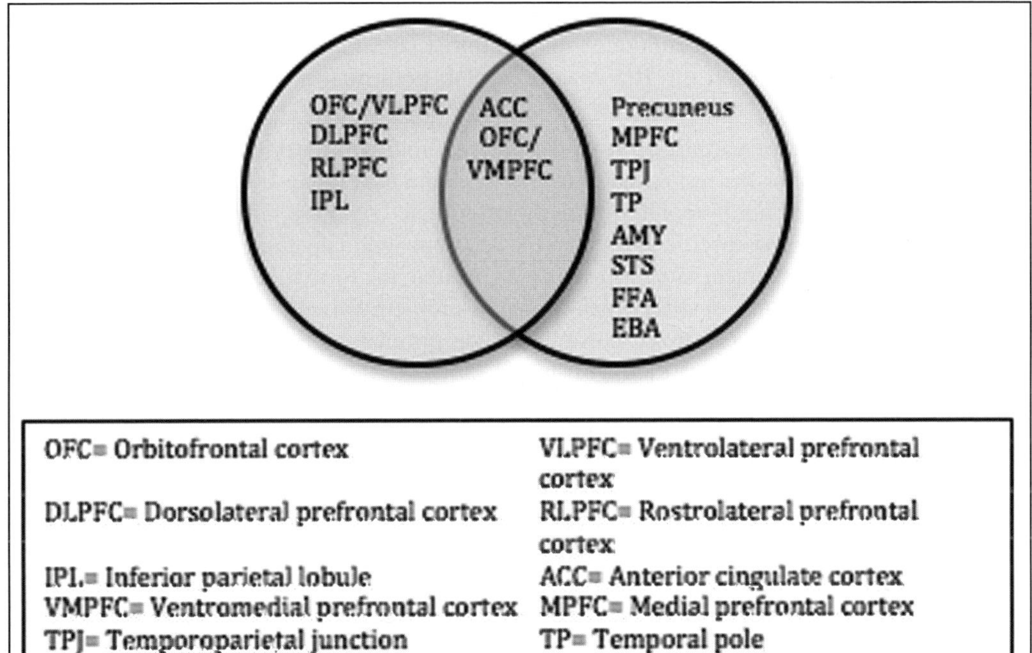

Fig. 2. Brain regions that overlap both executive function and social-cognitive networks, and those distinctly involved in one or the other network as described in recent reviews.

in youth after TBI as compared to typically-developing peers; these impairments include less accurate emotional processing, and reduced conversational and comprehension skills (Dennis & Barnes, 2001; Turkstra *et al.*, 2001). In general, studies to date have emphasized the relatively greater impairment of more complex skills rather than basic skills.

The ability of children with severe TBI to engage in age-appropriate social problem-solving was found to be impaired by Yeates and colleagues, who used the Interpersonal Negotiations Strategies Questionnaire (INS). The original INS was developed to integrate two theoretical approaches to social development, the structural approach (Kohlberg, 1969). informed by Piagetian developmental theory, and the functional approach (Dodge, 1985), which is based more on information processing theory. In the INS interview, the subject is presented an interpersonal conflict scenario in narrative form, and then is queried for a solution to the conflict based on four problem-solving steps: identifying the problem, generating possible solutions, selecting the best solution, and evaluating the likely outcome. Here is an example of a scenario:

Steve and Carl are friends. One day at school, they are trying to decide what to do on the weekend. Steve wants to invite the new kid in their class to see a movie with them, but Carl says he doesn't feel like having the new kid along.

Responses are rated on maturational level of the proposed solutions, with levels tied to developmental stages (impulsive, unilateral, reciprocal, collaborative). Reliability of the INS has been illustrated in several studies, with a test-retest of $r = .68$ across a 4-month interval (Yeates *et al.*, 1990). Using this paradigm, studies have reported that the children with TBI used less developmentally mature strategies to resolve conflicts than did children without head injury (Hanten *et al.*, 2008; Yeates *et al.*, 2004). This impairment, which was greatest at later steps of problem-solving, rather than at the initial step of identifying the problems, did not improve over a year relative to results in children without brain injury. Further, studies in our laboratory revealed that performance on the INS was related to performance on tasks of memory and language (Hanten *et al.*, 2008).

Although the presence of social-cognitive deficits in children after TBI has been established, the ecological validity of the tests used to assess outcome is at issue. For example, in real life, a child or adolescent is rarely required to perform discrete cognitive operations in daily activities. In the INS interview specifically, given the relations with language and consistent reports of higher language impairment after TBI, it is possible that the format of the original test allows for the underrepresentation of difficulties in social problem-solving encountered by children after TBI by providing an organized narrative of the problem as a starting point for the test. This, of course, is very different than it is in real life.

Recent advances in virtual reality (VR) gaming technology provide an opportunity to combine the specificity of neuropsychological tests with mundane realism to mimic the actions and activities of daily experience, which allows a more ecologically valid assessment of socio-cognitive skills. Because of this advantage, virtual environments (VEs) are now being used to study social cognition. Research with functional neuroimaging has shown that the medial prefrontal cortex is activated when participants observe social communication of virtual others via facial expressions, and also when perceiving personal involvement in a virtual situation through direct eye contact with virtual characters (Schilbach *et al.*, 2006). In another study, Riva *et al.* (2007a, 2007b) used college-age participants (19–25 years old) to estimate the effectiveness of VEs in inducing specific emotional responses by varying the setting of VR environments visited by the subjects (*i.e.*, 'anxious', 'relaxed', or 'neutral' settings). The study confirmed the efficacy of VR environments in eliciting the target emotion. The above studies demonstrate the promise of VR technology in facilitating understanding of social-cognitive deficits.

We took advantage of this technology to create a VR social problem-solving task (VR–SPS), which is an analogue of the INS interview. In the virtual task, participants are asked to watch six scripted, computerized VR scenarios involving four people (VR avatars), two of whom are in conflict. Figure 3 depicts a scene from one scenario. Different from the narrative form of the task, in the VR task, as in real life, the problem is revealed through naturalistic dialogue between the avatars. To explore the possibility that the cognitive processing load might have an effect on social problem-solving, we varied the type and amount of information processed by the participant in order to resolve the conflict by manipulating the number of people who speak, and the amount of irrelevant or relevant information communicated within the conflict scenario. (For detailed description of the task and procedures, please see Hanten *et al.*, 2011). An example of dialogue for one of the low-processing load scenarios is shown below. Note that the social conflict shown here corresponds to the INS narrative given previously:

Luis: *Hey, Devin. What are you up to this weekend?*
Devin: *Not much. What about you?*
Luis: *Well, I was thinking we could go see that movie that just came out. Maybe we could invite that new kid, Brandon, from Biology.*
Devin: *A movie sounds cool, but I don't know about Brandon.*
Luis: *That movie looks awesome. Why don't you want Brandon to go?*
Devin: *Brandon gets on my nerves.*
Luis: *I hung out with him last week and he was pretty cool.*
Devin: *I don't know.*
Luis: *Dude, give him a chance.*

After each scenario, participants are administered a structured interview. Responses to the interview questions are scored according to developmental level and a score is calculated for each of the four social problem-solving steps (Define Problem, Generate Solutions, Select Solution, Evaluate Outcome), with higher scores indicating better social perspective taking and desire to sustain relationships (Yeates *et al.*, 1990, 1991).

In addition to investigating social problem-solving in a naturalistic environment, we were also interested in looking at the neural correlates that related to specific aspects of performance on the task. In a preliminary study using the VR–SPS task on 15 youths with moderate to severe brain injury and 12 typically developing youths, as expected, we found that social problem-solving was impaired after TBI. Different from our previous findings using the narrative version of the task, with the VR–SPS task we found significant impairment at the initial stage of problem-solving (Defining Problem) across all three levels of processing load. In contrast, in the other three steps of problem-solving (Generate Solutions, Select Solution, Evaluate Outcome), the TBI group showed impairment, but only when burdened with the highest processing load. The typically developing youths were not affected by processing load. From these findings, we suggest that when faced with a social conflict, the initial hurdle for children and adolescents may be in merely understanding the nature of the problem. Further, even when the child with TBI correctly identifies the problem, the number of people involved in the situation and the amount of information that must be processed may affect other steps of social problem-solving, which may have social consequences for children and youths with TBI.

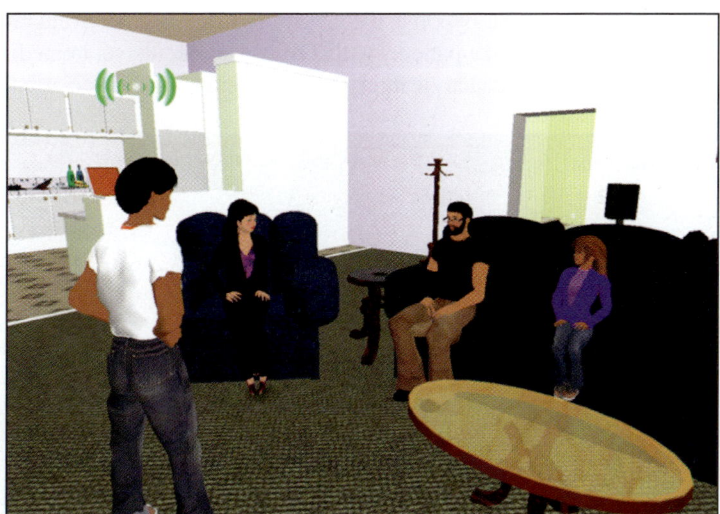

Fig. 3. Screenshot of a scenario from the Virtual Reality–Problem-Solving Task. Shown is a scene from the high-processing load condition.

With these findings in mind, we examined the relation of cortical thinning to performance on the VR–SPS task. We found that, consistent with the literature on brain development in adolescents (Giedd *et al.*, 1999a,b), performance in typically developing children was inversely related to cortical thickness, that is, cortical thinning was associated with improved performance. However, the pattern was the opposite for youth with TBI: better performance was related to greater cortical thickness. These differences were most pronounced in the medial orbitofrontal regions and the cuneus. For example, Figure 4 shows within-group correlations of cortical thickness with performance on the VR–SPS task in typically developing youth (on left) and youth with TBI (on right) for the most demanding task condition. The pattern of significant relations between cortical thickness and performance, as indicated by colored areas (blue = positive, red = negative), demonstrates that although the TBI group showed minimal apparent relations, for the typically developing group significant relations were found in the frontal regions, particularly in the frontal pole, with decreases in cortical thickness associated with better performance.

The orbitofrontal cortex is associated with emotion- and reward-based decision-making (Bechara *et al.*, 1994, 2005; Kringelbach, 2005; Rolls *et al.*, 1994). The mechanism involved appears to be the signaling of the affective value of stimuli, encoding expectations of future reward and updating expectations (O'Doherty, 2007). Further, the medial orbitofrontal cortex becomes activated with exposure to future rewards, both actual and imagined (Bray *et al.*, 2010). Theories of social decision making suggest the interplay of at least two neurologic systems: an amygdala-mediated system that provides positive or negative signals for immediate consequences and a reflective prefrontal system that provides positive or negative signals for future consequences. When the prefrontal system is immature or impaired, decisions favoring immediate rewards are more likely (Bechara *et al.*, 2005). The cuneus is associated with visual processing and is implicated in cognitive control in clinical populations, with studies suggesting that gray matter volume in the cuneus is positively associated with better inhibitory control (Haldane *et al.*, 2008). Interestingly, pathologic gamblers have demonstrated increased activity in the dorsal visual stream (including the cuneus) relative to controls (Crockford *et al.*, 2005). Given the high probability of prefrontal and orbitofrontal region compromise in children and adolescents with moderate to severe TBI, our data provide tentative support for the hypothesis that group differences in evaluating the outcome of a problem-solving strategy show that patients with TBI use an impulsive, immediately rewarding strategy, which may be the consequence of injury to key regions of the social brain.

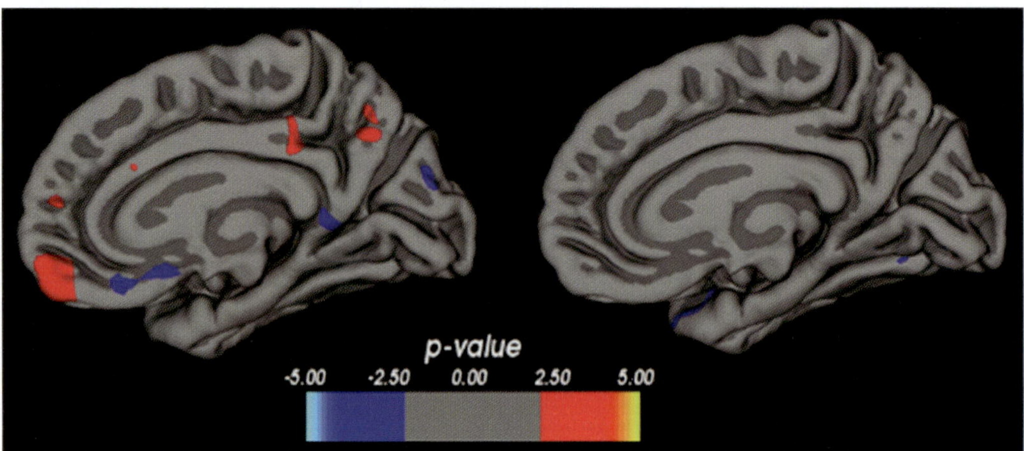

Fig. 4. Relation of performance on the VR–SPS task to cortical thickness in typically developing children (left) and children with severe TBI (right). A statistical threshold of p *<. 01 was used, and values displayed are either positive relations (in blue) or negative relations (in red).*

Conclusions

Clinicians and investigators have long recognized that peer relations and psychosocial development in general are impaired after severe traumatic brain injury in children and youth. These observations have been confirmed by controlled studies of social problem-solving by children occurring after moderate to severe TBI. Initial findings obtained by presenting social narratives to children with TBI have been confirmed using more realistic VR technology. This VR technology which more closely simulates real-life peer interactions, has confirmed and extended the finding that social problem-solving is persistently impaired after TBI in children and youth. Recent investigations using functional brain imaging have identified brain regions and circuitry linked to social cognition in typically developing children and youth. At the same time, clinical investigators using structural MRI and DTI have shown that development of these brain regions and connecting white matter tracts is disrupted by moderate to severe TBI. Both focal lesions and shearing of white matter tracts ostensibly contribute to the persistent impairment of social problem-solving, which does not appear to resolve over time in children and adolescents following moderate to severe TBI.

Acknowledgments: Research conducted in our laboratory as reported here was supported by NIH Grant NS-21889. We gratefully acknowledge the assistance of Alyssa P. Ibarra in preparing this manuscript.

References

Adelson, P.D. & P.M. Kochanek. (1998): Head injury in children. *J. Child Neurol.* **13,** 2–15.

Adolphs, R., Tranel, D. & Damasio, H. (2001): Emotion recognition from faces and prosody following temporal lobectomy. *Neuropsychology* **15,** 396–404.

Anderson, B., Southern, B.D. & Powers R.E. (1999): Anatomic asymmetries of the posterior superior temporal lobes: a postmortem study. *Neuropsychiatry Neuropsychol. Behav. Neurol.* **12,** 247–254.

Anderson S.W., Bechara A., Damasio H., Tranel D. & Damasio, A. R. (1999): Impairment of social and moral behavior related to early damage in human prefrontal cortex. *Nat. Neurosci.* **2,** 1032–1037.

Bechara, A. (2005): Decision making, impulse control and loss of willpower to resist drugs: a neurocognitive perspective. *Nat. Neurosci.* **8,** 1458–1463.

Bechara, A., Damasio, A.R., Damasio, H. & Anderson, S.W. (1994): Insensitivity to future consequences following damage to human prefrontal cortex. *Cognition* **50,** 7–15.

Bray, S., Shimojo, S. & O'Doherty, J. P. (2010): Human medial orbitofrontal cortex is recruited during experience of imagined and real rewards. *J. Neurophysiol.* **103,** 2506–2512.

Crockford, D. N., Goodyear, B., Edwards, J., Quickfall, J. & el-Guebaly, N. (2005): Cue-induced brain activity in pathological gamblers. *Biol. Psychiatry* **58,** 787–795.

Dennis, M. & Barnes, M.A. (2001); Comparison of literal, inferential, and intentional text comprehension in children with mild or severe closed head injury. *J. Head Trauma Rehabil.* **16,** 456–468.

D'Esposito, M. (2007): From cognitive to neural models of working memory. *Phil. Trans. R. Soc. Lond. B Biol. Sci.* **362,** 761–772.

D'Esposito, M. (2008): From cognitive to neural models of working memory. In: *Mental Processes in the Human Brain*, eds. J. Driver, P. Haggard & T. Shallice, pp. 7–25. New York: Oxford University Press.

Dodge, K. (1985): Facets of social interaction and the assessment of social competence in children. In: *Children's Peer Relations: Issues in Aassessment and Intervention*, eds. B. Schneider, H. Rubin & J. Ledingham, pp. 3–22. New York: Springer-Verlag.

Giedd, J.N., Blumenthal, J., Jeffries, N.O., Castellanos, F.X., Liu, H., Zijdenbos, A., *et al.* (1999): Brain development during childhood and adolescence: a longitudinal MRI study. *Nat. Neurosci.* **2,** 861–863.

Haldane, M., Cunningham, G., Androutsos, C. & Frangou, S. (2008): Structural brain correlates of response inhibition in bipolar disorder I. *J. Psychopharmacol.* **22,** 138–143.

Hanten, G., Scheibel, R.S., Li, X., Oomer, I., Stallings-Roberson, G., Hunter, J.V. & Levin, H.S. (2006): Decision-making after traumatic brain injury in children: a preliminary study. *Neurocase* **12,** 247–251.

Hanten, G., Wilde, E., Menefee, D., Li, X., Lane, S., Vasquez, C., *et al.* (2008): Correlates of social problem-solving during the first year after traumatic brain injury in children. *Neuropsychology* **22,** 357–370.

Hanten, G., Cook, L., Orsten, K., Chapman, S.B., Li, X., Wilde, E.A., *et al.* (2011): Effects of traumatic brain injury on a virtual reality social problem-solving task and relations to cortical thickness in adolescence. *Neuropsychologia* **49,** 486–497.

Johnson, M., Griffin, R., Csibra, G., Halit, H., Farroni, T. & De Haan, M. (2005): The emergence of the social brain network: evidence from typical and atypical development, *Dev. Psychopathol.* **17,** 599–619.

Kim, J., Avants, B., Patel, S., Whyte, J., Coslett, B.H., Pluta, J., Detre, J. A. & Gee, J.C. (2008): Structural consequences of diffuse traumatic brain injury: a large deformation tensor-based morphometry study. *NeuroImage* **39,** 1014–1026.

Kohlberg, L. (1969): Stage and sequence: the cognitive- developmental approach to socialization. In: *Handbook of Socialization Theory and Research*, eds. D. Goslin. Chicago: Rand McNally.

Kringelbach, M.L. (2005): The human orbitofrontal cortex: linking reward to hedonic experience. *Nat. Rev. Neurosci.* **6,** 691–702.

Levine, B., Kovacevic, N., Nica, E., Cheung, G., Gao, F., Schwartz, M.L. & Black, S.E. (2008): The Toronto traumatic brain injury study: injury severity and quantified MRI. *Neurology* **70,** 771–778.

McCauley, S.R., Wilde, E. A., Merkley, T.L., Schnelle, K.P., Bigler, E.D., Hunter, J., *et al.* (2010): Patterns of cortical thinning in relation to event-based prospective memory performance three months after moderate to severe traumatic brain injury in children. *Dev. Neuropsychol.* **35,** 318–332.

Merkley, T.L., Bigler, E.D., Wilde, E.A., McCauley, S.R., Hunter, J.V. & Levin, H.S. (2008): Diffuse changes in cortical thickness in pediatric moderate-to-severe traumatic brain injury. *J. Neurotrauma* **25,** 1343–1345.

Newsome, M.R., Steinberg, J.L., Scheibel, R.S., Troyanskaya, M., Chu, Z., Hanten, G., *et al.* (2008): Effects of traumatic brain injury on working memory-related brain activation in adolescents. *Neuropsychology* **22,** 419–425.

O'Doherty, J.P. (2007): Lights, camembert, action! The role of human orbitofrontal cortex in encoding stimuli, rewards, and choices. *Ann. N.Y. Acad. Sci.*. **1121,** 254–272.

Oni, M.B., Wilde, E.A., Bigler, E.D., McCauley, S.R., Wu, T.C., Yallampalli, R., *et al.* (2010): Diffusion tensor imaging analysis of frontal lobes in pediatric traumatic brain injury. *J. Child Neurol.* **25,** 976–984.

Riva, G., Mantovani, F., Capideville, C.S., Preziosa, A., Morganti, F., Villani, D., *et al.* (2007): Affective interactions using virtual reality: the link between presence and emotions. *CyberPsychol. Behav.* **10,** 45–56.

Rolls, E.T., Hornak, J., Wade, D. & McGrath, J. (1994): Emotion-related learning in patients with social and emotional changes associated with frontal lobe damage. *J. Neurol. Neurosurg. Psychiatry* **57,** 1518–1524.

Schilbach, L., Wohlschlaeger, A.M., Kraemer, N.C., Newen, A., Shah, N.J., Fink, G.R. & Vogeley, K. (2006): Being with virtual others: neural correlates of social interaction. *Neuropsychologia* **44,** 718–730.

Stewart, L., Meyer, B., Frith, U. & Rothwell, J. (2001): Left posterior BA37 is involved in object recognition: a TMS study. *Neuropsychologia* **39,** 1–6.

Tranel, D. & Eslinger, P.J. (2000): Effects of early onset brain injury on the development of cognition and behavior: introduction to the special issue. *Dev. Neuropsychol.* **18,** 273–280.

Turkstra, L.S., McDonald, S. & DePompei, R. (2001): Social information processing in adolescents: data from normally developing adolescents and preliminary data from their peers with traumatic brain injury. *J. Head Trauma Rehabil.* **16,** 469–483.

Wilde, E.A., Hunter, J.V., Newsome, M.R., Scheibel, R.S., Bigler, E.D., Johnson, J.L., *et al.* (2005): Frontal and temporal morphometric findings on MRI in children after moderate to severe traumatic brain injury. *J. Neurotrauma* **22,** 333–344.

Yeates, K.O., Schultz, L.H. & Selman, R.L. (1990): Bridging the gaps in child-clinical assessment: toward the application of social-cognitive developmental theory. *Clin. Psychol. Rev.* **10,** 567–588.

Yeates, K., Schultz, L. & Selman, R. (1991): The development of interpersonal negotiation strategies in thought and action: a social cognitive link to behavioral adjustment and social status. *Merrill-Palmer Q.* **37,** 369–406.

Yeates, K.O., Swift, E., Taylor, H.G., Wade, S.L., Drotar D., Stancin T. & Minich, N. (2004): Short- and long-term social outcomes following pediatric traumatic brain injury. *J. Int. Neuropsychol. Soc.* **10,** 412–426.

Yeates, K.O., Bigler, E.D., Dennis, M., Gerhardt, C.A., Rubin, K.H., Stancin, T., Taylor, H.G. & Vannatta, K. (2007): Social outcomes in childhood brain disorder: a heuristic integration of social neuroscience and developmental psychology. *Psychol. Bull.* **133,** 535–556.

Brain Lesion Localization and Developmental Functions, D. Riva, C. Njiokiktjien and S. Bulgheroni (eds.)

Chapter 8

The role of phonological working memory in specific language impairment

Daniela Brizzolara*,°, Claudia Casalini°, Anna Chilosi° and Chiara Pecini°

**Division of Child Neurology and Psychiatry, University of Pisa, Italy;*
°Department of Developmental Neurosciences, 'Stella Maris' Scientific Institute, via Dei Giacinti 2, 56018 Calambrone, Pisa, Italy
dbrizzolara@inpe.unipi.it
achilosi@inpe.unipi.it

Summary

Specific language impairment (SLI) is a developmental disorder which affects a large number of children in the preschool years and may present long-term effects, putting children at risk of developing specific reading and spelling difficulties at school age. At the level of underlying cognitive processes, deficits of phonological working memory (PhWM), which is part of the complex network of the executive functions, have been considered the genetic 'marker' of SLI: phonological working memory, in fact, has been found to be faulty in children affected by SLI. After describing the cognitive model of PhWM and the literature on its development, we present data from our laboratory on PhWM in children with SLI. In particular, we focus on the means of evaluating PhWM in SLI children; then we describe different PhWM profiles in children with different types of SLI and discuss the role played by PhWM in the continuity between oral and written language impairment in this population.

Introduction

Specific language impairment (SLI) is a selective failure to develop language at a normal rate, occurring in the absence of frank cognitive, neurologic, sensory deficit, and psychiatric disorders, and in spite of adequate social and educational opportunities for learning language (American Psychiatric Association, 1994 [DSM–IV]). It occurs in about 3 per cent of children in preschool years and may present long-term effects: a number of studies have shown that children with SLI are at risk of developing specific reading and spelling difficulties at school age (Bishop & Adams, 1990; Botting *et al.*, 2006; Brizzolara *et al.*, 2006a, 2007; Catts *et al.*, 2002; Snowling *et al.*, 2000).

The pathophysiology of SLI is still poorly defined: it is recognized that genetic mechanisms play a major role in causing SLI (Bishop, 2000), but it is still unknown how this genetic influence operates. However there is an emergent literature suggesting that different phenotypic markers of SLI may be due to different genetic influences (SLI Consortium, 2004); in particular two quantitative trait loci on chromosomes 16q and 19q have been identified (Falcaro *et al.*, 2008; Monaco, 2007).

As children with SLI are frequently characterized by a deficit in phonological working memory (PhWM) (Archibald & Gathercole, 2006; Botting & Conti-Ramsden, 2001; Conti-Ramsden *et al.*, 2001; Dollaghan & Campbell, 1998; Monaco, 2007; Weismer *et al.*, 2000), some authors have proposed that, at the level of underlying cognitive processes, the genetic 'marker' of SLI involves a specific deficit in PhWM (Bishop *et al.*, 1996; Bortolini *et al.*, 2006).

In the following sections we describe the cognitive model of PhWM and the recent literature on its development; then we present data from our laboratory on PhWM in children with SLI. In particular, we focus on the means of evaluating PhWM in these children with SLI; we then describe different PhWM profiles in children with different types of SLI and discuss the role played by PhWM in the continuity between oral and written language impairment.

Phonological Working Memory

PhWM is one domain-specific system of working memory (the 'phonological loop' or PL) specialized for the processing of verbal material, which is thought to represent the ability to temporally store and manipulate verbal information held 'on-line' in the course of complex cognitive tasks (Baddeley, 1990).

In the first version of his model, Baddeley (1986) proposed that the phonological loop consists of two components: a phonological short-term store, which can hold speech-related information for about 2 seconds, and an articulatory system, which serves to sub-vocally refresh the contents of the phonological store. The functioning of the two components has been supported by a great deal of experimental evidence on the 'phonological similarity' and the 'word length' effects: in verbal serial recall tasks it is more difficult to remember phonologically similar than dissimilar material and longer than shorter words. The first effect has been ascribed to difficulty in retrieving information registered in the phonological store, while the second is ascribed to the fact that longer words take more time than shorter to be processed by the articulatory system. Other effects have been described: 'unattended speech' and 'articulatory suppression', confirming the hypothesized functioning of the PL. The model has proved successful in accounting for the PhWM memory deficits of neuropsychological patients (*e.g.*, Baddeley & Wilson, 1993).

More recently it has been found that verbal short-term memory (STM) recall is also dependent on long-term memory (LTM) knowledge: several experimental studies have shown that phonological, lexical, and semantic LTM knowledge might be used as a mean for supporting the PhWM demands of temporarily retaining verbal information (Dollaghan *et al.*, 1995; Gathercole *et al.*, 1999; Turner *et al.*, 2000). This fact has contributed to modify the original model of PhWM, with the addition of another component, the 'episodic buffer', which reflects the operation of LTM mechanisms and explains experimental results such as the 'frequency' (Roodenrys *et al.*, 1993), 'imageability', 'phonotactic frequency' (Edwards *et al.*, 2004; Majerus & Van der Linden, 2003), and 'wordlikeness' (Gathercole *et al.*, 1991) effects.

Functional MRI studies have shown that a distributed network of regions in the prefrontal and in the temporoparietal cortex (Wagner & Smith, 2003) together with the cerebellar hemispheres (Kirschen *et al.*, 2005; Marvel & Desmond, 2010; Misciagna *et al.*, 2010) are associated with PhWM functioning. Several neuroimaging studies have identified neural correlates for the two components of the PL: the phonological store has been associated with the left inferior parietal regions and the superior cerebellum, whereas the articulatory system has been functionally related to the left inferior frontal regions and the inferior cerebellum. Both the cortical and cerebellar regions associated with the PL show increased activation with parametrically increasing memory load (Grasby *et al.*, 1994; Awh *et al.*, 1996; Cohen *et al.*, 1997; Kirschen *et al.*, 2005; Veltman *et al.*, 2003).

Phonological Working Memory in normal development

The phonological loop model has also proved highly successful at characterizing the nature of PhWM in the developmental period (Gathercole, 1998), and many studies have tapped the functioning of PL components in children, documenting the effects of phonological similarity and word length (Hulme & Tordoff, 1989) and of LMT linguistic representations on STM recall (Gathercole *et al.*, 1991, 2001; Majerus & Van der Linden, 2003; Roodenrys *et al.*, 1993) from the preschool years.

Development of PhWM parallels structural changes in the frontoparietal association cortices. The cerebellum, along with frontal and parietal cortices, has been shown to exhibit linear PhWM load-dependent activation in developmental populations, although linear load-dependency effects have been found to change with age. In a recent fMRI study O'Hare *et al.* (2008) suggest that, while children, adolescents, and young adults activate similar cerebro-cerebellar PhWM networks, the extent to which parietal and cerebellar regions respond to increasing task difficulty changes significantly between childhood and adolescence. During normal development, PhWM plays a critical role in some aspects of language acquisition, including language comprehension (Bowey, 1996) and reading (Cain *et al.*, 2004; Gathercole *et al.*, 2006; Mann, 1984), acting as a 'language learning device' (Baddeley *et al.*, 1998), especially in the lexical domain (Gathercole & Baddeley, 1993), although other cognitive abilities are implicated in vocabulary learning (Morra & Camba, 2009). PhWM relates to native and foreign vocabulary in the early phases of acquisition (Gathercole *et al.*, 1992, 1997; Service, 1992) and, later on, under conditions that do not favour the use of a lexical mediation strategy (Carroll & Snowling, 2004; Palladino & Ferrari, 2008). PhWM is assumed to be important not only for lexical acquisition but also for the storage of phonological, grammatical, and semantic knowledge in LTM, supporting receptive and expressive language skills (Edwards & Lahey, 1998; Montgomery, 2004). Among the different measures of PhWM, word serial recall and nonword repetition tasks have been most frequently used in children. These tasks are assumed to measure primarily PhWM: the listeners, in fact, after perceiving the verbal stimuli, have to encode and maintain the word strings or the novel phonological sequence for a sufficiently long time and in a sufficiently fine-grained form to support its articulatory output (Gathercole, 1995).

In our laboratory, we constructed and standardized on Italian children two PhWM tasks: a word serial recall task (WSRT) and a nonword repetition task (NWRT).

The WSRT, requires the child to repeat six lists of Italian words varying for lexical frequency (high *vs.* low), length (two *vs.* four syllables) and phonological similarity (phonologically similar *vs.* dissimilar). According to the model of the PL, the frequency effect (better recall for high- than low-frequency words) can be explained by the influence of LTM lexical knowledge on short-term recall, whereas the phonological similarity and the length effects (better recall for dissimilar than for similar and for short than for long words, respectively) reflect phonological coding processes and articulatory rehearsal mechanisms in PhWM. The lists, for a total of 60 strings of words, are presented on a tape recorder at the rate of one word every 2 seconds, and the child has to repeat the words of each string in the same order of presentation. Two strings are given at each length (two to six words); one point is assigned for each correctly repeated string. The list presentation is interrupted when the child fails on two strings of the same length. Each child obtains a score that is calculated by summing the number of strings correctly repeated for each list. Normative data from a large sample of 280 Italian children, aged from 4 to 10 years, are available for this test (Brizzolara & Casalini, 2002), which demonstrated the increasing PhWM capacity across ages and the sensibility of the STM recall to the frequency, phonological similarity, and word length effects from age 4.

More recently a new version of the WSRT has been standardized (Brizzolara *et al.*, 2006b). The task's structure is identical to that of the previous version. Stimuli presentation is controlled by a PC using dedicated software. For each list, sequences of increasing length are presented (two to seven words); five strings are given at each length. The list presentation is interrupted when the child fails on four out of five strings of the same length. For each subject (in each condition), a characteristic performance is defined as the length at which he or she gives 50 per cent correct answers. Scores being discrete numbers, an exact 50 per cent is not always hit; in such cases the expected estimate is given by linear interpolation. This scoring allows for a more fine-grained evaluation of individual performance than do standard span measures. For example, a child who has repeated correctly five sequences of two and three words, three sequences of four, and one of five words obtains a score of 4.21. The software transforms the raw score into a standard score with mean = 100 and SD = 15. After the mean and the SD of the control group are calculated, the above characteristic value then can be converted to a z score with reference to a normative sample of 190 children between 5 and 17 years of age. In the example reported, a score of 4.21 yielded a z score of 0.07.

The NWRT (Casalini *et al.*, 2007) consists of two sets of 20 nonwords each and one set of 20 words, for a total of 60 stimuli. The nonwords in the first set (morphologic nonwords) are composed of a root plus a derivational suffix, resulting in a new combination which does not exist in Italian. The nonwords in the second set (nonmorphologic or simple nonwords) are matched for orthographic-phonological properties to the nonwords in the first set, but do not include existing morphemes, neither a root nor a suffix. The roots in the first set of nonwords have a high frequency in the Italian children's lexicon, and the related suffixes are among the most frequent and productive in Italian nominal and adjectival derivatives. The nonsuffix final strings in the simple nonwords have the same mean frequency in word-final position as the suffixes in the morphologic nonwords. Words in the third set are matched across the two sets of nonwords on consonant-vowel structure, length, and phonotactic frequency. Stimuli, pronounced by a female voice, were recorded in digital audiotape modality; each item was successively sampled through a digital Sound Blaster hard-disk recording for PC. Children are instructed to repeat, as accurately as possible, each phoneme string they hear. Answers are tape-recorded and the number of correct repetitions for words (W), simple nonwords (NW), and morphologic nonwords (MNW) is scored. The score in the repetition of NW is used as a 'pure' measure of PhWM. The differences between W and the two types of nonwords (NW and MNW), and the difference between MNW and NW, are both considered measures of LTM facilitation (lexical and morpho-lexical effects, respectively). The test has been standardized on two groups of 40 children, one in preschool (mean age = 5.6; range = 5.3–5.9) and one in school years (mean age = 6.6; range = 6.4–6.9). Children's performances increase from the preschool to the school level and show a significant lexical advantage for W over NW and MNW, and a morpho-lexical advantage for MNW over NW. The presence of lexical and morpho-lexical effects in children from age 4 is a proof that they make use of lexical and morpho-lexical representations to aid PhWM recall.

Phonological working memory in specific language impairment

The documented PhWM's role in language acquisition in normally developing children soon paved the way for the hypothesis that impaired PhWM skills might be a core factor in developmental language disorders. First, Gathercole and Baddeley (1990) proposed that a primary impairment in PhWM would be the basis for the language difficulties of SLI children; later a PhWM dysfunction was considered as the core deficit and the most probable heritable cause of SLI and the nonword repetition impairment as the behavioural marker of such a disease (Bishop *et al.*, 1996; Conti-Ramsden, 2003).

However, because SLI is a heterogeneous disorder, it is not clear whether a PhWM deficit characterizes all types of SLI. Studies on cognitive processes in SLI have generally not taken into account the different clinical manifestations of the disorder, treating SLI as a unitary condition, but the clinical and linguistic profiles of children with SLI are highly variable, as extensively described (*e.g.*, Leonard, 1998; Plante, 1998). Based on international classification criteria (DSM–IV, American Psychiatric Association, 1994), three different types of SLI can be diagnosed clinically: mixed receptive-expressive language disorder (RE) when both comprehension and production are impaired; expressive language disorder (Ex), when only production is impaired; and phonological disorder (Ph), when the expressive deficit selectively affects the use of speech sounds and phonological rules. The interest in studying cognitive abilities in different subtypes of SLI is quite recent (Pecini *et al.*, 2005; Nickisch & von Kries *et al.*, 2009).

The question of whether PhWM is differently affected in different types of SLI is still open, but the answer to it gains importance for another matter: although it is recognized that SLI can show different clinical manifestations, the question of whether the different types of SLI are clearly separable entities or one common disorder with different grades of quantity and quality (Bishop, 1997) is much debated. Indeed, children with Ph and Ex SLI show better therapy results compared to children with RE SLI (*e.g.*, Boyle *et al.*, 2007) and show different long-term outcomes (Brizzolara *et al.*, 2006a, 2007); the potential causes for these apparent differences in outcome are poorly understood and could be traced back to different deficits in PhWM.

Moreover, the relationship between PhWM deficits and language impairment in SLI is far from clear: PhWM impairment in children with SLI, in fact, might reflect a primary deficit in PhWM as well as a limitation in LTM verbal knowledge (Snowling *et al.*, 1991).

Experimental evidence is controversial. Van der Lely and Howard (1993), Howard and Van der Lely (1995), and Sahlén *et al.* (1999) demonstrated that children with SLI show a sensitivity to the semantic characteristics of the to-be-remembered items, suggesting that they can make use of stored verbal knowledge to aid STM recall. Conversely, Gathercole and Baddeley (1993, 1995) and Montgomery (1995) showed that the nonword repetition of children with SLI is affected to a greater extent by stimulus length rather than by linguistic factors such as prosodic structure or wordlikeness, although more recently Archibald and Gathercole (2007) recognized the role of linguistic factors on nonword repetition deficit in SLI.

Finally, although many experimental findings indicate that there is a continuity between oral and written language disorders, the nature of the relationship between different types of SLI and literacy difficulties remains unclear: it is not yet known whether there is a subtype of SLI where the child is at higher risk of developing reading and spelling difficulties at school age or what cognitive deficits makes SLI children at risk of learning disabilities; nor is it clear whether there is a common cognitive factor underlying both SLI and literacy difficulties. So far PhWM abilities have been studied in SLI children as a factor contributing to their reading/spelling difficulties, as it has been showed that PhWM deficits have been frequently described in developmental dyslexia (Bishop & Snowling, 2004; Goulandris *et al.*, 2000; Hulme & Snowling, 1992; Snowling, 2008; Van der Leij & Van Daal, 1999).

In the next part of this chapter, we present data from our laboratory reviewing some of our research about PhWM in children aimed to clarify the aforementioned questions.

Data from our laboratory

PhWM in specific language impairment

We administered the WSRT to thirteen SLI children (mean age = 5.5 years, range = 5.0–5.11; mean PIQ = 112, range 98–125) and compared their performances with those of two groups of 40 normal control children, one group matched on chronological age and the other matched on language age (Casalini & Brizzolara, 1998).

SLI children showed poor PhWM abilities when compared to typical peers in the chronological age control group, while their performances were similar to those of children in the language age control group (Figs. 1, 2 and 3). PhWM performances of SLI children, like those of their typical control-group peers, was, however, sensitive to the phonological similarity, the word length, and the frequency effects, suggesting a problem in the capacity (span), but not in the nature of the processes of their PhWM.

In a second study (Brizzolara *et al.*, 1999), we followed, in the early stages of written language acquisition, a group of 18 SLI children diagnosed in their preschool years. The children have been divided into two groups comparable for age and Performance IQ (PIQ): they differed in the level attained in language development at the beginning of first grade: one group (8 children; mean age = 6.9, mean PIQ = 104) had resolved the language problem, while the other (10 children; mean age = 6.6, mean PIQ = 102) still showed persistent problems, mostly in phonological and morphosyntactic production.

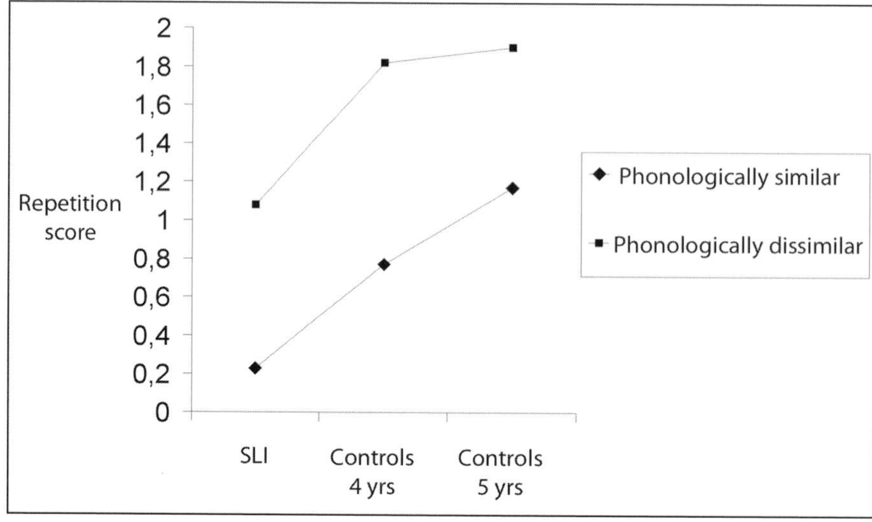

Fig. 1. Scores in repetition of phonologically similar and dissimilar words.

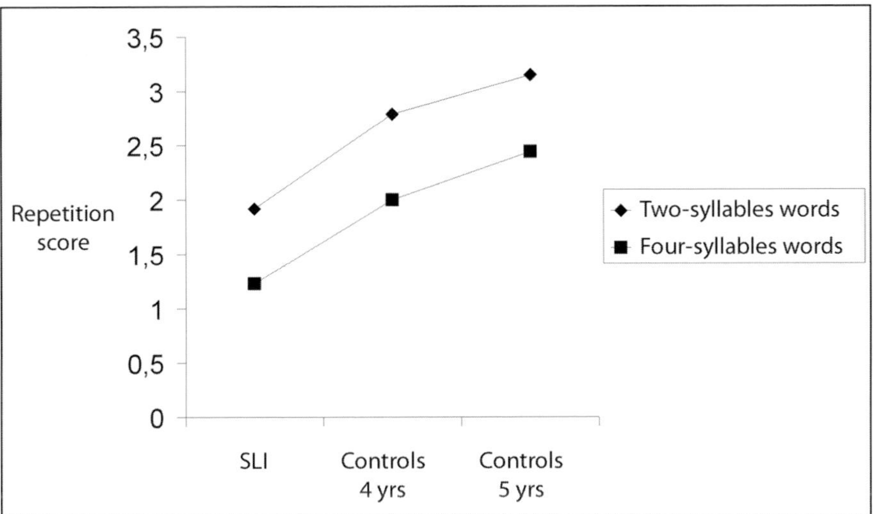

Fig. 2. Scores in repetition of short and long words.

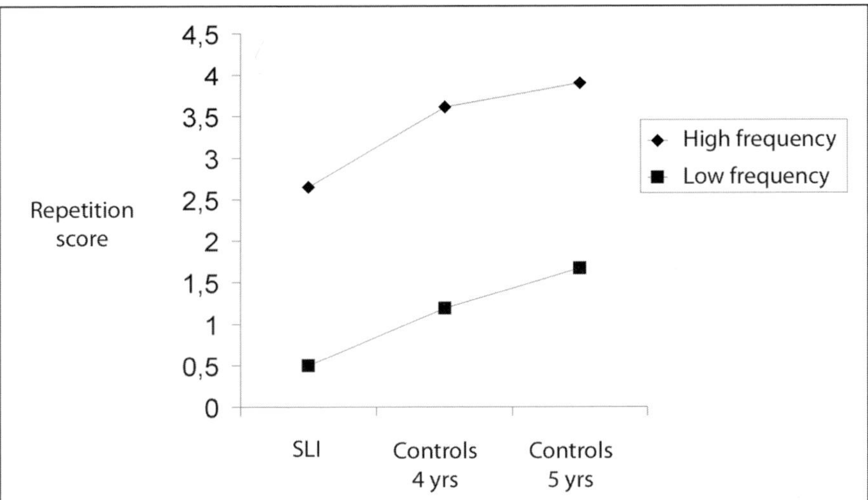

Fig. 3. Scores in repetition of high-frequency and low-frequency words.

The two groups differed in terms of written language abilities at the end of the first and second grades. The group with good language recovery showed an initial delay in reading and writing in first grade, accompanied by a delay in PhWM (evaluated with the WSRT) and in metaphonological abilities, but reached a normal reading and writing level at the end of second grade. The group with persistent language deficits also had impaired PhWM and a metaphonological disorder, and reading and writing proficiency was still very low at the end of second grade compared to normal controls. PhWm performances are reduced, but sensitive to the phonological similarity, the word length, and the frequency effects, confirming the previous result that SLI children show a problem in the capacity (span), but not in the nature of the processes of their PhWM.

These results support the view that a PhWM deficit characterizes more severe and persistent forms of SLI and that it may be a cause of these children's problems in learning to read and write at a normal rate.

PhWM in different types of SLI

PhWM is differently affected not only in how it appears in clinical manifestations of SLI varying in severity, but also in clinically different types of SLI.

We conducted a study (Pecini *et al.*, 2005) administering the WSRT to a group of 24 children with SLI divided into the Ph, Ex, and RE subgroups. An effect of SLI type on PhWM was found, whereby all children with RE and most with the Ex form of the disorder had a deficient performance in the WSRT, children with a Ph disorder were not impaired in this test. Mean z scores and percentages of delayed (1 SD below the mean) and deficient performances (at least 2 SDs below the mean) in the three groups are shown in Table 1.

Table 1. Phonological working memory in the three subtypes of SLI

	RE	Ex	Ph	Total
Mean	– 2,57	– 1.29	– 0.34	– 1.25
SD	(0.83)	(1.56)	(1.26)	(1.5)
Delay (%)	0	23	57	28
Deficit (%)	100	61	0	52

Moreover while Ph and Ex SLI children showed the length and the phonological similarity effects in a proportion equal to that found in the normal population (Brizzolara & Casalini, 2002), in the RE group the length effect and particularly the phonological similarity effect were less frequent than in the other groups (40 per cent and 20 per cent, respectively). This result suggests that PhWM abilities vary in relation to different types of SLI.

PhWM deficit and LTM knowledge in specific language impairment

We investigated the relationship between PhWM and LTM verbal knowledge in SLI by testing a sample of 32 preschool (7 girls and 25 boys) and 22 school-age (7 girls and 15 boys) SLI children in the NWRT. (The SLI sample was subdivided into three subgroups on the basis of the type of language disorder [RE, Ex, and Ph]. The three groups did not differ for performance IQ.)

The main purpose of the study (Casalini *et al.*, 2007) was to examine the effects of LTM verbal knowledge on STM verbal recall in Italian SLI children. We investigated whether a deficient performance in verbal STM recall in SLI children is partially due to a reduced contribution of LTM verbal knowledge and whether an impairment in lexical processing and representation may contribute to the impaired performance in STM recall. Moreover, we also examined whether and how PhWM abilities and the contribution of LTM verbal knowledge were differently affected in the different subtypes of SLI. We expected that RE and Ex disorders, in which lexical and PhWM abilities are often reported to be more impaired, would be associated with reduced lexical and morpho-lexical effects.

The results indicated that SLI children, as a group, showed significantly lower scores in the repetition task, compared to those of normal controls, although, as in normal children, their performance improved from preschool age to first grade (Fig. 4).

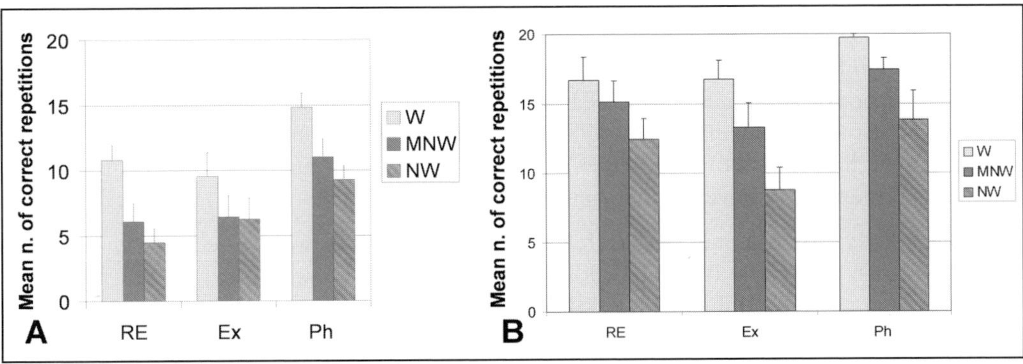

Fig. 4. Nonword repetition in the three subtypes of SLI in preschool (A) and first grade (B).

However, in spite of the significantly reduced overall scores, the qualitative profiles of the SLI patients were quite similar to those of typically developing children. Both SLI and controls repeated words more accurately than both types of nonwords (simple and morphologic), and MNW better than NW, thus showing the expected facilitative lexical and morpho-lexical effects.

SLI children's sensitivity to the linguistic characteristics of the items varied in relation to grade: in preschoolers, but not in first-graders with SLI, the magnitude of the lexical and morpho-lexical effects was significantly smaller compared to those of normal controls. SLI children showed smaller differences, with respect to controls, between W and NW and between MNW and NW; that is, SLI children had reduced lexical and morpho-lexical effects on repetition performance.

These results seem to corroborate the hypothesis that the impairment of PhWM can be considered as a marker (Bishop *et al.*, 1996) of SLI. Moreover, it may persist across ages and can be found in the context of preserved LTM verbal knowledge, at least in school-age children.

The reduced contribution of LTM verbal knowledge that has been suggested (*e.g.*, Van der Lely & Howard, 1993) might be more evident in preschoolers and become more limited with increasing exposure to spoken and written language, such as in first-graders with SLI.

The SLI type had a significant effect on PhWM: preschoolers with Ph SLI scored significantly higher than the other two groups, whereas sensitivity to lexical and morpho-lexical information did not significantly differ among groups.

These findings provide further support to the hypothesis that memory abilities may be differently affected in different subtypes of SLI and that the facilitative effects of LTM verbal knowledge are operative in most children with SLI (Pecini *et al.*, 2005).

Moreover, we found that children with an isolated Ph language disorder showed better PhWM abilities in retaining and processing verbal information. This might be one of the reasons explaining the better clinical prognosis and academic outcome in children affected by an isolated Ph SLI, as has been reported by several authors (*e.g.*, Bird *et al.*, 1995; Snowling *et al.*, 2000; Stothard *et al.*, 1998).

The role of PhWM deficit in the continuity between oral and written language disorders

Studying the problem of differential literacy outcomes in children with different types of SLI, we showed that not all children with SLI in the preschool years have problems with reading and writing (Brizzolara *et al.*, 2006a, 2007): children with morphosyntactic and phonologic deficits have a higher risk of difficulties in literacy acquisition than those with isolated phonological problems who have a better outcome.

In a recent study (Brizzolara *et al.*, 2011; Gasperini *et al.*, 2009) we focused on the long-term literacy outcome of a group of Italian adolescents with a documented history of SLI relative to both actual and previous oral language skills. Sixteen Italian adolescents diagnosed in our clinic in the preschool years as having SLI and 32 controls were submitted to an extensive assessment of oral and written language skills. At a group level, adolescents with SLI had weak oral and written language skills in almost all tests. Nonword repetition tasks best distinguished the participants of our study from their schoolmates, confirming that PhWM is weak in these students and that phonological processing deficits are a marker of language impairment, although they are not necessarily associated with literacy difficulties. In agreement with these data, in a previous study of Italian dyslexic children, we had shown that phonological processing deficits were not markers of all Italian dyslexics, but characterized only those with a previous history of language delay (Brizzolara *et al.*, 2006b; Chilosi *et al.*, 2009): children with a history of language impairment performed significantly worse than children without a history of language delay in PhWM and spoonerism tests. This finding indicates that, at least in a subgroup of Italian dyslexic children, reading disabilities may occur in the absence of clear PhWM and metaphonological deficits.

The deficient PhWM abilities found in our group of dyslexics with previous language delay may have been be a residual sign of their early language impairment, often persisting in children in whom the language problems have apparently been resolved.

Conclusions

Taken together, the results of our studies seem to demonstrate that PhWM is primarily disordered in SLI and that the severity of the deficit may vary in relation to the type of language impairment. However, some caution might be necessary because of possible misclassifications of the language disorder. As pointed out by Laws and Bishop (2004), if experts now agree that SLI is a heterogeneous condition, there is little consensus about how it should be subclassified. The three DSM–IV SLI subtypes are largely based on exclusionary criteria and are usually defined in terms of behavioural characteristics which do not take into consideration the severity and the pervasiveness of the linguistic impairment. The foregoing dimensions may be clinically relevant and give additional information for subtyping SLI children. If we take into account the severity of language impairment, in our samples, Ph SLI children appear to be the best group on a possible continuum, with mixed RE children being the most severely impaired. As already outlined by some authors, classification based on DSM–IV criteria may be responsible for some variability within the Ex and mixed RE subgroups, which may have attenuated the differences between them (see Tomblin [2008] and Tomblin *et al.* [1996] for a thorough discussion). In fact, some Ex children have low, though not defective, receptive abilities, while mixed RE children may show a variable degree of expressive and receptive impairment. A suggestion for future research is to study PhWM in SLI children classified according to multiple criteria, which would include the pervasiveness and/or the severity of the linguistic impairment (Bishop & Clarkson, 2003).

As a concluding remark, our data may have clinical implications for the early treatment of late-talking and SLI children. Since PhWM deficits tend not to completely resolve with age, and may contribute to the continuity between SLI and learning disabilities, it could be useful to increase PhWM capacities through specific training aimed at reducing the load on the PhWM system, which appears to be primarily impaired in SLI children (Gathercole & Alloway, 2006).

References

American Psychiatric Association (1994): *Diagnostic and Statistical Manual of Mental Disorders*, 4th ed. Washington, DC: American Psychiatric Association.

Archibald, L.M.D. & Gathercole, S.E. (2006): Short-term and working memory in SLI. *Int. J. Lang. Commun. Dis.* **41,** 675–693.

Archibald, L.M.D. & Gathercole, S.E. (2007): Nonword repetition in specific language impairment: more than a phonological short-term memory deficit. *Psychon. Bull. Rev.* **14,** 919–924.

Awh, E., Jonides, J., Smith, E.E. & Schumacher, E.H. (1996): Dissociation of storage and rehearsal in verbal working memory: evidence from positron emission tomography. *Psychol. Sci.* **7,** 25–31.

Baddeley, A.D. (1986): *Working Memory*. Oxford: Oxford University Press.

Baddeley, A.D. (1990): *Human Memory: Theory and Practice*. London: Lea Ltd.

Baddeley, A.D. & Wilson, B.A. (1993): A developmental deficit in short-term phonological memory: implications for language and reading. *Memory* **1,** 65–78.

Baddeley, A.D., Gathercole, S.E. & Papagno, C. (1998): The phonological loop as a language learning device. *Psychol. Rev.* **105,** 158–173.

Bird, J., Bishop, D.V.M. & Freeman, N.H. (1995): Phonological awareness and literacy development in children with expressive phonological impairments. *J. Speech Hearing Res.* **38,** 446–462.

Bishop, D.V.M. (1997): Cognitive neuropsychology and developmental disorders: uncomfortable bedfellows. *Q. J. Exp. Psychol.* **50,** 899–923.

Bishop, D.V.M. (2000): How does the brain learn language? Insights from the study of children with and without language impairment. *Dev. Med. Child Neurol.* **42,** 133–142.

Bishop, D.V.M. & Adams, C. (1990): A prospective study of the relationship between specific language impairment, phonological disorders, and reading retardation. *J. Child Psychol. Psychiatry* **21,** 1027–1050.

Bishop, D.V.M. & Clarkson, B. (2003): Written language as a window into residual language deficits: a study of children with persistent and residual speech and language impairments. *Cortex* **39,** 215–237.

Bishop, D.V.M. & Snowling, M.J. (2004): Developmental dyslexia and specific language impairment: same or different? *Psychol. Bull.* **130,** 858–886.

Bishop, D.V.M., North, T. & Donlan, C. (1996): Nonword repetition as a behavioural marker for inherited language impairment: evidence from a twin study. *J. Child Psychol. Psychiatry* **37,** 391–403.

Bortolini, U., Arfé, B., Caselli, C.M., Degasperi, L., Deevy, P. & Leonard, L.B. (2006): Clinical markers for specific language impairment in Italian: the contribution of clitics and non-word repetition. *Int. J. Lang. Commun. Dis.* **41,** 695–712.

Botting, N. & Conti-Ramsden, G. (2001): Non-word repetition and language development in children with specific language impairment (SLI). *Int. J. Lang. Commun. Dis.* **36,** 421–432.

Botting, N., Simkin, Z. & Conti-Ramsden, G. (2006): Associated reading skills in children with a history of Specific Language Impairment (SLI). *Reading & Writing: Interdisc. J.* **19,** 77–98.

Bowey, J.A. (1996): On the association between phonological memory and receptive vocabulary in five-year olds. *J. Exp. Child Psychol.* **63,** 44–88.

Boyle, J., McCartney, E., Forbes, J. & O'Hare, A. (2007): A randomised controlled trial and economic evaluation of direct versus indirect and individual versus group modes of speech and language therapy in children with primary language impairment. *Health Technol. Assess.* **11,** 1–139.

Brizzolara, D. & Casalini, C. (2002): Memoria di lavoro e difficoltà di apprendimento. In: *I Disturbi dello Sviluppo: Neuropsicologia Clinica e Ipotesi Riabilitative,* eds. S.Vicari & M.C. Caselli, pp. 241–260. Bologna: Il Mulino.

Brizzolara, D., Casalini, C., Sbrana, B., Chilosi, A.M. & Cipriani, P. (1999): Memoria di lavoro fonologica e difficoltà di apprendimento della lingua scritta nei bambini con disturbo specifico di linguaggio. *Psicol. Clin. Sviluppo* **3,** 465–488.

Brizzolara, D., Casalini, C., Gasperini, F., Roncoli, S., Mazzotti, S., Cipriani, P. & Chilosi, A.M. (2006a): A follow-up study of reading and writing in Italian children with specific language impairment. In: *Language: Normal and Pathological Development*, eds. D. Riva, I. Rapin & G. Zardini, pp. 239–252. Mariani Foundation Paediatric Neurology Series – XVI. Paris: John Libbey Eurotext.

Brizzolara, D., Chilosi, A.M., Cipriani, P., Di Filippo, G., Gasperini, F., Mazzotti, S., *et al.* (2006b): Do phonologic and rapid automatized naming deficits differentially affect dyslexic children with and without a history of language delay? A study of Italian dyslexic children. *Cogn. Behav. Neurol.* **19,** 141–149.

Brizzolara, D., Casalini, C., Gasperini, F., Mazzotti, S., Roncoli, S., Cipriani, P. & Chilosi, A.M. (2007): L'apprendimento della lingua scritta nei bambini con Disturbo Specifico di Sviluppo del Linguaggio: uno studio di follow-up. *Saggi, Child Dev. Disabil.* **33,** 53–69.

Brizzolara, D., Gasperini, F., Pfanner, L., Cristofani, P., Casalini, C. & Chilosi, A.M: (2011): Long-term reading and spelling outcome in Italian adolescents with a history of Specific Language Impairment. *Cortex* **47,** 955–973.

Cain, K., Oakhill, J. & Bryant, P. (2004): Children's reading comprehension ability: concurrent prediction by working memory, verbal ability, and component skills. *J. Educ. Psychol.* **96,** 31–42.

Carroll, J.M. & Snowling, M.J. (2004): Language and phonological skills in children at high risk of reading difficulties. *J. Child Psychol. Psychiatry* **45,** 631–640.

Casalini, C. & Brizzolara, D. (1998): La memoria di lavoro fonologica nei bambini con disturbo specifico del linguaggio. *Ciclo Evolutivo Disabilità* **1,** 249–264.

Casalini, C., Brizzolara, D., Cipriani, P., Chilosi, A., Marcolini, S., Pecini, C., *et al.* (2007): Non-word repetition in children with Specific Language Impairment: a deficit in phonological working memory or in long-term knowledge? *Cortex* **43,** 769–776.

Catts, H., Fey, M., Tomblin, J. & Zhang X. (2002): A longitudinal investigation of reading outcomes in children with language impairment. *J. Speech Lang. Hearing Res.* **45,** 1142–1157.

Chilosi, A.M., Brizzolara, D., Lami, L., Pizzoli, C., Gasperini, F., Pecini, C., *et al.* (2009): Reading and spelling disabilities in children with and without a history of early language delay: a neuropsychological and linguistic study. *Child Neuropsychol.* **2,** 1–23.

Cohen, J.D., Perlstein, W.M., Braver, T.S. & Nystrom, L.E. (1997): Temporal dynamics of brain activation during a working memory task. *Nature* **386,** 604–608.

Conti-Ramsden, G. (2003): Processing and linguistic markers in young children with specific language impairment (SLI). *J. Speech Lang. Hear. Res.* **46,** 1029–1037.

Conti-Ramsden, G., Botting, N. & Faragher, B. (2001): Psycholinguistic markers for specific language impairment (SLI). *J. Child Psychol. Psychiatry* **42,** 741–748.

Dollaghan, C. & Campbell, T.F. (1998): Nonword repetition and child language impairment. *J. Speech Lang. Hear. Res.* **41,** 1136–1146.

Dollaghan, C., Biber, M. & Campbell, T. (1995): Lexical influences on nonword repetition. *Appl. Psycholinguistics* **16,** 211–222.

Edwards, J. & Lahey, M. (1998): Nonword repetition of children with specific language impairment. *Appl. Psycholinguistics* **19,** 279–309.

Edwards, J., Beckman, M.E. & Munson, B. (2004): The interaction between vocabulary size and phonotactic probability effects on children's production accuracy and fluency in nonword repetition. *J. Speech Lang. Hear. Res.* **47,** 421–436.

Falcaro, M., Pickles, A., Newbury, D.F., Addis, L., Banfield, E., Fisher, S.E., Monaco, A.P., Simkin, Z. & Conti-Ramsden, G. (2008): Genetic and phenotypic effects of phonological short-term memory and grammatical morphology in specific language impairment. *Genes Brain Behav.* **7,** 393–402.

Gasperini, F., Brizzolara, D., Casalini, C., Cristofani, P. & Chilosi, A.M. (2009): Disturbo Specifico del Linguaggio e apprendimento della lingua scritta: uno studio di follow-up in adolescenza. *Dislessia* **6,** 93–124.

Gathercole, S.E. (1995): Is nonword repetition a test of phonological memory or long-term knowledge? It all depends on the nonwords. *Memory Cognit.* **23,** 83–94.

Gathercole, S.E. (1998): The development of memory. *J. Child Psychol. Psychiatry* **39,** 3–27.

Gathercole, S.E. & Alloway, T.P. (2006b): Practitioner review: short-term and working memory impairments in neurodevelopmental disorders: diagnosis and remedial support. *J. Child Psychol. Psychiatry* **47,** 4–15.

Gathercole, S.E. & Baddeley, A.D. (1990): Phonological memory deficits in language-disordered children: is there a causal connection? *J. Mem. Lang.* **29,** 336–360.

Gathercole, S.E. & Baddeley, A.D. (1993): *Working Memory and Language*. Hove, UK: Lawrence Erlbaum Associates.

Gathercole, S.E. & Baddeley, A.D. (1995): Short-term memory may yet be deficient in children with language impairments: a comment on Van der Lely and Howard (1993). *J. Speech Hear. Res.* **38,** 463–466.

Gathercole, S.E., Willis, C., Emslie, H. & Baddeley, A.D. (1991): The influences of number of syllables and word-likeness on children's repetition of nonwords. *Appl. Psycholinguistics* **12,** 349–367.

Gathercole, S.E., Willis, C., Emslie, H. & Baddeley, A.D. (1992): Phonological memory and vocabulary development during the early school years: a longitudinal study. *Dev. Psychol.* **28,** 887–898.

Gathercole, S.E., Hitch, G.J., Service, E. & Martin, A.J. (1997): Phonological short-term memory and new word learning in children. *Dev. Psychol.* **33,** 966–979.

Gathercole, S.E., Frankish, C.R., Pickering, S. & Peaker, S. (1999): Phonotactic influences on short-term memory. *J. Exp. Psychol. Learn. Mem. Cognit.* **25,** 84–95.

Gathercole, S.E., Pickering, S.J., Hall, M. & Peaker, S.M. (2001): Dissociable lexical and phonological influences on serial recognition and serial recall. *Q. J. Exp. Psychol.* **54A,** 1–30.

Gathercole, S.E., Alloway, T.P., Willis, C. & Adams,. A.M. (2006a): Working memory in children with reading disabilities. *J. Exp. Child Psychol.* **93,** 265–281.

Goulandris, N., Snowling, M. & Walker, I. (2000): Is dyslexia a form of specific language impairment? A comparison of dyslexic and language impaired children as adolescents. *Ann. Dyslexia* **50,** 103–120.

Grasby, P.M., Frith, C.D., Friston, K.J. & Simpson, J. (1994): A graded task approach to the functional mapping of brain areas implicated in auditory verbal memory. *Brain* **117,** 1271–1282.

Howard, D. & Van der Lely, H. (1995): Specific language impairment in children is not due to a short-term memory deficit: response to Gathercole and Baddeley. *J. Speech Hear. Res.* **38,** 466–472.

Hulme, C. & Tordoff, V. (1989): Working memory development: the effects of speech rate, word length and acoustic similarity on serial recall. *J. Exp. Child Psychol.* **47,** 72–87.

Hulme, C. & Snowling, M. (1992): Deficits in output phonology: an explanation of reading failure? *Cogn. Neuropsychol.* **4,** 321–366.

Kirschen, M.P., Chen, S.A., Schraedley Desmond, P. & Desmond, J.E. (2005): Load and practice dependent increases in cerebrocerebellar activation in verbal working memory: an fMRI study. *Neuroimage* **24,** 462–472.

Laws, G. & Bishop, D.V.M. (2004): Pragmatic language impairment and social deficits in Williams syndrome: a comparison with Down's syndrome and specific language impairment. *Int. J. Lang. Commun. Dis.* **39,** 45–64.

Leonard, LB. (1998): *Children with Specific Language Learning Impairment.* Cambridge, MA: MIT Press.

Majerus, S. & Van der Linden, M. (2003): Long-term memory effects on verbal short-term memory: a replication study. *Br. J. Devel. Psychol.* **21,** 303–310.

Mann, V.A. (1984): Longitudinal prediction and prevention of early reading difficulty. *Ann. Dyslexia* **34,** 117–136.

Marvel, C.L. & Desmond, J.E. (2010): The contributions of cerebro-cerebellar circuitry to executive verbal working memory. *Cortex* **46,** 880–895.

Misciagna, S., Iuvone, L., Mariotti, P. & Silveri, M.C. (2010): Verbal short-term memory and cerebellum: evidence from a patient with congenital cerebellar vermis hypoplasia. *Neurocase* **16,** 119–124.

Monaco, A.P. (2007): Multivariate linkage analysis of specific language impairment (SLI). *Ann. Hum. Genet.* **71,** 660–673.

Montgomery, J.W. (1995): Examination of phonological working memory in specifically language-impaired children. *Appl. Psycholinguistics* **16,** 355–378.

Montgomery, J.W. (2004): Sentence comprehension in children with specific language impairment: effects of input rate and phonological working memory. *Int. J. Lang. Commun. Disord.* **39,** 115–134.

Morra, S. & Camba, R. (2009): Vocabulary learning in primary school children: working memory and long-term memory components. *J. Exp. Child Psychol.* **104,** 156–178.

Nickisch, A. & von Kries, R. (2009): Short-term memory (STM) constraints in children with Specific Language Impairment (SLI): are there differences between Receptive and Expressive SLI? *J. Speech Lang. Hear. Res.* **52,** 578–596.

O'Hare, E.D., Lu, L.H., Houston, S.M., Bookheimer, S.Y. & Sowell, E.R. (2008): Neurodevelopmental changes in verbal working memory load-dependency: an fMRI investigation. *Neuroimage* **42,** 1678–1685.

Palladino, P. & Ferrari, M. (2008): Phonological sensitivity and memory in children with a foreign language learning difficulty. *Memory* **16,** 604–625.

Pecini, C., Casalini, C., Brizzolara, D., Cipriani, P., Pfanner, L. & Chilosi, A.M. (2005): Hemispheric specialization for language in children with different types of specific language impairments. *Cortex* **41,** 157–167.

Plante, E. (1998): Criteria for SLI. *J. Speech Lang. Hear. Res.* **41,** 951–957.

Roodenrys, S., Hulme, C. & Brown, G. (1993): The development of short-term memory span: Separable effects of speech rate and long-term memory. *J. Exp. Child Psychol.* **56,** 431–442.

Sahlén, B., Reuterskiöld-Wagner, C., Nettelbladt, U. & Radeborg, K. (1999): Non-word repetition in children with language impairment: pitfalls and possibilities. *Int. J. Lang. Commun. Dis.* **34,** 337–352.

Service, E. (1992): Phonology, working memory and foreign-language learning. *Q. J. Exp. Psychol.* **45A,** 21–50.

SLI Consortium (2004): Highly significant linkage to the SLI locus in an expanded sample of individuals affected by Specific Language Impairment. *Am. J. Hum. Genet.* **74,** 1225–1238.

Snowling, M.J. (2008): Specific disorders and broader phenotypes: the case of dyslexia. *Q. J. Exp. Psychol.* **61,** 142–156.

Snowling, M.J., Chiat, S. & Hulme, C. (1991): Words, nonwords, and phonological processes: some comments on Gathercole, Willis, Emslie, and Baddeley. *Appl. Psycholinguistics* **12,** 369–373.

Snowling, M.J., Bishop, D.V.M. & Stothard, S.E. (2000): Is preschool language impairment a risk factor for dyslexia in adolescence? *J. Child Psychol. Psychiatry* **41,** 587–600.

Stothard, S.E., Snowling, M.J., Bishop, D.V.M., Chipchase, B.B. & Kaplan, C.A. (1998): Language impaired preschoolers: a follow-up into adolescence. *J. Speech Lang. Hear. Res.* **41,** 407–418.

Tomblin, J.B. (2008): Validating diagnostic standards for specific language impairment using adolescent outcomes. In: *Understanding Developmental Language Disorders*, eds. C.F. Norbury, J.B. Tomblin & D.V.M. Bishop, pp. 93–114. New York: Psychology Press.

Tomblin, J.B., Records, N.L. & Zhang, X. (1996): A system for the diagnosis of Specific Language Impairment in kindergarten children. *J. Speech Hear. Res.* **39,** 1284–1294.

Turner, J.E., Henry, L.A. & Smith, P.T. (2000): The development of the use of long-term knowledge to assist short-term recall. *Q. J. Exp. Psychol.* **53A,** 457–78.

Van der Leij, A. & Van Daal, V.H. (1999): Automatization aspects of dyslexia: speed limitations in word identification, sensitivity to increasing task demands, and orthographic compensation. *J. Learn. Disabil.* **32,** 417–281.

Van der Lely, H.K.J. & Howard, D. (1993): Children with specific language impairment: linguistic impairment or short-term memory deficit? *J. Speech Hear. Res.* **36,** 1193–1207.

Veltman, D.J., Rombouts, S.A. & Dolan, R.J. (2003): Maintenance versus manipulation in verbal working memory revisited: an fMRI study. *NeuroImage* **18,** 247–256.

Wagner, T.D. & Smith, E.E. (2003): Neuroimaging studies of working memory: a meta-analysis. *Cogn. Affect. Behav. Neurosci.* **3,** 255–274.

Weismer, S.E., Tomblin, J.B., Zhang, X., Buckwalter, P., Chynoweth, J.G. & Jones, M. (2000): Nonword repetition performance in school-age children with and without language impairment. *J. Speech Lang. Hear. Res.* **43,** 865–878.

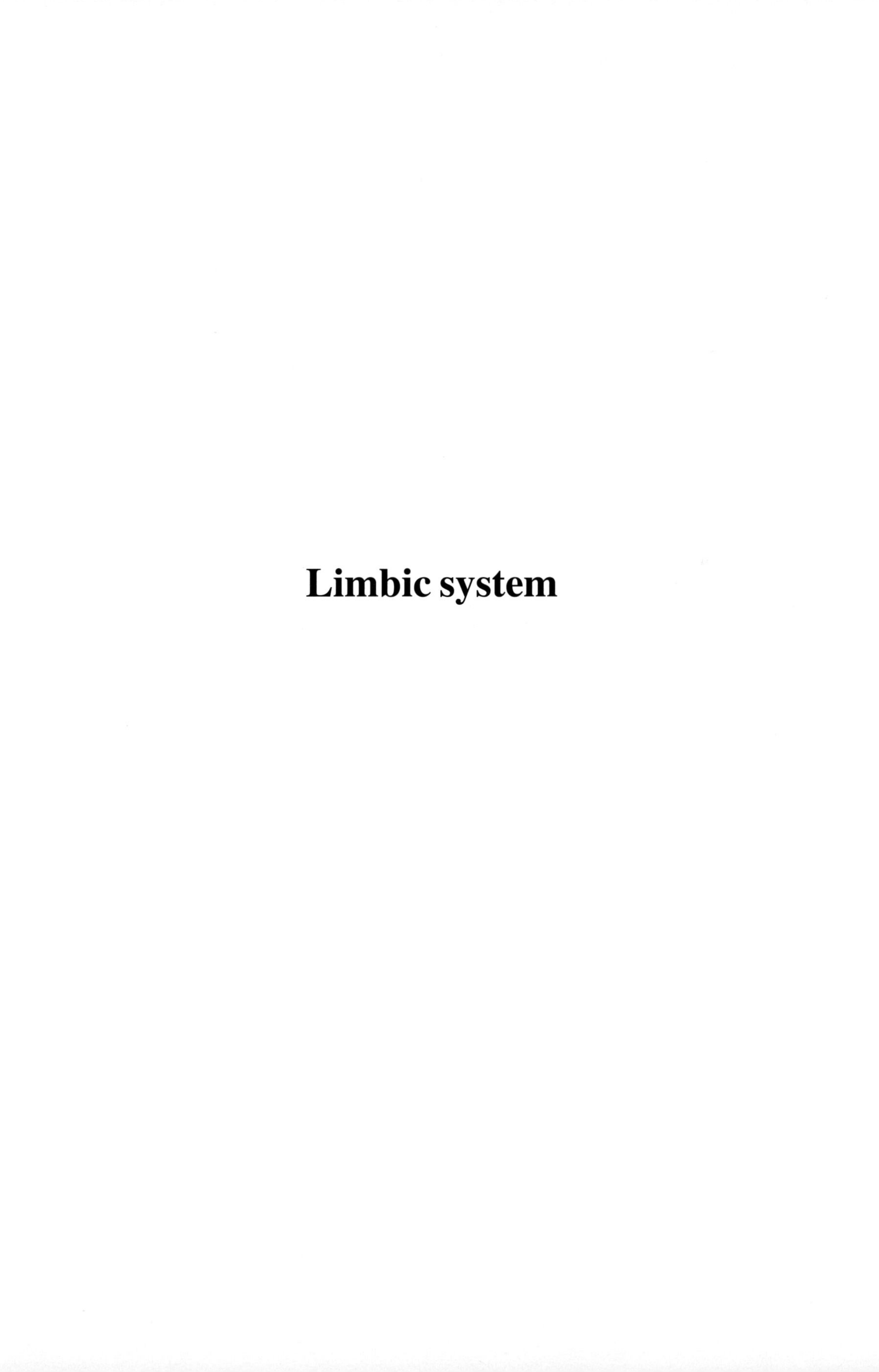

Limbic system

Brain Lesion Localization and Developmental Functions, D. Riva, C. Njiokiktjien and S. Bulgheroni (eds.)

Chapter 9

Neuroanatomic organization and fundamental functions of the hippocampus and amygdala

Pierre Lavenex

Laboratory of Brain and Cognitive Development, Department of Medicine, University of Fribourg, chemin du Musée 5, CH-1700 Fribourg, Switzerland
pierre.lavenex@unifr.ch

Summary

The hippocampus and the amygdala are two distinct brain structures located in the human medial temporal lobe, which are included in the so-called limbic system. In this chapter, it is considered that the limbic system *per se* does not exist, because these different brain structures contribute to disparate functional processes. Rather, this chapter focuses on the neuroanatomic organization and the fundamental functions of the hippocampal formation and the amygdaloid complex. First, the overall structural organization of these brain regions in adult humans and animals is described. Second, the basic functional processes carried out by these structures – memory for the hippocampal formation, and fear for the amygdaloid complex – is discussed. Findings from functional studies demonstrating, for both the hippocampus and the amygdala, that damage to these structures occurring either early in life or in adulthood has a differential impact on the functional processes that they normally subserve are presented. Third, a discussion of how the differential development of distinct hippocampal circuits might contribute to the emergence and maturation of different types of 'hippocampus-dependent' memory processes is presented. Finally, a discussion is proposed about the results of genome-wide analyses of gene expression in the postnatal, developing monkey hippocampal formation, which suggest that a developmental decrease in astrocytic processes may underlie the selective vulnerability of the hippocampus during hypoxic-ischaemic episodes in adulthood and its decreased susceptibility to febrile seizures with age, as well as contribute to the emergence of selective, adult-like memory function.

Introduction

The hippocampus and the amygdala are two distinct brain structures included in a group of brain regions called the limbic system, which was thought to be involved in the elaboration of emotional experience and expression. In this chapter, as others have already done before, the term 'limbic system' is considered obsolete because the different brain structures included in this so-called system contribute to disparate functional processes.

The term *limbic lobe* was first coined in 1877 by Broca to characterize a group of cortical brain regions located in the medial surface of the two hemispheres, which included the cingulate gyrus, the parahippocampal gyrus, and the olfactory bulb (Broca, 1877, 1878). Broca mainly described the overall organization of this brain region in different species (*'le grand lobe limbique, formé par la réunion du lobe olfactif, du lobe de l'hippocampe et du lobe du corps calleux'*). However, he also surmised that the function of the limbic lobe was characterized by mental abilities that predominate in beasts (and remains rather constant in different species), whereas the rest of the cortical mantle subserves the superior mental abilities of intelligent animals (which evolve and become predominant with the development of the cortex). He wrote: *'Le grand lobe limbique... est le siège des facultés inférieures qui prédominent chez la brute'*, *'le reste du manteau... est le siège des facultés supérieures qui prédominent chez l'animal intelligent'* (Broca, 1877, 1878). He did not specify, however, the mental abilities that were characteristics of beasts or of intelligent animals. In 1937, James Papez considered some of the brain regions included in Broca's limbic lobe to be part of a functional brain circuit thought to contribute to the experience and expression of emotions (Papez, 1937). *Papez's circuit* comprised the hippocampal formation, the cingulate gyrus, the mammillary bodies, the anterior thalamic nuclei, and their interconnections. The amygdala was not an integral part of the circuit: 'Concerning the olfactory centers and the amygdala, the case is simple... The stria terminalis connects the amygdala, the function of which is unknown, with the pars optica hypothalami...' (Papez, 1937, p. 742). In 1952, McLean formalized the concept of a *limbic system*, which contributed to the elaboration and expression of emotional experience: '[T]he limbic system represents an early neural development involved in the elaboration of emotional experience and expression', 'The limbic system is comprised of the cortex contained in the great limbic lobe of Broca together with its subcortical cell stations.' (MacLean, 1952, p. 407). Thus, according to MacLean's definition, the limbic system comprises the cortex adjacent to the olfactory striae, pyriform area, hippocampal gyrus, hippocampus, parasplenial, cingulate, subcallosal gyri, amygdala, septal nuclei, hypothalamus, epithalamus, anterior thalamic nuclei, and parts of the basal nuclei. Over the years, a number of researchers have questioned the existence or even the usefulness of such a concept (*e.g.*, Brodal, 1982; Kotter & Meyer, 1992; LeDoux, 1987, 1991). LeDoux provided detailed arguments against the concept of a limbic system in a review article in which he concluded: '[T]he limbic system continues to survive... [partly because] both the anatomical concept and the emotional function it was supposed to mediate were defined so vaguely as to be irrefutable' (LeDoux, 2000).

Here, it will be shown that the basic structural organization and functions of the hippocampal formation and the amygdaloid complex are clearly distinct. The amygdaloid complex is fundamental for the regulation of fear and emotional behavior, whereas the hippocampal formation plays a fundamental role in memory processes. Selective damage to the amygdala in adult humans leads to an inability to perceive and express negative emotions such as fear. In contrast, selective damage to the hippocampus in adult humans results in amnesia without having an impact on fear and emotional behavior. In this chapter, first the fundamental neuroanatomic and functional characteristics of these two brain regions are discussed (Fig. 1). Then the differential impacts of early *versus* late lesions of the amygdala or the hippocampus on the functional processes normally carried out by these brain structures are considered. Finally, a discussion focused on the hippocampal formation considers how the regulation of gene expression and the neuroanatomic changes occurring during postnatal development contribute to the emergence of memory processes. Understanding the normal development of the hippocampal formation also helps to further our understanding of the pathologic conditions affecting this brain region across the life span.

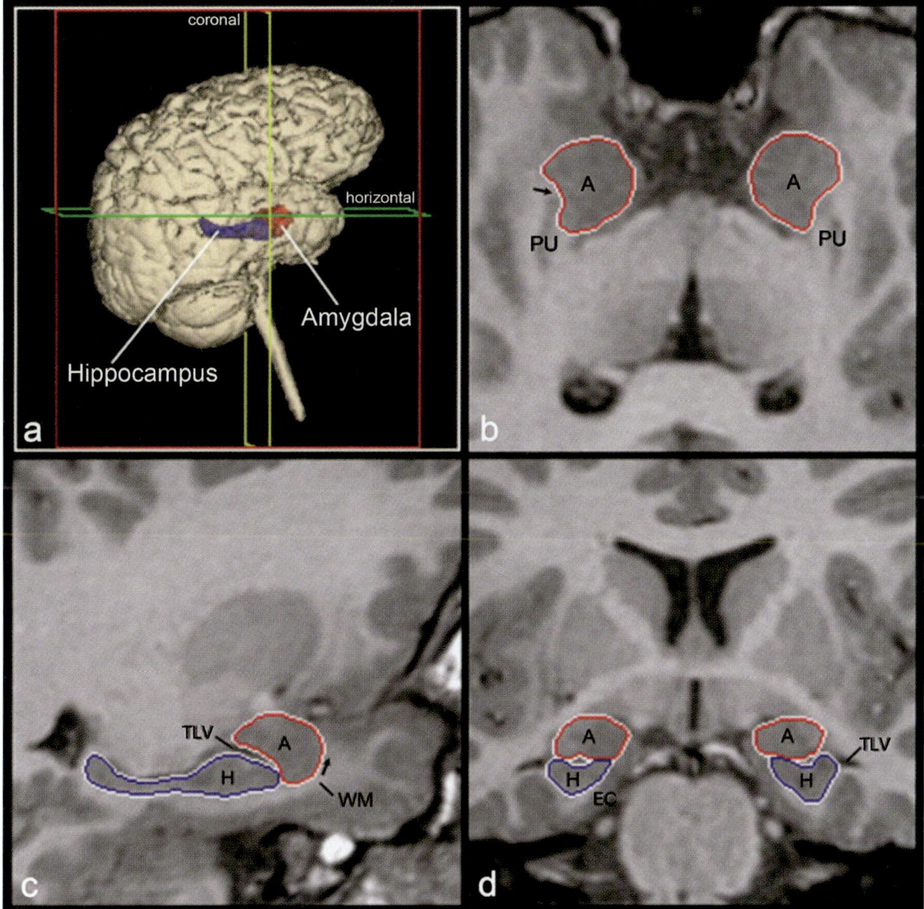

Fig. 1. Magnetic resonance imaging (MRI) representations of the hippocampus and amygdala in the human brain. A: amygdala; H: hippocampus; EC: entorhinal cortex; PU: putamen; TLV: lateral ventricle; WM: white matter. From Schumann et al. *(2004); reproduced by permission of the Society for Neuroscience.*

Neuroanatomic characteristics

The hippocampus

The terms *hippocampus* and *hippocampal formation* are often used interchangeably, yet they refer to and include different brain structures, depending on the context in which they are used. Detailed descriptions of the structural characteristics of the hippocampal formation have been provided elsewhere (Amaral & Lavenex, 2007; Lavenex, 2012), so only the basic aspects of its functional neuroanatomy are considered in this chapter. The term *hippocampus* typically refers to the bulge occupying the floor of the temporal horn of the lateral ventricle in the human brain (Fig. 2). The term *hippocampal formation* refers to a group of cortical regions located in the medial temporal lobe that includes the dentate gyrus, hippocampus proper (cornu Ammonis: CA3, CA2, CA1), subiculum, presubiculum, parasubiculum, and entorhinal cortex (Fig. 3). Each of these structures contains a number of different cell types, and different sets of intrinsic

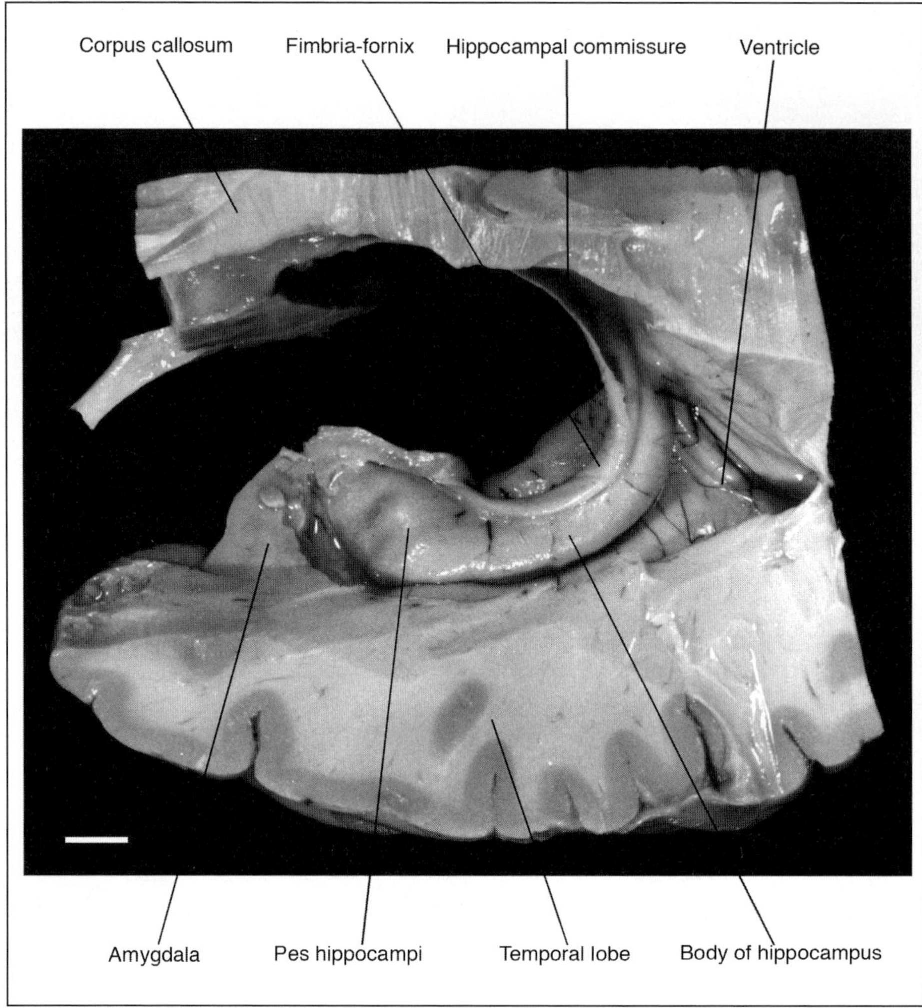

Fig. 2. Dorsolateral view of the human hippocampus after removing the overlying structures. The lateral ventricle has been opened, exposing the shape of the hippocampus. Scale bar = 1 cm. From The Hippocampus Book*; reproduced by permission from Oxford University Press.*

connections and interconnections with other brain regions, which exhibit clear and distinct topographic distributions. Altogether, these interconnected structures form a functional brain system essential for memory, which is particularly sensitive to a number of pathologic occurrences (Lavenex, 2012; Lavenex *et al.*, 2011).

The overall structural organization of the hippocampal formation is largely conserved across species, despite major species differences in the relative development of brain areas with which it interacts. This is largely due to the fact that very few cortical areas have direct interconnections with the hippocampus. Instead, cortical inputs are relayed through a hierarchy of associational cortices in which significant integration of information takes place before these inputs are forwarded to the next hierarchical level and finally reach the hippocampus (Fig. 4). Cortical regions send projections converging onto the hippocampal formation via three main structures: the perirhinal, parahippocampal, and entorhinal cortices. These different regions receive

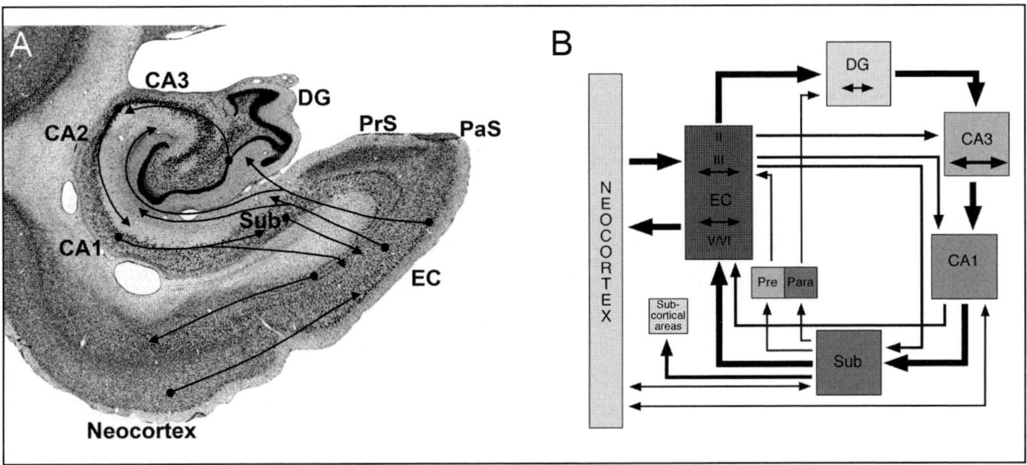

Fig. 3. Main serial and parallel pathways through the monkey hippocampal formation. Entorhinal cortex layer II neurons give rise to the perforant pathway projections reaching the molecular layer of the dentate gyrus and the stratum lacunosum-moleculare of the distal portion of CA3 and CA2, whereas entorhinal cortex layer III neurons give rise to the perforant and alvear pathways projections reaching CA1 stratum lacunosum-moleculare and the molecular layer of the subiculum. In contrast, entorhinal cortex layer V and VI neurons receive return projections from CA1 and the subiculum, and give rise to the cortical efferent projections of the entorhinal cortex. The other main output structure of the hippocampal formation is the subiculum, which gives rise to significant projections to a number of subcortical areas. (A) From Jabès et al. *(2011); reproduced by permission from Wiley-Liss. (B) From* The Hippocampus Book*; reproduced by permission from Oxford University Press.*

different sets of neocortical inputs and exhibit specific patterns of interconnections with the neocortex (Insausti & Amaral, 2008; Kobayashi & Amaral, 2003; Lavenex *et al.*, 2002; Munoz & Insausti, 2005; Suzuki & Amaral, 1994a). The perirhinal and parahippocampal cortices represent the first stage in the neocortical–hippocampal loop and provide about two-thirds of the neocortical input reaching the entorhinal cortex in monkeys (Suzuki & Amaral, 1994b). Other major neocortical projections reaching directly the entorhinal cortex originate in the cingulate and retrosplenial cortices, the insular and orbitofrontal cortices, the superior temporal gyrus, and the olfactory bulb (Insausti *et al.*, 1987). The retrosplenial cortex (Kobayashi & Amaral, 2003, 2007) has not been described explicitly in the classical view of the neocortical–hippocampal loop thought to be important for memory consolidation (Lavenex & Amaral, 2000). However, it also constitutes a relay between the neocortex and both the parahippocampal and entorhinal cortices, and there is increasing evidence linking the retrosplenial cortex to amnesia (Aggleton, 2010). The entorhinal cortex is the next stage in the neocortical–hippocampal loop and the first relay in the hippocampal formation. In humans, Insausti and colleagues (1995) delineated eight subdivisions for the entorhinal cortex: Eo, Er, Elr, Elc, Ei, Emi, Ec, and Ecl. The entorhinal cortex constitutes the main gateway for bidirectional communication between the neocortex and the hippocampal formation, and thus also constitutes the last stage for information processing within the hippocampal formation (see below). While some polymodal associational cortical areas, in particular the perirhinal and parahippocampal cortices, project directly to CA1 (Suzuki & Amaral, 1990), the entorhinal cortex is the only structure to transmit neocortical inputs to the dentate gyrus, CA3, and CA2. A schematic representation of the main serial and parallel pathways through the monkey hippocampal formation (Fig. 3), beginning and ending with the entorhinal cortex, helps to characterize the laminar organization of distinct

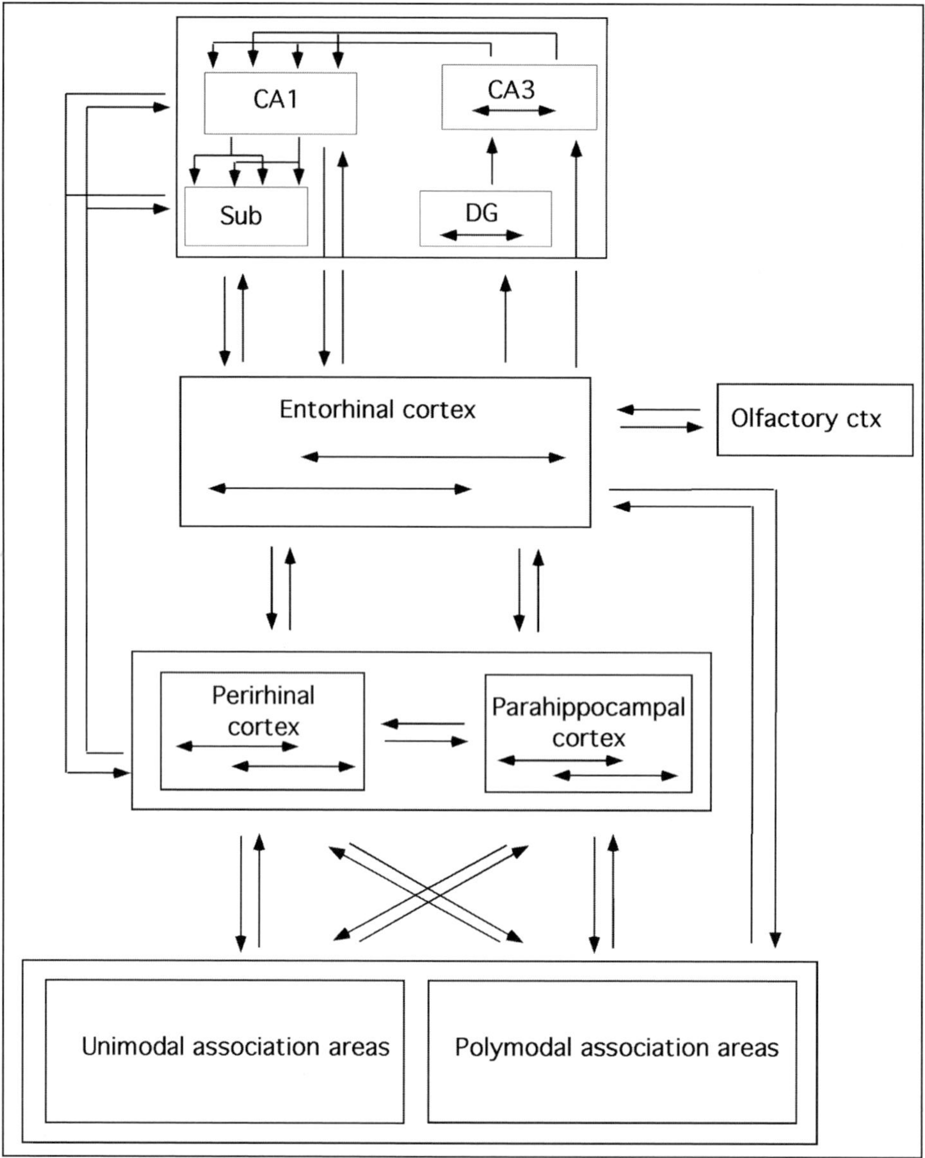

Fig. 4. Schematic representation of the hierarchical organization of projections within the medial temporal lobe. See main text for details. From Lavenex and Amaral (2000); reproduced by permission from Wiley–Liss.

hippocampal regions and functional circuits. Interestingly, these distinct regions exhibit different patterns of postnatal development that might underlie the emergence of different types of 'hippocampus-dependent' memory processes (Jabès *et al.*, 2011; see below).

Although the efferent projections from the hippocampal formation to the neocortex are generally of the feedback type, their laminar distribution differs in distinct cortical areas, and most importantly, these connections do not necessarily reciprocate the cortical afferents originating in defined brain regions (Lavenex *et al.*, 2002). Neither the dentate gyrus, nor CA3 or CA2 project toward cortical areas. In contrast, CA1, the subiculum, presubiculum, and parasubiculum send modest projections toward a limited number of cortical areas, which bypass the entorhinal cortex (Insausti & Munoz, 2001). Nevertheless, the vast majority of the efferent projections from the hippocampal formation to the neocortex originate in the deep layers of the entorhinal cortex and are relayed by the perirhinal and parahippocampal cortices (Lavenex *et al.*, 2002; Munoz & Insausti, 2005; Suzuki & Amaral, 1994b). As is observed for the parahippocampal–entorhinal cortex interconnections, parahippocampal area TF has largely reciprocal connections with the neocortex, whereas perirhinal area 36 has more asymmetric connections (Lavenex *et al.*, 2002). Thus, the organization of the cortical efferent projections of the perirhinal, parahippocampal, and entorhinal cortices has important implications for theories of memory consolidation. These theories were based on the observation that long-term declarative memories are only initially dependent on the integrity of the medial temporal lobe. The consolidation of long-term memories in cortical areas was thought to depend on reciprocal feedback projections from the medial temporal lobe to the neocortex. However, although the hippocampal–cortical projections are indeed of the feedback type, they differ and exhibit specific laminar patterns of termination in distinct brain areas. This suggests that different types of information processed by distinct cortical areas might require different types of feedback projections to enable memory consolidation (Lavenex *et al.*, 2002). In addition, these efferent projections do not necessarily reciprocate the cortical afferents to the medial temporal lobe structures. This further demonstrates the need to better take into account the structural organization of the brain in order to build realistic and valid models of the functions that it may subserve.

The amygdala

The amygdala, also known as the amygdaloid complex, is a brain region located in the rostral portion of the human medial temporal lobe (Fig. 1). In rodents and primates, including humans, the amygdala consists of 13 nuclei and cortical areas demarcated into several subdivisions (Fig. 5). Detailed descriptions of the nomenclature and morphologic characteristics of the amygdala nuclei can be found in the original descriptions by Price and colleagues (1987) and Freese and Amaral (2009). The fundamental organization of amygdala circuits is largely conserved between species, and the differences in the relative size and neuron numbers of the main amygdala nuclei observed between species is largely linked to their degree of connectivity with other brain structures (Chareyron *et al.*, 2011). The lateral, basal, and accessory basal nuclei are more developed in primates than in rodents, and they parallel the greater development of the neocortical areas with which these nuclei are interconnected in primates. Cortical information reaching the primate amygdala *via* the lateral, basal, and accessory basal nuclei can be processed within these nuclei and sent back to the neocortex to modulate cortical activity (Fig. 6). Intrinsic amygdala projections can further integrate these inputs and forward highly-processed information to influence the functions carried out by the central nucleus (see below). In addition, direct projections from the lateral, basal, and accessory basal nuclei can contribute to the modulation of neuronal activity in various subcortical structures (Fig. 7). In contrast, the central nucleus is connected mainly to visceral and autonomic systems (Freese & Amaral, 2009; Pitkänen, 2000). These systems are supposed to be conserved during the course of evolution leading to more limited species differences in the size of the central nucleus (Fig. 8). Similarly, the relatively small species differences in the volume and neuron number of the medial nucleus are paralleled by the highly conserved organization of the olfactory cortex with which it is interconnected (Chareyron *et al.*, 2011).

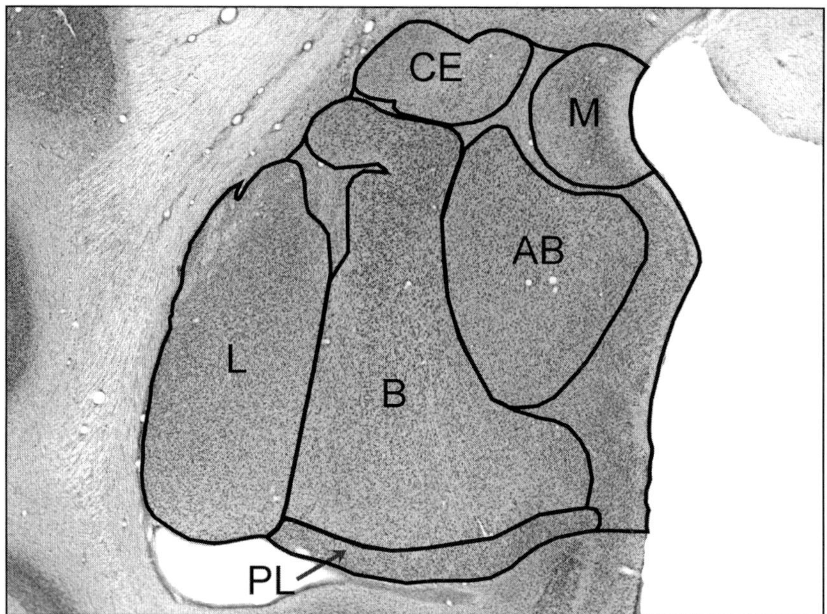

Fig. 5. Low-magnification photomicrograph of a coronal section at mid rostrocaudal level through the monkey amygdala, illustrating the locations of the six main nuclei. L, lateral; B, basal; AB, accessory basal; C, central; M: medial; PL, paralaminar. Unlabeled areas represent remaining nuclei of the amygdala. Other nuclei include the intercalated nuclei, anterior amygdaloid area, nucleus of the lateral olfactory tract, anterior cortical nucleus, periamygdaloid cortex, posterior cortical nucleus, and amygdalo-hippocampal area. Scale bar: 1 mm.

The main amygdala nuclei, including the lateral, basal, accessory basal, central, and medial nuclei, are also characterized by their unique sets of intra-amygdala connections (Fig. 9). Within the amygdala, the connections between these different nuclei are highly directional. The lateral nucleus projects to the basal, accessory basal, medial, and central nuclei, whereas the return projections are either very meager or totally nonexistent. The basal nucleus projects to the accessory basal, medial, and central nuclei, but the return projections are also either meager or nonexistent. The accessory basal nucleus projects most strongly to the central nucleus and sends moderate projections to the medial nucleus, whereas it returns only light projections to the lateral and basal nuclei. The medial nucleus receives its strongest afferents from the lateral nucleus and moderate projections from the accessory basal nucleus. The medial nucleus projects most heavily to the central nucleus and returns only light projections to the basal and accessory basal nuclei, but not to the lateral nucleus. Finally, the central nucleus is the site of convergence of projections originating in all the other main amygdala nuclei. In contrast, the central nucleus projects only lightly to the lateral, basal, and accessory basal nuclei.

In sum, although the basic circuitry of the amygdala is largely conserved between species, the amygdala likely exerts a greater modulation of cortical activity in primates, as compared to rodents. In addition, the primate amygdala integrates a greater number of cortical inputs that might also regulate the basic, visceral, and autonomic functions carried out by the central nucleus.

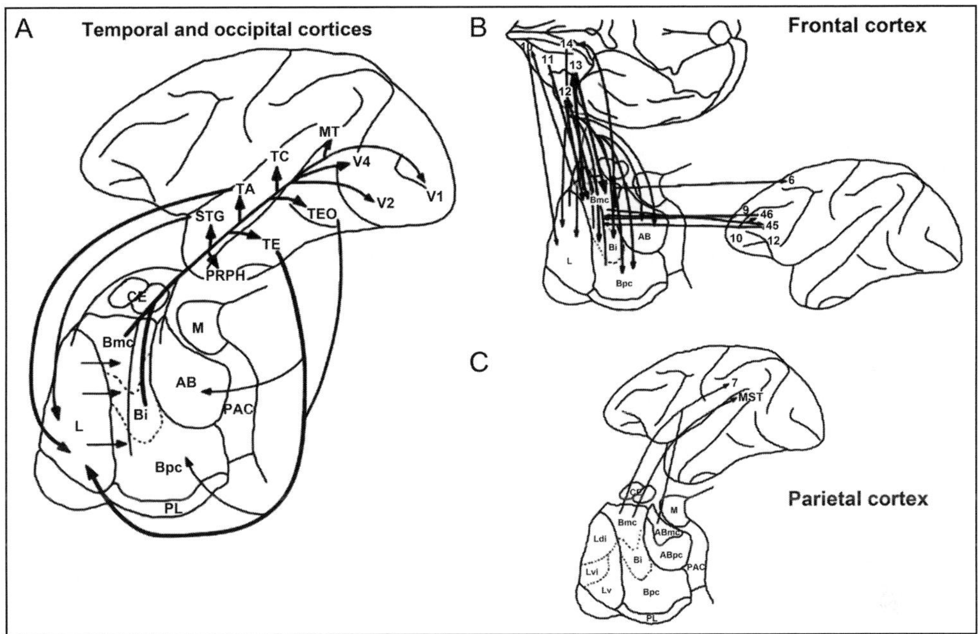

Fig. 6. Major amygdala connections with the neocortex. (A) Temporal and occipital cortices. (B) Frontal cortex. (C) Parietal cortex. Neocortical projections reaching the amygdala mainly via the lateral, basal, and accessory basal nuclei originate in higher-order associational cortical areas. Amygdala projections toward the neocortex originate mainly in the basal and accessory basal nuclei and terminate in various neocortical areas, incuding primary sensory areas that do not project directly to the amygdala. From Freese and Amaral (2009); reproduced by permission from Psychology Press.

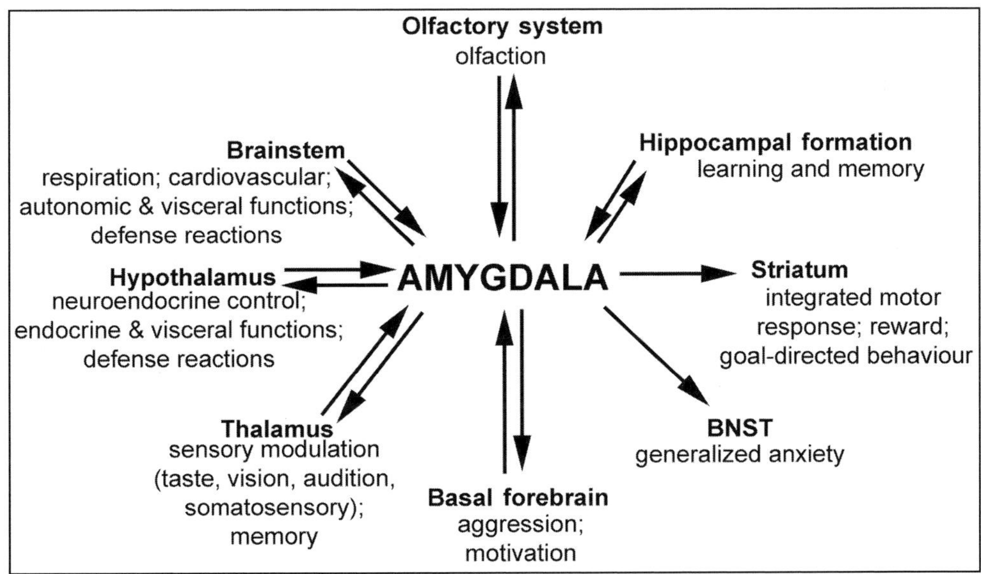

Fig. 7. Amygdala interconnections with subcortical structures. Amygdala nuclei have distinct sets of projections to subcortical structures. From Freese and Amaral (2009), who provide a detailed description; reproduced by permission from Psychology Press.

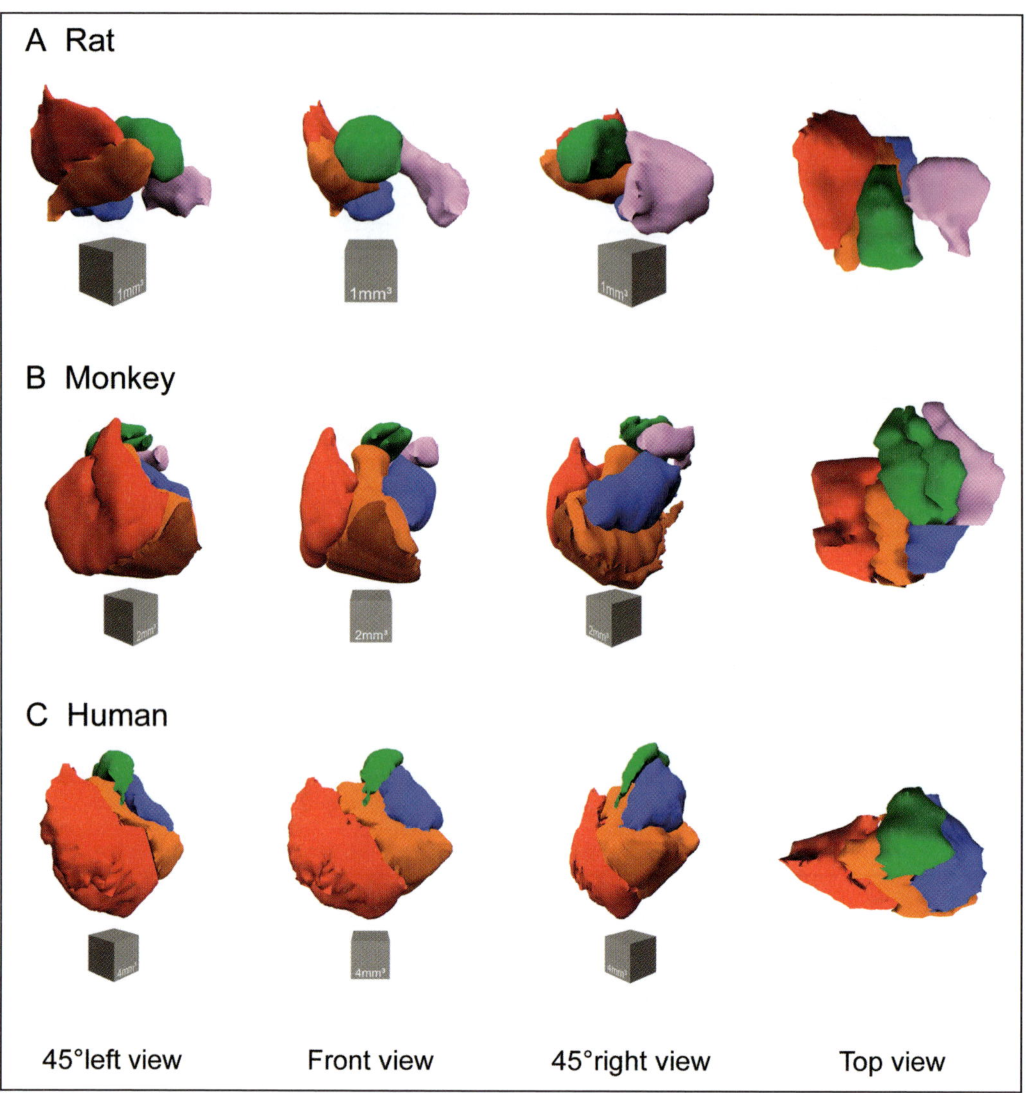

Fig. 8. Three-dimensional reconstruction of the main amygdala nuclei in rat (A), monkey (B) and human (C). Lateral nucleus is in red, basal nucleus in orange, paralaminar nucleus in dark orange (in monkeys only), accessory basal nucleus in blue, central nucleus in green, and medial nucleus in pink (not represented in humans). Scales: rat, grey cube is 1 mm^3; monkey, grey cube is 2 mm^3; human, grey cube is 4 mm^3. From Chareyron et al. *(2011); reproduced by permission from Wiley–Liss.*

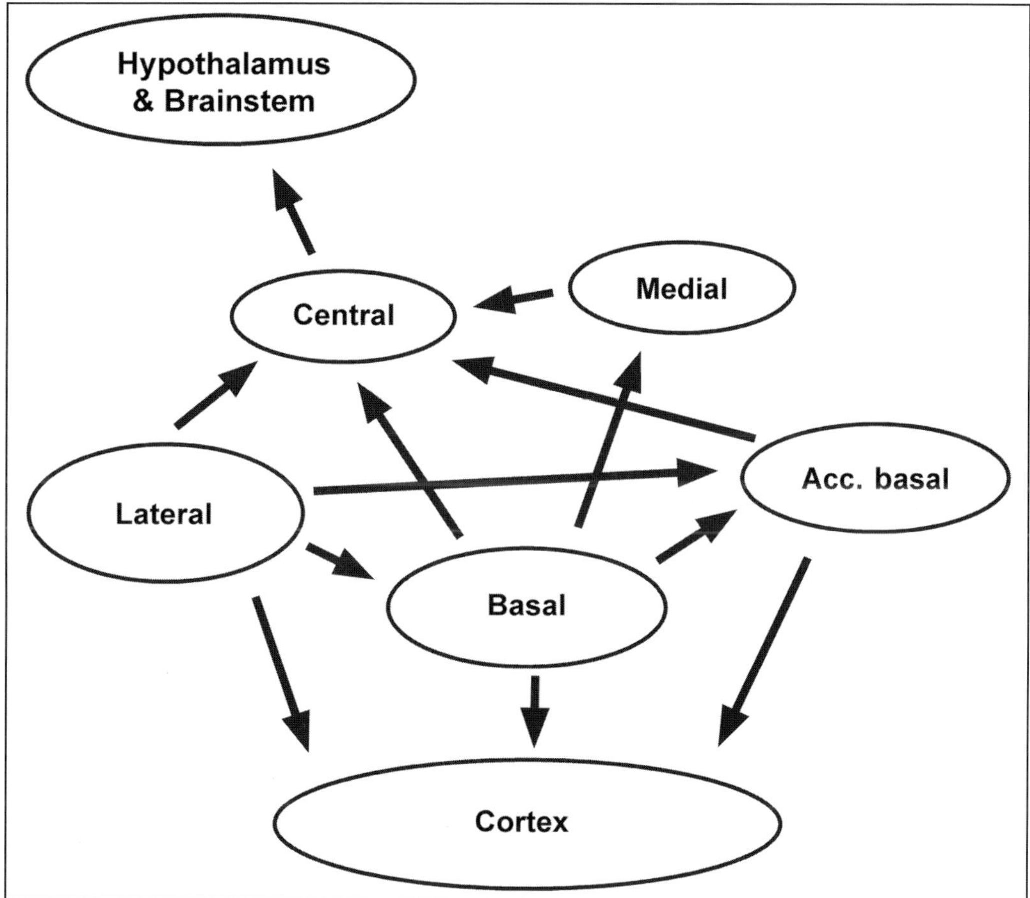

Fig. 9. Intrinsic connections of the amygdaloid complex. Connections are largely unidirectional. The lateral, basal, and accessory basal nuclei are highly interconnected with the neocortex and modulate cognitive processes; these nuclei also project toward the medial and central nuclei. Projections from the other amygdala nuclei converge onto the central nucleus, whose projections are mostly directed toward the hypothalamus and the brainstem and regulate the autonomic and visceral responses.

Fundamental functions

As briefly discussed in the introduction, the amygdala is fundamental for the regulation of fear and emotional behavior, whereas the hippocampal formation plays a fundamental role in memory processes. The literature on the functions of the amygdala is very extensive and a comprehensive review of this topic is beyond the scope of this chapter. Indeed, separate sets of studies have distinguished different functions assigned to the amygdala. Most work carried out in rodents associated amygdala function with the regulation of fear behavior (LeDoux, 2007). In contrast, work carried out in primates, including humans, considered the role of the amygdala in the regulation of social behavior (Adolphs, 2010). Interestingly, lesion studies in monkeys suggest that the amygdala is not an essential component of the neural network for social cognition (Amaral *et al.*, 2003). In addition, some studies evaluated amygdala function in relation to reward learning (Murray, 2007). All three approaches have provided significant information regarding the behaviors and psychological processes that are influenced by amygdala function. However, fear has been the behavior most consistently associated with the function of the amygdala (Amaral *et al.*, 2003; LeDoux, 2007). Consequently, the discussion below focuses on a limited number of studies carried out in monkeys, which considered the role of the amygdala in fear behavior in different contexts. In particular, a description of how lesions of the amygdala at different ages have a differential impact on the regulation of fear behavior will be made.

Since the description of the amnesic patient H.M. by Scoville and Milner (1957), the role of the hippocampus in memory processes has been clearly established (Milner *et al.*, 1998). The brain supports multiple memory systems, which are subserved by different neural systems (Fig. 10). Lesions of the hippocampus in adult humans generally impair both semantic (the memory for facts about the world) and episodic (the memory for autobiographical events) memory processes (Squire & Zola, 1996). It is also clear that, although the hippocampus plays a central role in declarative memory processes, other medial temporal lobe structures, including the entorhinal, perirhinal, and parahippocampal cortices, contribute actively to normal memory function. However, a comprehensive review of this topic is beyond the scope of this chapter. Consequently, only a limited number of studies carried out in monkeys will be discussed, which considered the role of the hippocampus in spatial relational memory, a fundamental component of episodic memory (Banta Lavenex & Lavenex, 2009, 2010). Specifically, it will be shown how selective lesions of the hippocampus at different ages have a differential impact on spatial, relational learning and memory.

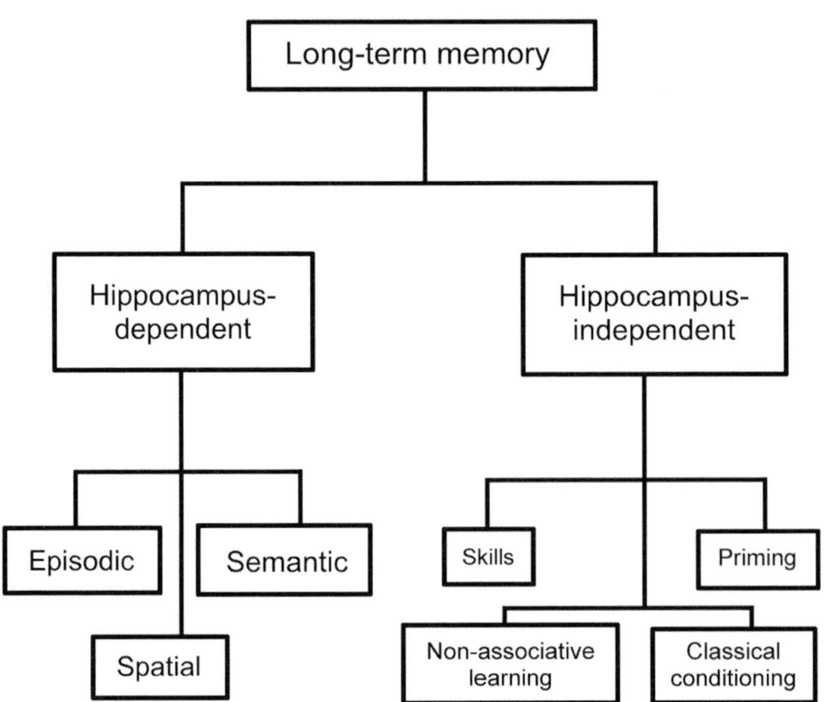

Fig. 10. Multiple memory systems. Long-term memory can be subdivided into different types of memories that are differentially sensitive to damage to the hippocampal formation. Allocentric or spatial relational memory is a fundamental component of episodic memory, memory that happened in a unique spatiotemporal context.

Differential effects of early *versus* late lesions

Brain plasticity after early injury is generally greater than after injury occurring in adulthood (Guzzetta *et al.*, 2010; Qi *et al.*, 2010; Rushmore *et al.*, 2008). However, the mechanisms underlying brain reorganization that might enable functional recovery after early injury are poorly understood (Kolb *et al.*, 2000; Thompson *et al.*, 2009). Moreover, it is also considered that different mechanisms might contribute to the recovery of function in distinct brain systems, which reflect differences in the normal maturation of these systems (Staudt, 2010). Here, two series of functional studies demonstrating, for both the amygdala and the hippocampus, that damage to these structures occurring either early in life or in adulthood has a differential impact on the functional processes that they normally subserve are discussed.

The amygdala

In a first study, Emery and colleagues (2001) evaluated the role of the amygdala in social behavior in adult rhesus monkeys (*Macaca mulatta*). Control monkeys and monkeys that underwent selective, bilateral lesioning of the amygdala in adulthood were evaluated in three different experiments testing dyadic social interactions. Across all experiments, the amygdalectomized monkeys exhibited increased social affiliation, decreased anxiety, and increased confidence compared with control monkeys, particularly during early encounters (Fig. 11A). Normal subjects also demonstrated increased social affiliation toward the amygdalectomized subjects. These results indicate that amygdala lesions in adult monkeys lead to a decrease in the species-normal reluctance to immediately engage a novel conspecific in social behavior. These findings were confirmed when these animals were tested in a larger group of familiar animals (Machado *et al.*, 2010). Monkeys interacted in four-member social groups over 32 test days. Amygdala-lesioned animals engaged in more affiliative social interactions with control group partners than did control animals. In the course of their interactions, amygdala-lesioned animals also displayed an earlier decrease in nervous and fearful personality qualities than controls. Findings from these two studies suggest that the amygdala plays a modulatory role in normal primate social behaviour, a role that is highly specialized for proper reactivity to threat as opposed to other facets of social behavior (Machado *et al.*, 2010).

Adult monkeys with selective, bilateral amygdala lesions were also compared with controls in several novel situations, including exposure to metal objects, toy animals and a person (Mason *et al.*, 2006). Early in testing, lesioned monkeys exhibited reduced inhibition of responsiveness (Fig. 11B). With continuing exposures, differences between groups diminished as inhibition waned in control monkeys. As the authors concluded, these findings were consistent with the idea that the amygdala mediates caution in initial reactions to ambiguous or threatening novel situations, which, in the absence of adverse consequences, diminishes with repetition. In sum, selective bilateral lesion of the amygdala in adult monkeys induces a decreased fear behavior in both social and nonsocial contexts. These findings are in agreement with the proposed role of the amygdala in the regulation of fear behavior (LeDoux, 2007).

Another set of studies evaluated the impact of neonatal damage to the amygdala on the development of social behavior. These studies were aimed at determining whether, while the amygdala is not necessary for generating social behavior, it might be essential for learning appropriate social behaviors. Monkeys that underwent selective bilateral amygdala lesion at two weeks of age were subsequently tested in response to the presentation of novel or fearful objects or

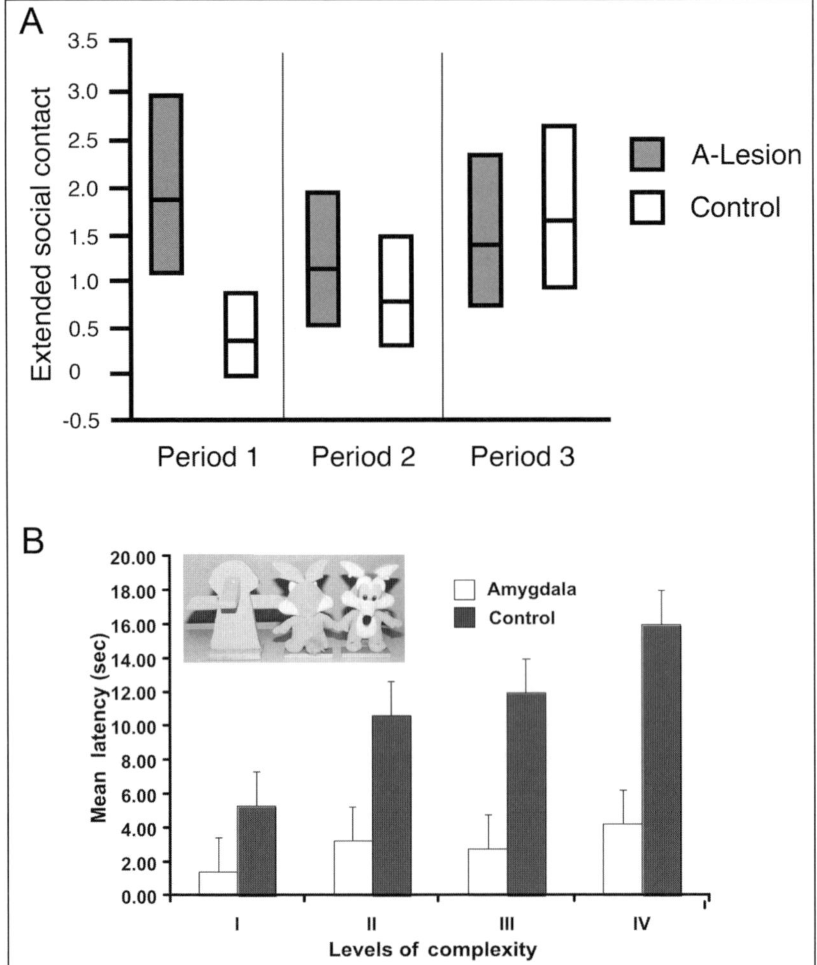

Fig. 11. Fear behaviour after selective amygdala lesioning in adult rhesus monkeys. (A) Social context: Amygdalectomized monkeys exhibited increased extended social interaction, especially during early encounters. From Emery et al. *(2001); reproduced by permission from the American Psychological Association. (B) Nonsocial context: lesioned monkeys exhibited reduced inhibition of responsiveness. See main text for details. From Mason* et al. *(2006); reproduced by permission from the American Psychological Association.*

during social encounters with conspecifics (Prather *et al.*, 2001). At six to eight months of age, amygdala-lesioned animals demonstrated less fear of novel objects, such as rubber snakes, than age-matched controls (Fig. 12a). However, they displayed substantially more fear behaviour than controls during dyadic social interactions (Fig. 12b). These results suggest that neonatal amygdala lesions dissociate a system that mediates social fear from one that mediates fear of inanimate objects (Prather *et al.*, 2001). Most interestingly, amygdala lesions early in development had a different effect on social behaviour than lesions produced in adulthood. These results were confirmed in a more comprehensive study (Bauman *et al.*, 2004), which revealed that neonatally-amygdala-lesioned subjects developed a species-typical repertoire of social behaviours. Similar to adult lesioned monkeys, they displayed more affiliative behaviours,

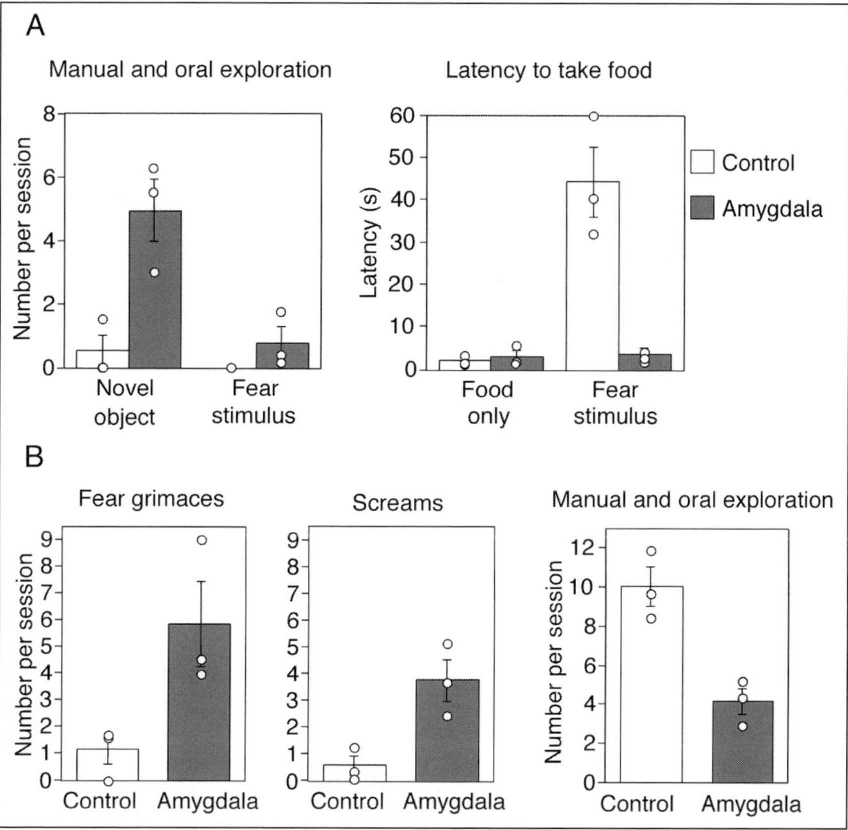

Fig. 12. Fear behaviour after selective amygdala lesioning in neonate rhesus monkeys. (A) Nonsocial context: Average number (per session) of manual and oral explorations of a novel object during trial 1 (neutral object only). Latency to take the food during 'food only' trials and during trials where food was placed adjacent to a fear stimulus on day 4 of responsiveness testing. (B) Social context: Average number (per session) of fear grimaces and screams produced during dyadic social interactions. Average number (per session) of manual and oral explorations of the cage and objects placed in the cage during dyadic social interactions. From Prather et al. *(2001); reproduced by permission from Elsevier.*

including follows, coos, and grunts during familiar and novel dyads (Fig. 13A). However, despite the development of a normal social repertoire, the neonatally-amygdala-lesioned subjects consistently produced more fear behaviors (*i.e.*, fear grimacing, fleeing, freezing, screaming) during social interactions than either control or hippocampus-lesioned subjects (Fig. 13B).

In sum, this series of studies in monkeys revealed that the amygdala is not directly involved in developing or expressing basic components of the social repertoire (Amaral *et al.*, 2003), but instead plays a central role in developing and expressing appropriate fear responses (LeDoux, 2007). As the amygdala is clearly a central component of the brain network involved in the regulation of fear, early lesion studies raise questions about the other brain regions that might be supporting the animals' fear response in the absence of a functioning amygdala. Brain regions that may not normally be involved in fear processing may assume this function after early amygdala damage. This questions remains to be investigated experimentally.

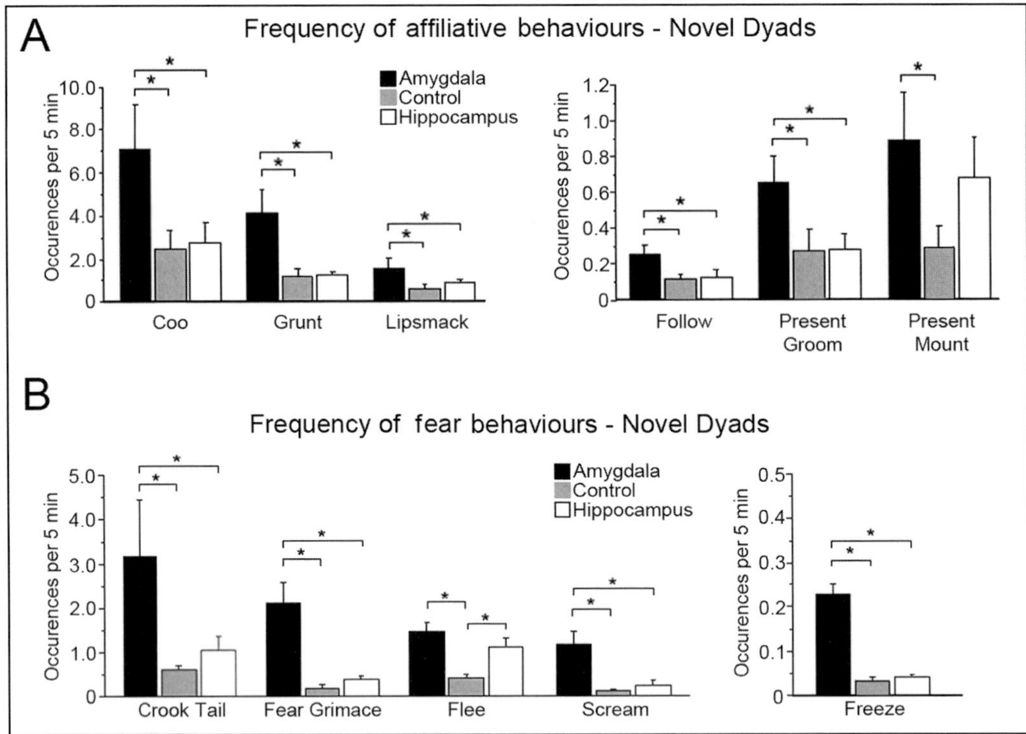

Fig. 13. Fear behaviour following selective amygdala lesioning in neonate rhesus monkeys. (A) Frequency of affiliative behaviours during encounters with novel partners. (B) Frequency of fear behaviours during encounters with novel partners. See main text for details. Modified from Bauman et al. *(2004) by permission from MIT Press Journals.*

The hippocampus

It is well established that lesions of the hippocampus in adult humans impair both semantic and episodic memory processes (Milner *et al.*, 1998). In contrast, patients who sustained hippocampal damage early in life exhibit memory impairments preferentially affecting episodic memory, whereas semantic memory is somehow preserved (Vargha-Khadem *et al.*, 1997). We have recently shown similar functional plasticity in monkeys that received hippocampal lesions early in life. Hippocampal lesions prevent spatial relational learning in adult-lesioned monkeys (Banta Lavenex *et al.*, 2006), whereas spatial relational learning persists following neonatal lesions (Lavenex *et al.*, 2007b).

In a first experiment (Banta Lavenex *et al.*, 2006), we evaluated the role of the monkey hippocampus in spatial relational learning and memory, a fundamental component of episodic memory (Banta Lavenex & Lavenex, 2010). Prior to that study, numerous studies in rodents had established the role of the hippocampus in spatial learning and memory (Morris *et al.*, 1982; Schenk *et al.*, 1995). In contrast, comparable studies in nonhuman primates were few and findings were often contradictory. This was likely attributable to the failure to distinguish between allocentric and egocentric spatial representations in experimental designs (see Banta Lavenex & Lavenex, 2009, for a detailed discussion). For this experiment, six adult monkeys received selective bilateral hippocampal lesions and six control subjects underwent sham surgery. Freely moving monkeys then foraged for food located in two arrays of three distinct locations among 18 locations distributed in an open-field arena (Fig. 14). Multiple goals and

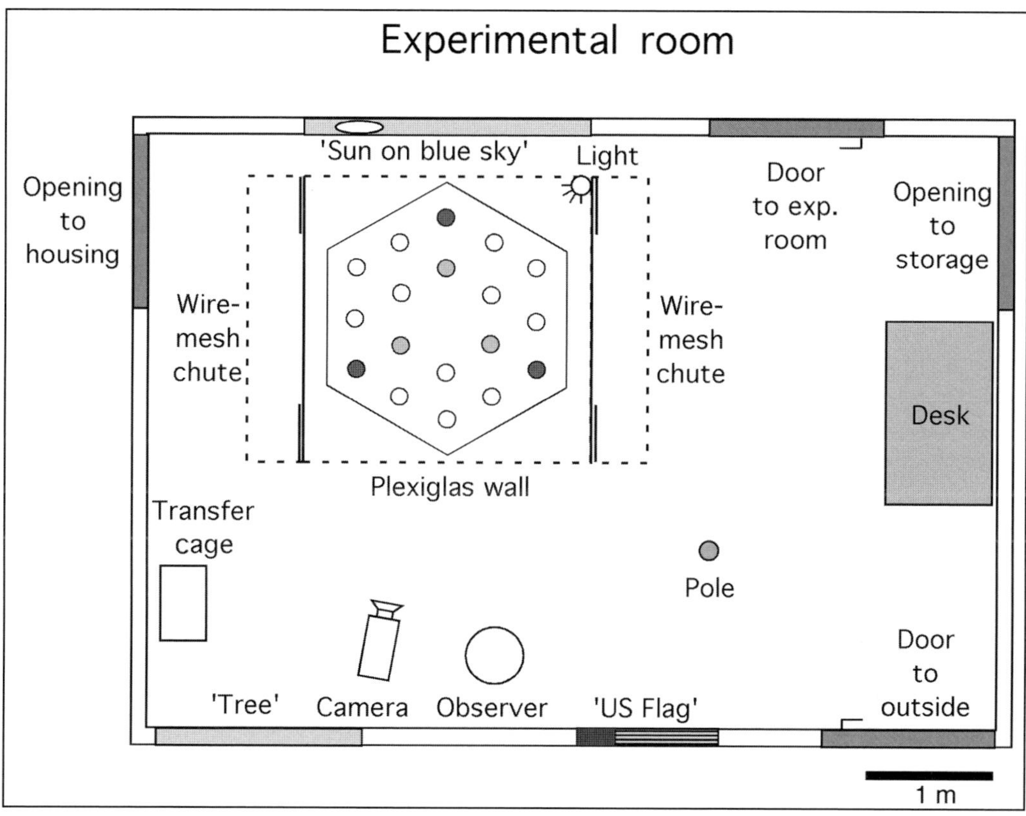

Fig. 14. Schematic representation of the testing environment and experimental conditions. Eighteen plastic cups were regularly distributed on a hexagonal board (210 cm in diameter) placed in a square testing arena (220 cm W × 220 cm D × 220 cm H). Remotely operated sliding doors at each corner of the arena (double solid lines) allowed the animals to go in and out of the area from wire-mesh chutes located along both sides. The front panel, the roof, and the top half of the back panel (dashed lines) were made of Plexiglas, allowing a clear view of distant environmental cues; two opaque side panels (solid lines) provided visual barriers between the open-field area and the wire-mesh holding chutes. The ability of monkeys to rely on an egocentric representation of space was precluded by alternating pseudorandomly between four different entrances into the open-field area and using multiple goal locations. From Banta Lavenex et al. *(2006); reproduced by permission from the Society for Neuroscience.*

four pseudorandomly chosen entrance points precluded the monkeys' ability to rely on an egocentric strategy to identify food locations. Monkeys were tested in two conditions. First, local visual cues marked the food locations. Second, no local cues marked the food locations, so that monkeys had to rely on an allocentric (spatial relational) representation of the environment to discriminate these locations. Both hippocampal-lesioned and control monkeys were able to determine the food locations in the presence of local cues (Fig. 15A). However, in the absence of local cues, control subjects could find the food locations, whereas hippocampal-lesioned monkeys were unable to do so (Fig. 15B). Most interestingly, histologic analysis of the brain of one control monkey whose behavior was identical to that of the experimentally lesioned animals revealed a bilateral ischaemic lesion restricted to the hippocampus (Fig. 16). The inclusion of this animal was fortuitous because extensive histologic analysis of its brain indicated that it had a circumscribed lesion of portions of the hippocampus bilaterally. The

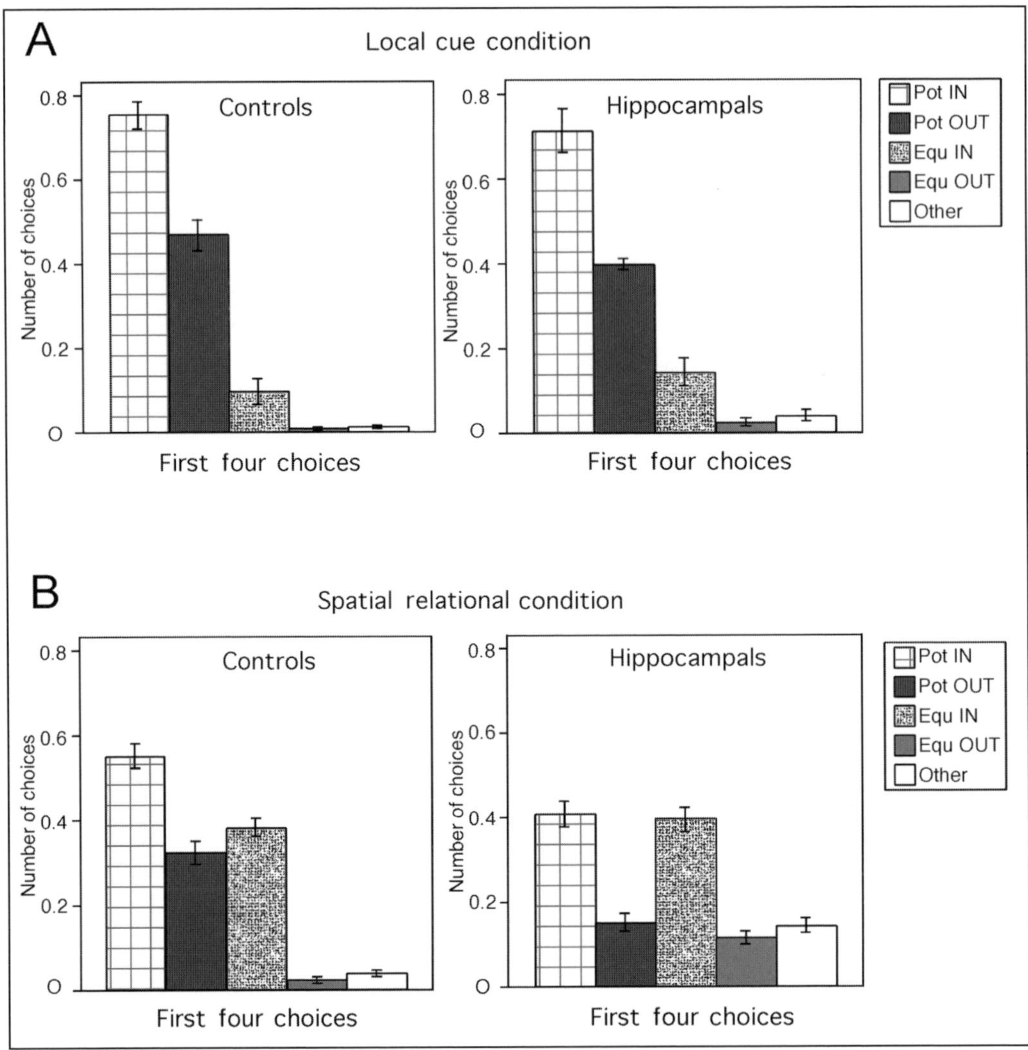

Fig. 15. (A) Hippocampal-lesioned and control monkeys' strategy in the local cue condition. Pot IN, potentially-baited locations at the corners of the inner hexagon; Pot OUT, potentially-baited locations at the corners of the outer hexagon; Equ IN, never-baited locations at the corners of the inner hexagon; Equ OUT, never-baited locations at the corners of the outer hexagon; Other, never-baited locations on the sides of the outer hexagon. The number of choices in each category (n) *is normalized according to the probability of making that choice* (n *of 3 for Pot IN, Pot OUT, Equ IN, and Equ OUT;* n *of 6 for Other). (B) Hippocampal-lesioned (A) and control (B) monkeys' strategy in the spatial relational condition. From Banta Lavenex* et al. *(2006); reproduced by permission from the Society for Neuroscience.*

cause of the lesion is unknown, and the animal had an unremarkable medical history. The location of the lesion in the CA fields is reminiscent of experimentally induced ischaemic lesions (Zola-Morgan *et al.*, 1992). Although the extent of the damage appears more restricted than in experimentally induced ischaemic lesions (*i.e.*, we did not observe a decrease in the volume of the CA fields and the lesion was undetectable with modern magnetic resonance imaging technology), we suspect that a hypoxic-ischaemic episode may have been the cause

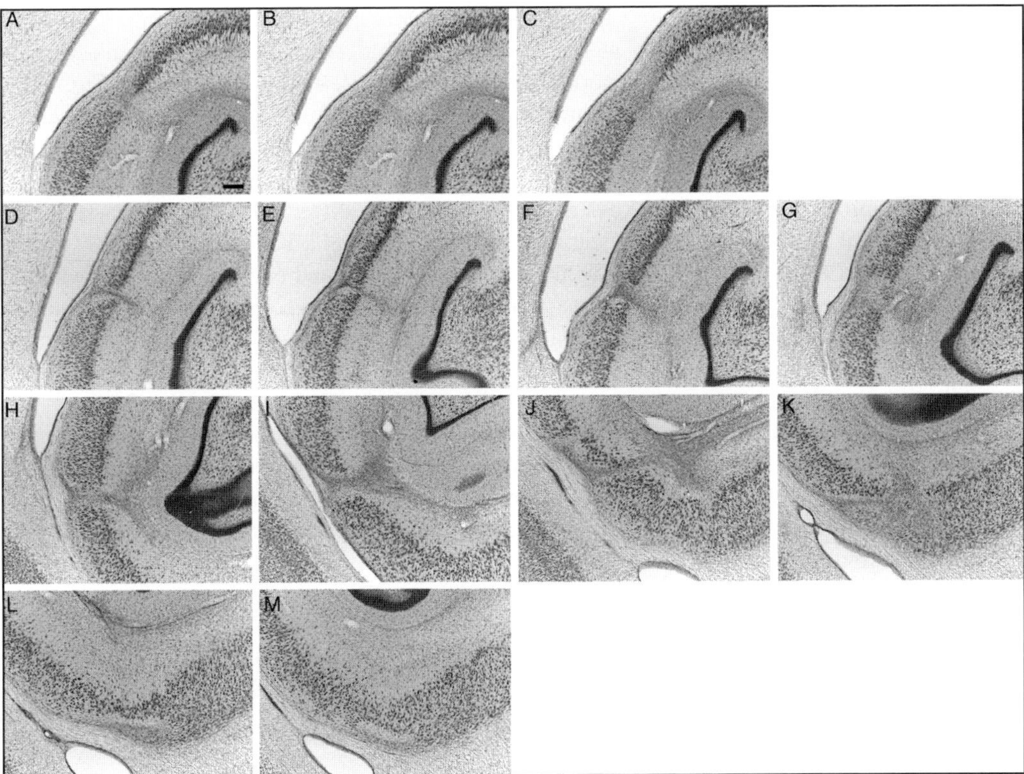

Fig. 16. Photomicrographs illustrating the extent of the lesioned area on the left side of the brain in the control monkey, whose behaviour was identical to that of experimentally lesioned monkeys. (A–C) Rostral area exhibiting neuronal damage, gliosis, and neuropil disorganization. (D–M) Caudal area exhibiting neuronal damage, gliosis, and neuropil disorganization. Individual panels represent adjacent sections separated by 240 μm. All Nissl-stained sections on which signs of damage were visible are presented. There was an area of about 1.44 mm between C and D, with no visible neuron loss, gliosis, or disorganization of the neuropil. Scale bar, 250 μm (applies to all panels). The area exhibiting cell loss extended for 21 per cent of the entire rostrocaudal extent of the left hippocampus. The lesion observed on the right side of the brain was similar, and extended for 31 per cent of the entire rostrocaudal extent of the right hippocampus. From Banta Lavenex et al. *(2006); reproduced by permission from the Society for Neuroscience.*

of the brain damage observed in this monkey. The finding that this animal was unable to discriminate the baited locations in the spatial relational condition supports the idea that damage entirely restricted to the CA fields of the hippocampus is sufficient to produce clinically significant memory impairments (Zola-Morgan *et al.*, 1986). In sum, these findings demonstrate that the adult monkey hippocampal formation is critical for the establishment or use of allocentric spatial representations and that selective damage of the hippocampus prevents spatial relational learning in adult nonhuman primates.

In a second experiment, we tested the ability of juvenile monkeys that received hippocampal lesions shortly after birth to learn new spatial relational information (Lavenex *et al.*, 2007b). Neonatally lesioned monkeys were tested in the same experimental design as the monkeys lesioned in adulthood. Consistent with the hyperactivity observed following bilateral hippocampal damage in rats, we found that neonatally lesioned monkeys were hyperactive compared with sham-operated control monkeys. During an acclimation phase, they 'locomoted' more than controls did; and during testing they generally opened more cups than control monkeys (Fig. 17A). However, in contrast to monkeys with adult hippocampal lesions, monkeys with neonatal hippocampal lesions showed normal spatial relational learning and memory (Fig. 17B). These findings suggest that early hippocampal damage leads to functional brain reorganization that enables spatial information to be acquired through the use of brain regions that normally do not subserve this function. The differential effect of early *versus* late hippocampal lesions on spatial relational learning in monkeys is reminiscent of the differential effect of early *versus* late hippocampal lesions on semantic learning in humans (Vargha-Khadem *et al.*, 1997). Hippocampal lesions in adult human subjects impair both semantic and episodic memory, whereas individuals with early hippocampal damage have deficits in episodic memory, but not in semantic memory. In humans, electrophysiologic evidence suggested that early hippocampal injury induces structural reorganization of interconnected brain regions, which might support learning and memory processes normally carried out by hippocampal circuits (Duzel *et al.*, 2001). We also hypothesized that, in monkeys, cortical regions normally specialized for the maintenance and retrieval of long-term spatial memory undergo functional reorganization to enable the acquisition of these memories following neonatal hippocampal damage. The plasticity mechanisms that support recovery of function following early but not late lesions are the subject of ongoing investigation in our laboratory. We hope to provide experimental answers to these questions in future editions of this series.

Genes, development, memory and pathology

Postnatal development of the hippocampus

Understanding the normal development of the hippocampal formation can provide invaluable information about its functions and its susceptibility to pathologies across the life span (Lavenex, 2012; Lavenex *et al.*, 2007a). In this section, recent studies on the normal postnatal development of the monkey hippocampus (Jabès *et al.*, 2010, 2011; Lavenex *et al.*, 2011) are described, which help to establish links between the maturation of distinct hippocampal circuits and the emergence of different 'hippocampus-dependent' memory processes.

Neurogenesis in the dentate gyrus

The dentate gyrus is one of only two regions of the mammalian brain where substantial neurogenesis occurs postnatally: rats (Altman & Das, 1965), monkeys (Rakic & Nowakowski, 1981), and humans (Eriksson *et al.*, 1998). We recently demonstrated that about 40 per cent of the total number of granule cells found in 5–10-year-old monkeys are added to the granule cell layer postnatally, with a peak (about 25 per cent) in the first 3 months after birth (Jabès *et al.*, 2010). We also found significant levels of cell proliferation, neurogenesis, and cell death in the context of an overall stable number of granule cells in mature monkeys (Fig. 18). Importantly, we established that the developmental period during which a significant number of neurons are added to the monkey granule cell layer is longer than previously thought. Indeed, although we observed a significant decrease in the rate of neuron addition at about 3 months of age, we calculated that about 3,100 neurons are added to the granule cell layer each day between 3 months and 1 year of age in monkeys. These data, which are derived from stereological counts of neurons in Nissl-stained preparations, are supported by immunohistochemical findings on cell proliferation, neurogenesis, and cell death (Jabès *et al.*, 2010). Indeed, the number of Ki-67-labeled cells decreased strongly between birth and 3 months of age, but

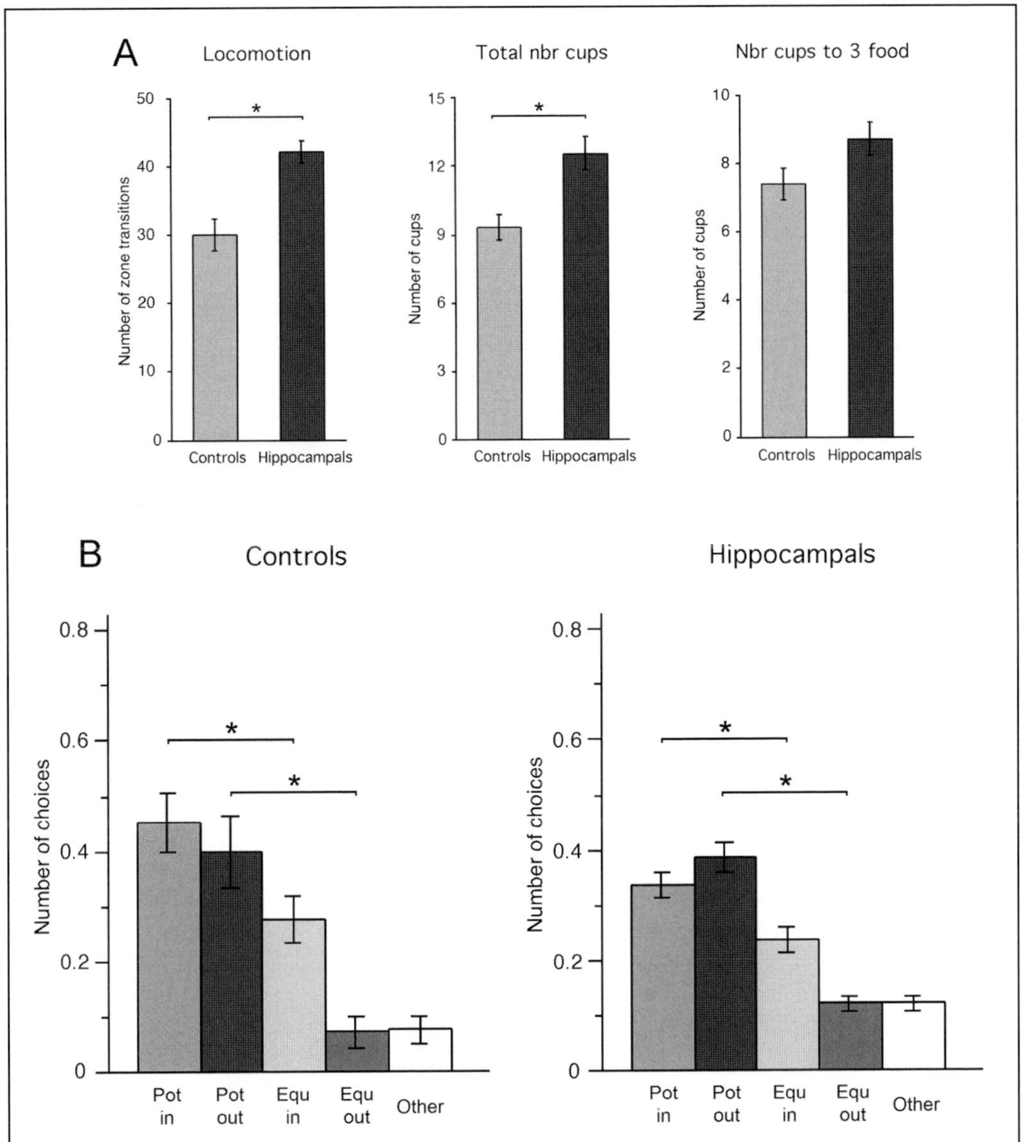

Fig. 17. (A) Indices of the overall activity level for sham-operated control and hippocampus-lesioned monkeys. (top) Number of zone transitions per session during 5-min acclimation sessions and number of cups opened per trial across the local cue and spatial relational conditions. Data are given as mean ± SEM. (B) Monkeys' first four choices during standard trials in the spatial relational condition. From Lavenex et al. *(2007); reproduced by permission from the Nature Publishing Group.*

remained at an intermediate level, which was ten times higher than that observed in mature monkeys, between 6 months and 1 year of age. The overall distribution of Ki-67-labeled cells that we described in newborn monkeys was similar to that observed in newborn humans (Seress, 2001). In humans, cell proliferation also seems to persist until at least the end of the first year after birth, the latest age examined immunohistochemically by Seress and colleagues (2001). In the absence of strict quantification of older human cases, our findings in monkeys suggest

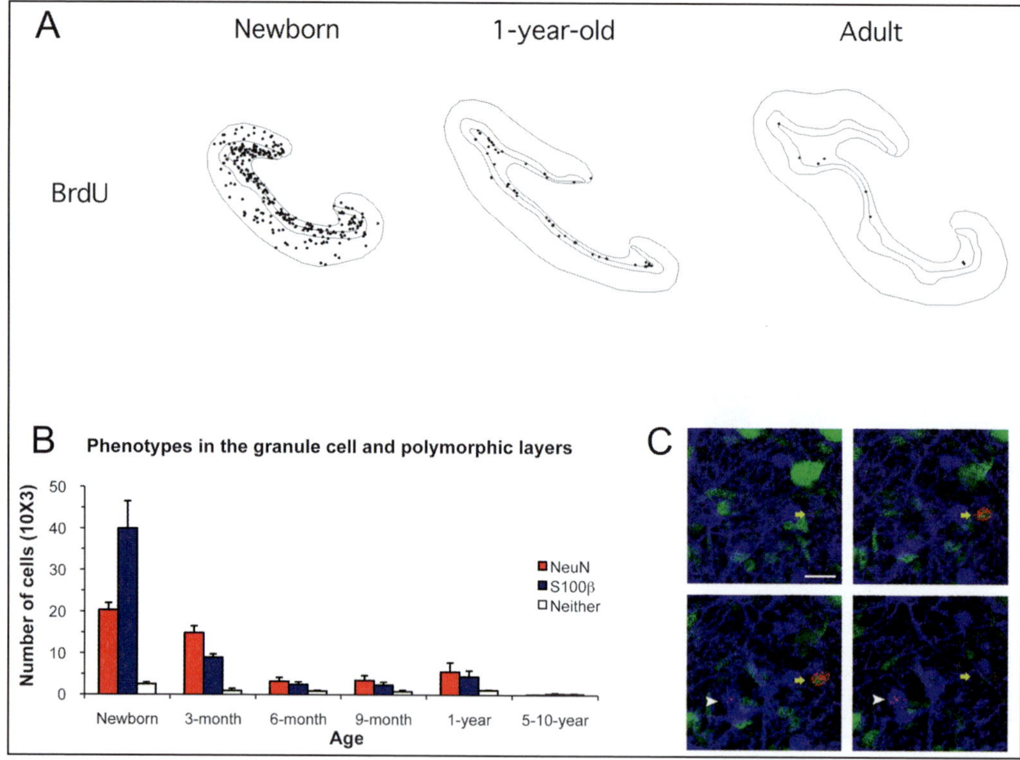

Fig. 18. Postnatal neurogenesis in the primate dentate gyrus. (A) Representative coronal sections through the monkey dentate gyrus illustrating the location of 5′-bromo-2-deoxyuridine (BrdU)–positive cells 4 weeks after BrdU injection, at different ages through postnatal life (newborns; 1-year-olds; 5–10-year-olds). (B) Phenotypes of BrdU-labeled cells in the monkey granule cell and polymorphic layers, 4 weeks following BrdU injection (150 mg/kg). (C) Confocal images of BrdU/NeuN-positive (yellow arrow) and BrdU/S100 beta-positive (white arrowheads) cells at the border between the granule cell and polymorphic layers. Scale bar: 10 μm (applies to all panels). From Jabès et al. *(2010); reproduced by permission from Blackwell.*

that sustained levels of developmental neurogenesis might continue and have an impact on the dentate gyrus structure until about 4 years of age in humans. Importantly, we also estimated the number of new neurons that could potentially be integrated into the granule cell layer of mature monkeys to be about 1,300 per day or 0.02 per cent of total neuron number (7.21 million). This daily rate of adult neurogenesis is about ten times lower, in percentage of total neuron number, than that reported for 9–10-week-old rats, where 2,250 new neurons are generated per day or 0.2 per cent of total neuron number [1.2 million (Cameron & McKay, 2001)]. However, considering that monkeys live 20–30 years and rats 2–3 years (Havenaar *et al.*, 1993), postnatal neurogenesis has a similar potential in rats and monkeys: that is the renewal of the entire population of granule cells during an individual's lifetime. It is therefore likely to be the case in humans as well.

Maturation of distinct hippocampal circuits

The protracted period of neuron addition in the dentate gyrus described above is accompanied by a concomitant late maturation of the granule cell population and individual dentate gyrus layers that extend beyond the first year of life (Fig. 19A) (Jabès *et al.*, 2010, 2011). Together with the late maturation of the granule cells, it has been reported that the mossy cells, the major targets of the granule cell projections in the polymorphic layer, exhibit clear morphologic changes in soma and dendritic structure until at least nine 9 months of age in monkeys (qualitative data: Seress & Ribak, 1995a) and at least 30 months of age in humans (qualitative data: Seress & Mrzljak, 1992). Our analyses revealed a 25 per cent increase in volume of the polymorphic layer between 1 year and 5–9 years of age. Although the mossy cells and the axons of granule cells represent a major component of the polymorphic layer, there are a variety of other neuronal types and afferent projections targeting this area (Amaral & Lavenex, 2007; Amaral *et al.*, 2007; Lavenex, 2012). Thus, although the postnatal development of the polymorphic layer circuits is likely delayed, as compared to that of the dentate gyrus afferents reaching the molecular layer, detailed analyses of the postnatal maturation of the different cell types contained in the dentate gyrus will be necessary to provide a definite answer regarding the functional consequences of this delayed maturation.

Although the development of CA3 generally parallels that of the dentate gyrus, the distal portion of CA3, which receives direct entorhinal cortex projections, matures earlier than the proximal portion of CA3 (Fig. 19B). At the cellular level, we found that the proximal CA3 pyramidal neurons exhibit significant changes in soma size within the first 3 to 6 postnatal months (Jabès *et al.*, 2011). In contrast, the size of distal CA3 pyramidal neurons does not vary during postnatal development. Our quantitative data are thus in agreement with the qualitative report by Seress

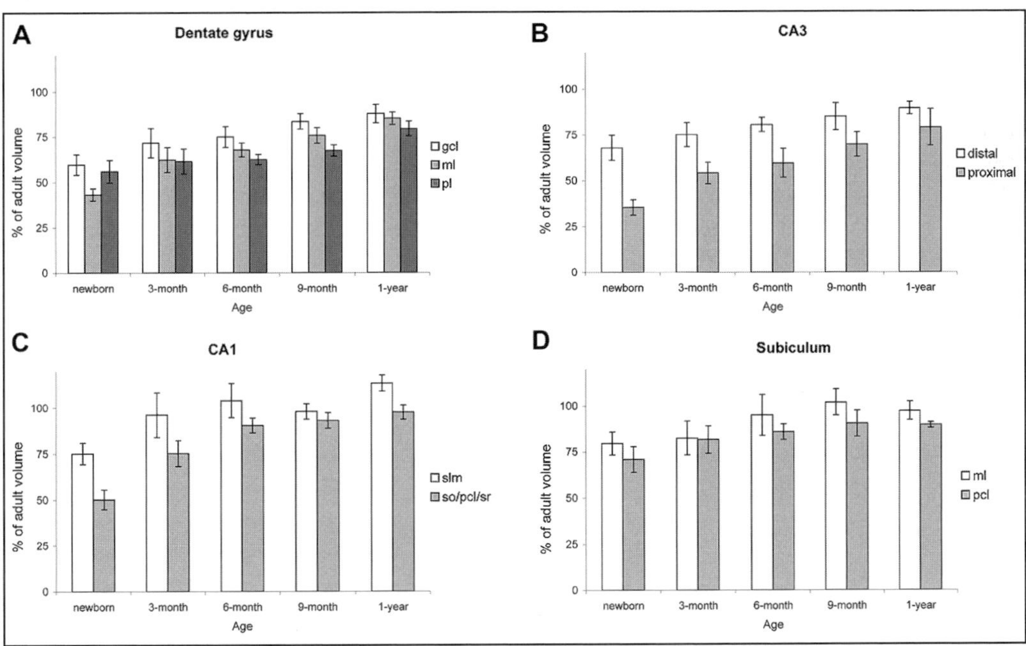

Fig. 19. Volumes of individual layers/regions of the monkey hippocampal formation at different ages during early postnatal development (expressed as percentage of the volume of the layer/region observed in 5–9-year-old monkeys: average ± standard error of the mean). (A) Dentate gyrus: granule cell layer (gcl), molecular layer (ml), polymorphic layer (pl). (B) CA3: proximal and distal portions. (C) CA1: strata oriens, pyramidale and radiatum (so/pcl/sr), stratum lacunosum-moleculare (slm). (D) Subiculum: stratum pyramidale (pcl), stratum moleculare (ml). From Jabès et al. *(2011); reproduced by permission from Wiley–Liss.*

and Ribak (1995b) showing that the somas and dendrites of distal CA3 pyramidal neurons exhibit adult-like ultrastructural features at birth. There is, unfortunately, no published information on the ultrastructural characteristics of developing proximal CA3 pyramidal neurons.

CA1 matures relatively earlier than the dentate gyrus and CA3, despite the fact that CA3 pyramidal neurons contribute the largest projection to CA1 pyramidal neurons (Lavenex, 2012). Interestingly, the CA1 stratum lacunosum-moleculare, in which direct entorhinal cortex projections terminate, matures earlier than CA1 strata oriens, pyramidale, and radiatum, in which the CA3 projections terminate (Fig. 19C). Our quantitative measurements are in agreement with recent qualitative reports of a later myelination of fibers in strata pyramidale and radiatum, as compared to stratum lacunosum-moleculare, in CA1 of humans (Abraham *et al.*, 2010).

The subiculum develops earlier than does the dentate gyrus, CA3 and CA1, but not CA2. However, similar to CA1, the molecular layer of the subiculum, in which the entorhinal cortex projections terminate, is overall more mature in the first postnatal year, as compared to the stratum pyramidale in which most of the CA1 projections terminate (Fig. 19D). Unlike other hippocampal fields, volumetric measurements suggest regressive events in the structural maturation of presubicular neurons and circuits. Finally, areal and neuron soma size measurements reveal an early maturation of the parasubiculum. Two unique features of these structures, as compared to other hippocampal regions, are their reciprocal connections with the anterior thalamic nuclear complex and their heavy cholinergic innervation. Accordingly, cell circuits in the presubiculum and parasubiculum might contribute to some of the earliest functions subserved by the hippocampal formation (Jabès *et al.*, 2011).

In sum, the protracted period of neuronal addition and maturation in the dentate gyrus is accompanied by the late maturation of specific layers in distinct hippocampal regions that are located downstream from the dentate gyrus within the hippocampal loop of information processing. This suggests that the developmental regulation of neurogenesis might be a limiting factor in the maturation of defined hippocampal circuits and specific memory functions. In contrast, the early maturation of defined layers in distinct hippocampal regions, which receive direct projections from the entorhinal cortex, suggests that specific circuits and certain 'hippocampus-dependent' memory functions might appear earlier than others during postnatal development. The early structural development of the subiculum, presubiculum, and parasubiculum might contribute to the early functional maturation of 'head-direction cells' and 'place cells' found in these structures (Langston *et al.*, 2010; O'Keefe, 2007). Together with their reciprocal connections with the anterior thalamic nuclear complex and their direct inputs from the retrosplenial cortex, early maturation of neurons of the subicular complex might contribute to the early emergence of one type of 'hippocampus-dependent' spatial memory system, dead reckoning. The subsequent maturation of direct inputs from the entorhinal cortex to CA1 might enable the elaboration of a basic allocentric, spatial relational representation of the environment. Indeed, we have previously shown that spatial relational memory processes are present in 9-month-old monkeys (Lavenex & Banta Lavenex, 2006), an age at which some functional circuits within CA1, but not CA3 or the dentate gyrus, might already be mature. Finally, episodic memory might be one of the last types of 'hippocampus-dependent' memory processes to emerge around 3–5 years of age in humans (Rubin, 2000). The prolonged period of developmental neurogenesis, granule cell addition, and a further protracted maturation of distinct dentate gyrus circuits beyond one year of age in monkeys might explain the inability to form enduring episodic memories until the dentate gyrus has become fully structurally mature. A more detailed discussion of the implications of these findings with respect to the role of the hippocampal formation in memory can be found in Jabès *et al.* (2011).

Molecular analyses

In an effort to understand the molecular basis of the normal development of the hippocampal formation and its susceptibility to a number of different pathologies, we recently launched a series of experiments examining the regulation of gene expression in distinct regions of the monkey hippocampal formation during postnatal development. In a first study (Lavenex *et al.*, 2011), we characterized the molecular signature of individual hippocampal regions in an attempt to understand the paradox that, although the hippocampus plays a central role in the brain network essential for memory function (Banta Lavenex *et al.*, 2006; Morris, 2007), it is also the brain structure that is most sensitive to hypoxic-ischaemic episodes (Banta Lavenex *et al.*, 2006; Nedergaard & Dirnagl, 2005; Sommer, 1880; Spielmeyer, 1925; Zola-Morgan *et al.*, 1986). We found that the expression of genes associated with glycolysis and glutamate metabolism in astrocytes, and the coverage of excitatory synapses by astrocytic processes, undergo significant decreases in the CA1 field of the monkey hippocampus during postnatal development (Fig. 20). Our findings at the gene, protein, and structural levels therefore suggest that the developmental decrease in astrocytic processes and functions may be the critical factor underlying the selective vulnerability of CA1 to hypoxic-ischaemic episodes in adulthood. They also provide an explanation for the relative resistance of this brain structure to hypoxia in the perinatal period, and, in particular, during the birth process. Indeed, hypoxia reduces glycolysis, which in turn leads to a decrease in ATP (Pellerin & Magistretti, 1994). As a consequence, the sodium–potassium gradient necessary for the co-transport of glutamate from the synaptic cleft into astrocytes dissipates. This reduces glutamate clearance from the synapse, increasing neuronal depolarization and the potential for neuronal death via excitotoxicity (Swanson, 2005). High astrocytic coverage, as we have shown in the newborn, likely maintains sufficient glutamate reuptake to limit neuronal depolarization and excitotoxicity during mild to moderate hypoxic-ischaemic events. In the adult, however, a lower expression level of genes associated with glycolysis or glutamate uptake and metabolism (Rao *et al.*, 2001), as well as a lower astrocytic coverage of excitatory synapses in CA1, render the system more vulnerable to a reduction in oxygen concentration.

In contrast, a major benefit that derives from decreased astrocytic coverage is the regulation of synaptic efficacy, leading to an increase in synaptic selectivity advantageous for learning (Karlsson & Frank, 2008). Indeed, reduction of glutamate clearance associated with a relative decrease in astrocytic processes in the vicinity of synapses can affect transmitter release through modulation of presynaptic metabotropic glutamate receptors (Oliet *et al.*, 2001). Reduced glutamate clearance results in increased glutamate concentration in the extracellular space (Bergles & Jahr, 1998; Tanaka *et al.*, 1997), which in turn increases the activation of presynaptic metabotropic glutamate receptors (Scanziani *et al.*, 1997), thus leading to a lower probability of glutamate release by the presynaptic terminal (Oliet *et al.*, 2001). Presynaptic inhibition can be overcome by high-frequency bursts of afferent synaptic potentials (Grover *et al.*, 2009), thus serving as a high-pass filter increasing the signal-to-noise ratio for information transmitted through these synapses (Oliet *et al.*, 2001). Thus, the decreased astrocytic coverage of excitatory synapses in the adult CA1 could serve to ensure that only the most salient information generates synaptic activity in the hippocampal circuits that contribute to learning and memory processes. A developmental decrease of astrocytic processes and functions may therefore contribute to the emergence of adult-like, selective memory function.

Finally, the relatively high astrocytic coverage of the neonatal synapses might also play a central role in the generation of febrile seizures. The highest incidence of seizures is in the first year of life in humans and is most often associated with a febrile illness (Hauser, 1994).

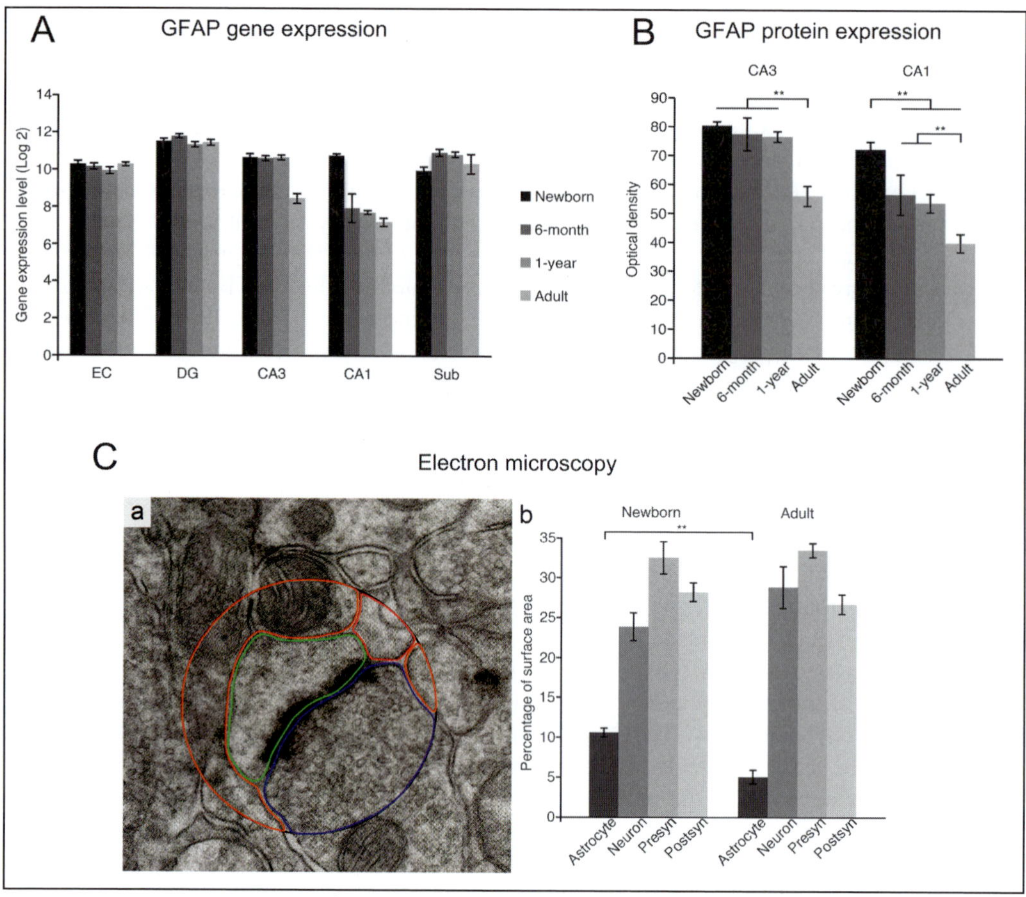

Fig. 20. (A) Microarray analysis of GFAP gene expression in the postnatally developing monkey hippocampal formation. (B) Immunohistochemical analysis of GFAP protein expression. (C) Electron microscopy evaluation of astrocytic processes around excitatory synapses in the stratum radiatum of CA1. (a) Blue outline, presynaptic neuronal element; green outline, postsynaptic neuronal element; orange outline, nonsynaptic neuronal elements; red outline, astrocytic elements; circle diameter, 1,000 nm. (b) The surface area occupied by astrocytic processes decreased between birth and adulthood. Modified from Lavenex et al. *(2011), with permission from Wiley–Liss.*

Fever begins with the activation of immune response cells that produce interleukin-1, which in turn increases prostaglandin E2 synthesis (Biddle, 2006). Prostaglandins act at the level of the hypothalamus to regulate body temperature and induce fever. Interestingly, prostaglandins also stimulate calcium-dependent glutamate release in astrocytes (Bezzi *et al.*, 1998; Volterra & Meldolesi, 2005), which can induce abnormal prolonged depolarization with repetitive spiking in CA1 pyramidal neurons leading to seizures (Kang *et al.*, 2005; Tian *et al.*, 2005). Thus, the relatively high astrocytic coverage of the dense network of CA1 excitatory synapses in the newborn (twice that of the adult) could explain why infants exhibit a higher incidence of febrile seizures. Conversely, the decrease in the astrocytic coverage of hippocampal excitatory synapses with development might provide the cellular basis for the decreased susceptibility to febrile seizures with age.

Conclusions

The hippocampus and the amygdala are two distinct brain structures located in the human medial temporal lobe. Functionally, the amygdala is fundamental for the regulation of fear and emotional behavior, whereas the hippocampal formation plays a fundamental role in memory processes. Of particular interest in the context of this book, damage to these structures occurring either early in life or in adulthood has a differential impact on the functional processes that these structures normally subserve. Selective bilateral lesioning of the amygdala in adult monkeys induces a decreased fear behavior in both social and nonsocial contexts, whereas neonatal amygdala lesions dissociate a system that mediates social fear from one that mediates fear of inanimate objects. Similarly, hippocampal lesions prevent spatial relational learning in adult lesioned monkeys, whereas spatial relational learning persists after neonatal lesions. Both sets of functional studies raise questions about the plasticity mechanisms that support recovery of function after early but not late lesions, which we will address in future experimental studies in animals. Finally, a discussion of recent studies on the normal postnatal development of the monkey hippocampal formation showed that understanding its normal development can provide invaluable information about its functions and its susceptibility to pathologic events across the human life span.

Acknowledgments: This work was supported by grants from the Swiss National Science Foundation (PP00A-106701, PP00P3-124536) and the National Alliance for Research on Schizophrenia and Depression (NARSAD).

References

Abraham, H., Vincze, A., Jewgenow, I., Veszpremi, B., Kravjak, A., Gomori, E. & Seress, L. (2010): Myelination in the human hippocampal formation from midgestation to adulthood. *Int. J. Dev. Neurosci.* **28,** 401–410.

Adolphs, R. (2010): What does the amygdala contribute to social cognition? *Ann. N.Y. Acad. Sci.* **1191,** 42–61.

Aggleton, J.P. (2010): Understanding retrosplenial amnesia: insights from animal studies. *Neuropsychologia* **48,** 2328–2338.

Altman, J. & Das, G.D. (1965): Autoradiographic and histological evidence of postnatal hippocampal neurogenesis in rats. *J. Comp. Neurol.* **124,** 319–336.

Amaral, D.G. & Lavenex, P. (2007): Hippocampal neuroanatomy. In: *The Hippocampus Book.* Oxford: Oxford University Press.

Amaral, D.G., Bauman, M.D., Capitanio, J.P., Lavenex, P., Mason, W.A., Mauldin-Jourdain, M.L. & Mendoza, S.P. (2003): The amygdala: is it an essential component of the neural network for social cognition? *Neuropsychologia* **41,** 517–522.

Amaral, D.G., Scharfman, H.E. & Lavenex, P. (2007): The dentate gyrus: fundamental neuroanatomical organization (dentate gyrus for dummies). *Prog. Brain Res.* **163,** 3–22.

Andersen, P., Morris, R.G., Amaral, D.G., Bliss, T. & O'Keefe, J. (2007): Historical perspective: proposed functions, biological characteristics, and neurobiological moels of the hippocampus. In: *The Hippocampus Book,* eds. P. Andersen, R.G.M. Morris, D.G. Amaral, *et al.* Oxford: Oxford University Press.

Banta Lavenex, P. & Lavenex, P. (2009): Spatial memory and the monkey hippocampus: not all space is created equal. *Hippocampus* **19,** 8–19.

Banta Lavenex, P. & Lavenex, P. (2010): Spatial relational learning and memory abilities do not differ between men and women in a real-world, open-field environment. *Behav. Brain Res.* **207,** 125–137.

Banta Lavenex, P., Amaral, D.G. & Lavenex, P. (2006): Hippocampal lesion prevents spatial relational learning in adult macaque monkeys. *J. Neurosci.* **26,** 4546–4558.

Bauman, M.D., Lavenex, P., Mason, W.A., Capitanio, J.P. & Amaral, D.G. (2004): The development of social behavior following neonatal amygdala lesions in rhesus monkeys. *J. Cogn. Neurosci.* **16,** 1388–1411.

Bergles, D.E. & Jahr, C.E. (1998): Glial contribution to glutamate uptake at Schaffer collateral-commissural synapses in the hippocampus. *J. Neurosci.* **18,** 7709–7716.

Bezzi, P., Carmignoto, G., Pasti, L., Vesce, S., Rossi, D., Rizzini, B.L., *et al.* (1998): Prostaglandins stimulate calcium-dependent glutamate release in astrocytes. *Nature* **391,** 281–285.

Biddle, C. (2006): The neurobiology of the human febrile response. *AANA J.* **74,** 145–150.

Broca, P. (1877): Sur la circonvolution limbique et la scissure limbique. *Bull. Soc. Anthropol. (Paris)* **12,** 646–657.

Broca, P. (1878): Étude sur le cerveau du gorille. *Rev. Anthropol.* **1,** 1–46.

Brodal, A. (1982): *Neurological Anatomy.* New York: Oxford University Press.

Cameron, H.A. & McKay, R.D.G. (2001): Adult neurogenesis produces a large pool of new granule cells in the dentate gyrus. *J. Comp. Neurol.* **435,** 406–417.

Chareyron, L.J. (2011): Stereological analysis of the rat and monkey amygdala. *J. Comp. Neurol.* May 25. doi: 10.1002/cne.22677.

Duzel, E., Vargha-Khadem, F., Heinze, H.J. & Mishkin, M. (2001): Brain activity evidence for recognition without recollection after early hippocampal damage. *Proc. Natl. Acad. Sci. USA* **98,** 8101–8106.

Emery, N.J., Capitanio, J.P., Mason, W.A., Machado, C.J., Mendoza, S.P. & Amaral, D.G. (2001): The effects of bilateral lesions of the amygdala on dyadic social interactions in rhesus monkeys (*Macaca mulatta*). *Behav. Neurosci.* **115,** 515–544.

Eriksson, P.S., Perfilieva, E., Bjork-Eriksson, T., Alborn, A.M., Nordborg, C., Peterson, D.A. & Gage, F.H. (1998): Neurogenesis in the adult human hippocampus. *Nature Med.* **4,** 1313–1317.

Freese, J.L. & Amaral, D.G. (2009): Neuroanatomy of the primate amygdala. In: *The Human Amygdala,* eds. P.J. Whalen & E.A. Phelps, E. A. New York: Guilford Press.

Grover, L.M., Kim, E., Cooke, J.D. & Holmes, W.R. (2009): LTP in hippocampal area CA1 is induced by burst stimulation over a broad frequency range centered around delta. *Learn. Mem.* **16,** 69–81.

Guzzetta, A., D'acunto, G., Rose, S., Tinelli, F., Boyd, R. & Cioni, G. (2010): Plasticity of the visual system after early brain damage. *Dev. Med. Child Neurol.* **52,** 891–900.

Hauser, W.A. (1994): The prevalence and incidence of convulsive disorders in children. *Epilepsia* 35, S1–S6.

Havenaar, R., Meijer, J.C., Morton, D.B., Ritskes-Hoitinga, J. & Zwart, P. (1993): Biology and husbandry of laboratory animals. In: *Principles of Laboratory Animal Science,* eds. L.F.M. Zutphen, V. Baumans & A.C. Beynen. Amsterdam: Elsevier Science.

Insausti, R. & Munoz, M. (2001): Cortical projections of the non-entorhinal hippocampal formation in the cynomolgus monkey (*Macaca fascicularis*). *Eur. J. Neurosci.* **14,** 435–451.

Insausti, R. & Amaral, D.G. (2008): Entorhinal cortex of the monkey: IV. Topographical and laminar organization of cortical afferents. *J. Comp. Neurol.* **509,** 608–641.

Insausti, R., Amaral, D.G. & Cowan, W.M. (1987): The entorhinal cortex of the monkey: II. Cortical afferents. *J. Comp. Neurol.* **264,** 356–395.

Insausti, R., Tunon, T., Sobreviela, T., Insausti, A.M. & Gonzalo, L.M. (1995): The human entorhinal cortex: a cytoarchitectonic analysis. *J. Comp. Neurol.* **355,** 171–198.

Jabès, A., Lavenex, P.B., Amaral, D.G. & Lavenex, P. (2010): Quantitative analysis of postnatal neurogenesis and neuron number in the macaque monkey dentate gyrus. *Eur. J. Neurosci.* **31,** 273–285.

Jabès, A., Lavenex, P.B., Amaral, D.G. & Lavenex, P. (2011): Postnatal development of the hippocampal formation: a stereological study in macaque monkeys. *J. Comp. Neurol.* **519,** 1051–1070.

Kang, N., Xu, J., Xu, Q., Nedergaard, M. & Kang, J. (2005): Astrocytic glutamate release-induced transient depolarization and epileptiform discharges in hippocampal CA1 pyramidal neurons. *J. Neurophysiol.* **94,** 4121–4130.

Karlsson, M.P. & Frank, L.M. (2008): Network dynamics underlying the formation of sparse, informative representations in the hippocampus. *J. Neurosci.* **28,** 14271–14281.

Kobayashi, Y. & Amaral, D.G. (2003): Macaque monkey retrosplenial cortex: II. Cortical afferents. *J. Comp. Neurol.* **466,** 48–79.

Kobayashi, Y. & Amaral, D.G. (2007): Macaque monkey retrosplenial cortex: III. Cortical efferents. *J. Comp. Neurol.* **502,** 810–833.

Kolb, B., Gibb, R. & Gorny, G. (2000): Cortical plasticity and the development of behavior after early frontal cortical injury. *Dev. Neuropsychol.* **18,** 423–444.

Kotter, R. & Meyer, N. (1992): The limbic system: a review of its empirical foundation. *Behav. Brain Res.* **52,** 105–127.

Langston, R.F., Ainge, J.A., Couey, J.J., Canto, C.B., Bjerknes, T.L., Witter, M.P., *et al.* (2010): Development of the spatial representation system in the rat. *Science* **328,** 1576–1580.

Lavenex, P. (2012): Functional anatomy, development and pathology of the hippocampus. In: *Clinical Neurobiology of the Hippocampus,* ed. T. Bartsch. Oxford: Oxford University Press.

Lavenex, P. & Amaral, D.G. (2000): Hippocampal-neocortical interaction: a hierarchy of associativity. *Hippocampus* **10,** 420–430.

Lavenex, P. & Banta Lavenex, P. (2006): Spatial relational memory in 9-month-old macaque monkeys. *Learn. Mem.* **13,** 84–96.

Lavenex, P., Suzuki W.A. & Amaral, D.G. (2002): Perirhinal and parahippocampal cortices of the macaque monkey: projections to the neocortex. *J. Comp. Neurol.* **447,** 394–420.

Lavenex, P., Banta Lavenex, P. & Amaral, D.G. (2007a): Postnatal development of the primate hippocampal formation. *Dev. Neurosci.***29,** 179–192.

Lavenex, P., Banta Lavenex, P. & Amaral, D.G. (2007b): Spatial relational learning persists following neonatal hippocampal lesions in macaque monkeys. *Nat. Neurosci.* **10,** 234–239.

Lavenex, P., Sugden, S.G., Davis, R.R., Gregg, J.P. & Banta Lavenex, P. (2011): Developmental regulation of gene expression and astrocytic processes may explain selective hippocampal vulnerability. *Hippocampus* **21,** 142–149.

LeDoux, J.E. (1987): Emotion. In: *Handbook of Physiology. 1: The Nervous System.* ed. F. Plum. Bethesda, MD: American Physiological Society.

LeDoux, J.E. (1991): Emotion and the limbic system concept. *Concepts Neurosci.* **2,** 169–199.

LeDoux, J.E. (2000): Emotion circuits in the brain. *Annu. Rev. Neurosci.* **23,** 155–184.

LeDoux, J.E. (2007): The amygdala. *Curr. Biol.* **17,** R868–R874.

Machado, C.J., Emery, N.J., Mason, W.A. & Amaral, D.G. (2010): Selective changes in foraging behavior following bilateral neurotoxic amygdala lesions in rhesus monkeys. *Behav. Neurosci.* **124,** 761–72.

MacLean, P.D. (1952): Some psychiatric implications of physiological studies on frontotemporal portion of limbic system (visceral brain). *Electroencephalogr. Clin. Neurophysiol.* **4,** 407–418.

Mason, W.A., Capitanio, J.P., Machado, C.J., Mendoza, S.P. & Amaral, D.G. (2006): Amygdalectomy and responsiveness to novelty in rhesus monkeys (*Macaca mulatta*): generality and individual consistency of effects. *Emotion* **6,** 73–81.

Milner, B., Squire, L.R. & Kandel, E.R. (1998): Cognitive neuroscience and the study of memory. *Neuron* **20,** 445–468.

Morris, R.G.M. (2007): Theories of hippocampal function. In: *The Hippocampus Book,* eds. P. Andersen, R.G.M. Morris, D.G. Amaral, *et al.* Oxford: Oxford University Press.

Morris, R.G., Garrud, P., Rawlins, J.N. & O'Keefe, J. (1982): Place navigation impaired in rats with hippocampal lesions. *Nature* **297,** 681–683.

Munoz, M. & Insausti, R. (2005): Cortical efferents of the entorhinal cortex and the adjacent parahippocampal region in the monkey (*Macaca fascicularis*). *Eur. J. Neurosci.* **22,** 1368–1388.

Murray, E. A. (2007): The amygdala, reward and emotion. *Trends Cogn. Sci.* **11,** 489–497.

Nedergaard, M. & Dirnagl, U. (2005): Role of glial cells in cerebral ischemia. *Glia* **50,** 281–286.

O'Keefe, J. (2007): Hippocampal neurophysiology in the behaving animal. In: *The Hippocampus Book,* eds. P. Andersen, R.G.M. Morris, D.G. Amaral, *et al.* Oxford: Oxford University Press.

Oliet, S.H., Piet, R. & Poulain, D.A. (2001): Control of glutamate clearance and synaptic efficacy by glial coverage of neurons. *Science* **292,** 923–926.

Papez, J.W. (1937) A proposed mechanism of emotion. *Arch. Neurol. Psychiatry* **38,** 725–743.

Pellerin, L. & Magistretti, P. J. (1994): Glutamate uptake into astrocytes stimulates aerobic glycolysis: a mechanism coupling neuronal-activity to glucose-utilization. *Proc. Natl. Acad. Sci. USA* **91,** 10625–10629.

Pitkänen, A. (2000): Connectivity of the rat amygdaloid complex. In: *The Amygdala: The Functional Analysis of the Amygdala,* ed. J.P. Aggleton. New York: Wiley–Liss.

Prather, M.D., Lavenex, P., Mauldin-Jourdain, M.L., Mason, W.A., Capitanio, J.P., Mendoza, S.P. & Amaral, D.G. (2001): Increased social fear and decreased fear of objects in monkeys with neonatal amygdala lesions. *Neuroscience* **106,** 653–658.

Price, J.L., Russchen, F.T. & Amaral, D.G. (1987): The limbic region. II: The amygdaloid complex. In: *Handbook of Chemical Neuroanatomy,* eds. A. Björklund, T. Hökfelt & L.W. Swanson. Amsterdam: Elsevier.

Qi, H.X., Jain, N., Collins, C.E., Lyon, D.C. & Kaas, J.H. (2010): Functional organization of motor cortex of adult macaque monkeys is altered by sensory loss in infancy. *Proc. Natl. Acad. Sci. USA* **107,** 3192–3197.

Rakic, P. & Nowakowski, R.S. (1981): The time of origin of neurons in the hippocampal region of the rhesus monkey. *J. Comp. Neurol.* **196,** 99–128.

Rao, V.L., Dogan, A., Todd, K.G., Bowen, K.K., Kim, B.T., Rothstein, J.D. & Dempsey, R. J. (2001): Antisense knockdown of the glial glutamate transporter GLT-1, but not the neuronal glutamate transporter EAAC1, exacerbates transient focal cerebral ischemia-induced neuronal damage in rat brain. *J. Neurosci.* **21,** 1876–1883.

Rubin, D.C. (2000): The distribution of early childhood memories. *Memory* **8,** 265–269.

Rushmore, R.J., Rigolo, L., Peer, A.K., Afifi, L.M., Valero-Cabre, A. & Payne, B.R. (2008): Age-dependent sparing of visual function after bilateral lesions of primary visual cortex. *Behav. Neurosci.* **122,** 1274–1283.

Scanziani, M., Salin, P.A., Vogt, K.E., Malenka, R.C. & Nicoll, R.A. (1997): Use-dependent increases in glutamate concentration activate presynaptic metabotropic glutamate receptors. *Nature* **385,** 630–634.

Schenk, F., Grobéty, M.-C., Lavenex, P. & Lipp, H.-P. (1995): Dissociation between basic components of spatial memory in rats. In: *Behavioural Brain Research in Naturalistic and Semi-Naturalistic Settings. NATO ASI Series D, Behavioural and Social Sciences.* eds. E. Alleva, A. Fasolo, H.P. Lipp, *et al.* Dordrecht, the Netherlands: Kluwer.

Schumann, C.M., Hamstra, J., Goodlin-Jones, B.L., Lotspeich, L.J., Kwon, H., Buonocore, M.H., *et al.* (2004): The amygdala is enlarged in children but not adolescents with autism; the hippocampus is enlarged at all ages. *J. Neurosci.* **24,** 6392–6401.

Scoville, W.B. & Milner, B. (1957): Loss of recent memory after bilateral hippocampal lesions. *J. Neurol. Neurosurg. Psychiatry* **20,** 11–21.

Seress, L. (2001): Morphological changes of the human hippocampal formation from midgestation to early childhood. In: *Handbook of Developmental Cognitive Neuroscience,* eds. C.A. Nelson & M. Luciana. Cambridge, MA: The MIT Press.

Seress, L. & Mrzljak, L. (1992): Postnatal development of mossy cells in the human dentate gyrus: a light microscopic Golgi study. *Hippocampus* **2,** 127–141.

Seress, L. & Ribak, C.E. (1995a): Postnatal development and synaptic connections of hilar mossy cells in the hippocampal dentate gyrus of rhesus monkeys. *J. Comp. Neurol.* **355,** 93–110.

Seress, L. & Ribak, C.E. (1995b): Postnatal development of CA3 pyramidal neurons and their afferents in the Ammon's horn of rhesus monkeys. *Hippocampus* **5,** 217–231.

Seress, L., Abraham, H., Tornoczky, T. & Kosztolanyi, G. (2001): Cell formation in the human hippocampal formation from mid-gestation to the late postnatal period. *Neuroscience* **105,** 831–843.

Sommer, W. (1880): Erkrankung des Ammonshorns als aetiologisches Moment der Epilepsie. *Arch. Psychiatr. Nervenkr.* **10,** 631–675.

Spielmeyer, W. (1925): Zur Pathogenese örtlich elektiver Gehirnveränderungen. *Z. Ges. Neurol. Psychiatr.* **99,** 756–776.

Squire, L.R. & Zola, S.M. (1996): Structure and function of declarative and nondeclarative memory systems. *Proc. Natl. Acad. Sci. USA* **93,** 13515–13522.

Staudt, M. (2010): Reorganization after pre- and perinatal brain lesions. *J. Anat.* **217,** 469–474.

Suzuki, W.A. & Amaral, D.G. (1990): Cortical inputs to the CA1 field of the monkey hippocampus originate from the perirhinal and parahippocampal cortex but not from area TE. *Neurosci. Lett.* **115,** 43–48.

Suzuki, W.A. & Amaral, D.G. (1994a): Perirhinal and parahippocampal cortices of the macaque monkey: cortical afferents. *J. Comp. Neurol.* **350,** 497–533.

Suzuki, W.A. & Amaral, D.G. (1994b): Topographic organization of the reciprocal connections between the monkey entorhinal cortex and the perirhinal and parahippocampal cortices. *J. Neurosci.* **14,** 1856–1877.

Swanson, R. A. (2005): Astrocyte neurotransmitter uptake. In: *Neuroglia,* eds. H. Kettenmann & B.R. Ransom. Oxford: Oxford University Press.

Tanaka, K., Watase, K., Manabe, T., Yamada, K., Watanabe, M., Takahashi, K., *et al.* (1997): Epilepsy and exacerbation of brain injury in mice lacking the glutamate transporter GLT-1. *Science* **276,** 1699–1702.

Thompson, K., Biddle, K.R., Robinson-Long, M., Poger, J., Wang, J., Yang, Q.X. & Eslinger, P.J. (2009): Cerebral plasticity and recovery of function after childhood prefrontal cortex damage. *Dev. Neurorehabil.* **12,** 298–312.

Tian, G.F., Azmi, H., Takano, T., Xu, Q., Peng, W., Lin, J., *et al.* (2005): An astrocytic basis of epilepsy. *Nat. Med.* **11,** 973–981.

Vargha-Khadem, F., Gadian, D.G., Watkins, K.E., Connelly, A., Van Paesschen, W. & Mishkin, M. (1997): Differential effects of early hippocampal pathology on episodic and semantic memory. *Science* **277,** 376–380.

Volterra, A. & Meldolesi, J. (2005): Astrocytes, from brain glue to communication elements: the revolution continues. *Nat. Rev. Neurosci.* **6,** 626–640.

Zola-Morgan, S., Squire, L.R. & Amaral, D.G. (1986): Human amnesia and the medial temporal region enduring memory impairment following a bilateral lesion limited to field CA1 of the hippocampus. *J. Neurosci.* **6,** 2950–2967.

Zola-Morgan, S., Squire, L.R., Rempel, N.L., Clower, R.P. & Amaral, D.G. (1992): Enduring memory impairment in monkeys after ischemic damage to the hippocampus. *J. Neurosci.* **12,** 2582–2596.

Brain Lesion Localization and Developmental Functions, D. Riva, C. Njiokiktjien and S. Bulgheroni (eds.)
© 2011 John Libbey Eurotext, pp. 119–128.

Chapter 10

Early hippocampal disease and memory disorders

Daria Riva, Arianna Usilla, Chiara Vago and Sara Bulgheroni

Developmental Neurology Division, Fondazione IRCCS Istituto Neurologico 'C. Besta', via Celoria 11, 20133 Milan, Italy
driva@istituto-besta.it

Summary

The complex system of human memory is processed in its various components not by a single brain structure, but by a complex system with a corresponding, equally complex neural network that is widely distributed throughout the brain. In this chapter the organization of cognitive or declarative memories is described. Cognitive memories are represented by memory for facts and events (semantic memory) and by memory of personal experiences in the temporo-spatial context (episodic memory). There is consensus that the hippocampus and related medial temporal lobe structures are crucial for adult declarative memories, but much less is known about their contribution during developmental age. We review here the developmental studies in this topic and their related models. The *model of unitary memory* claims that semantic knowledge is the result of amassing several episodic memories that lack contextual cues, and only retain their general feature, whereas the *functional hierarchy model* claims that there are two separate memory systems served by partially different neural circuits that process the learning of semantic memory, and afterwards of episodic memory. From studies conducted to date it is impossible to draw any final conclusions on the developmental competencies of the hippocampus and of the adjacent cortexes in processing declarative memory; for that, further studies are needed to clarify how this memory is processed.

Introduction

Human memory, defined as the capacity to acquire, retain, and recall experiences and/or information, is processed in its various components not by a single system, but by a complex system with a corresponding, equally complex neural network that is widely distributed throughout the brain.

Functional studies in normal individuals and evidence of neuropsychological double dissociations in patients have provided support for the model in which memory is distributed in systems and subsystems that are strongly interconnected even though they are functionally independent. In 1987 Squire proposed a model of mnemonic function that has proved useful not only for the theoretical systematization of other models, but also from a clinical standpoint. This model draws a first distinction between short-term (ST) and long-term (LT) memory. The independence of these two macro-systems has also been supported by double dissociations in pathologic conditions, for example, in patients with severe deficiencies in LT memory, but a practically normal ST memory (Baddeley & Warrington, 1970), and in patients with a severely impaired verbal span (a measure of STM) but normal behavior as regards their LT memory (Basso *et al.*, 1982).

The LT memory system can be further divided into explicit or declarative memories and implicit or procedural memories. Explicit or cognitive memory consists of the conscious and deliberate recall and recognition of previous experiences, facts, and information, and represents knowledge of the world that is shared more or less by everyone. The LT memory forming the subject of this chapter is also supported by double dissociations in patients with brain lesions. The pure amnesia seen in adults supports a dichotomous system represented by impairments in intentional recall of previously learned material coinciding with a normal procedural memory and repetition priming level (Schacter *et al.*, 1993).

Among the implicit memories, *priming* is defined as the implicit memory in which exposure to a stimulus influences response to a later stimulus. It can occur following the repetition of perceptual, semantic, or conceptual stimuli. For example, if persons read a list of words including the word *table*, and are later asked to complete a word starting with *tab*, the probability of their saying *table* is greater than if they had not been primed. Another example is when people see an incomplete sketch that they are unable to identify, and are then shown more of the sketch until they recognize the picture. After priming, they will identify the sketch at an earlier stage than they were able to do the first time. The effects of priming can be very salient and long lasting, even more so than simple recognition memory. Unconscious priming effects can affect word choice in a word-stem completion test long after the words have been consciously forgotten (Kolb & Whishaw, 2003; Tulving *et al.*, 1982).

Another type of implicit memory is facilitation (a gradual improvement in performance obtained after repeatedly administering a stimulus) in various types of perceptual, cognitive, or motor tasks, without any awareness of previous experiences. Procedural memory is typically based on implicit learning mechanisms and it is used mainly for learning motor skills that can only be improved through repetition, so it is unnecessary to form new explicit memories. The neural processing network depends on distributed structures, such as the basal ganglia, the cerebellum and the prefrontal cortex, which are distinct from the networks that process declarative memory.

The intentional and conscious storage and recall of information are part of our cultural heritage (or knowledge of the world) and are termed *semantic memory*, whereas *episodic memory* refers to experiences and events that are mainly autobiographical and located in a spatial and temporal context. Episodic memory is associated with the retrieval of contextual details relating to the encoding process (*I came to Turin to see my friend Charles*), while semantic memory is unrelated to contextual details *(Turin is in Piedmont)*; both involve explicit processes. The two macro-systems of LT memory are represented by complex networks that obviously differ from one another. While cognitive memory is mediated by the prefrontal cortex, the parietal lobe, the medial temporal lobe, the thalamic nuclei, and mammillothalamic tracts, the broader-scale network of episodic memory is based on interaction between the prefrontal and temporal areas, which work together to process the memories. On the formation of cognitive memory, there are two different theories. According to one, semantic memories are episodic memories cleansed of any contextual residues, in which case the first episodic encoding would subsequently become generalized as semantic. According to the other theory, the information would first enter as semantic and would subsequently be used to modify episodic memories, in which case the first encoding would be semantic and only afterwards, having been contextualized in a space/time frame, it would become episodic. The first theory has been formalized in the model of unitary memory, according to which semantic knowledge is the result of amassing several episodic memories that lack contextual cues, and only retain their general features. The second theory has been formalized in the functional hierarchy model, according to which there are two separate memory systems served by partially different neural circuits that process the learning of semantic memory, and afterwards of episodic memory.

Cognitive memories are mediated by the medial temporal lobe, a system of anatomically connected structures where the hippocampus and adjacent cortexes (the perirhinal, entorhinal, and posterior parahippocampal) work in series and/or in parallel.

According to the *unitary memory approach*, semantic and episodic memory are processed by the same circuit (Squire & Zola, 1998), whereas in the hierarchical model *two separate systems* are involved in processing semantic and episodic memory: this means that distinct (or at least partially distinct) circuits underlie these memories (Tulving *et al.*, 1991; Vargha-Kadhem *et al.*, 1997). According to this latter model, information processing develops in a hierarchical manner because perceptual information enters the parahippocampal regions, mediating semantic memory, and only afterwards enters the hippocampal regions needed for episodic memory. This functional hierarchical model (Eichenbaum, 1997; Mishkin *et al.*, 1998) places the hippocampus above the entorhinal, perirhinal, and parahippocampal cortexes, from which it receives the afferents and to which it transmits the output, respectively. The cortical representations are semantically associated on a level with the parahippocampal region by means of a very rigid link (mediated by a relationship of juxtaposition) and subsequently processed by the hippocampus, which relies on a more flexible type of association to enrich them with a spatiotemporal connotation. The hippocampus not only contributes to the encoding of single episodes, but is also capable of creating complex combinations of memories (Eichenbaum, 2001), giving rise to the cognitive map of personal experiences that each of us carries and uses in our daily lives (Riva *et al.*, 2000). The hippocampus is a complex structure divided into many substructures: the hippocampus proper is composed of CA fields and the dentate gyrus; the hippocampal formation contains the hippocampus proper and the subiculum; and the hippocampal complex comprises the parahippocampal regions (the entorhinal, perirhinal, and parahippocampal cortexes). Consistent with the hierarchy hypothesis, the hippocampus is crucial to the formation of episodic memories, but not of semantic memories. As a consequence, children with early brain injuries involving the hippocampus should be able to develop normal knowledge despite having a poor episodic memory. According to the unitary hypothesis, on the other hand, the hippocampus itself is involved in both semantic and episodic memory, so children with early brain injuries involving the hippocampus should be impaired in both semantic and episodic memory.

What is relevant is that patients with organic amnesia are significantly more severely impaired in learning new *episodic* information than in the case of *semantic* information, suggesting that semantic and episodic information follow (at least partially) independent memorization routes (Tulving & Markowitsch, 1998).

In adults, this discrepancy is still controversial. Some studies support the feasibility of at least some new semantic learning (Kitchener *et al.*, 1998; McKenna & Gerhand, 2002), while others fail to confirm this ability (Gabrieli *et al.*, 1988; Reed & Squire, 1998; Verfaellie *et al.*, 1995). In children, findings are even more controversial. Ostergaard (1987) described a 10-year-old boy who had multifocal brain damage with bilateral involvement of the hippocampus after an anoxic episode, and whose IQ and procedural memory were intact, while his semantic and episodic declarative memory were both equally impaired. He was able to progress in terms of academic skills, showing a partially preserved ability to store new semantic information.

Other studies in children with bilateral hippocampal lesions have shown a dissociation between good (or fairly good) semantic memory and impaired episodic memory. This dissociation was described by Wood *et al.* (1989) in a 9-year-old child after acute encephalopathy, as well as by Broman *et al.* (1997) in a 9-year-old child who showed a loss of medial temporal lobe volume bilaterally and a shortened hippocampus on MRI after respiratory arrest, and by Brizzolara (2003) in a 6-year-old girl with an acute encephalopathy that resulted in multifocal brain damage. Epileptic disease, as well as focal discrete lesions, can also generate memory impairments. De Renzi and Lucchelli (1990) described a 22-year-old, prematurely born, immature girl with an EEG characterized by delta and theta rhythms in the frontotemporal regions, difficulty in remembering things, a normal VIQ and PIQ, a poor semantic memory for past events or famous names, poor recognition of famous faces, and an impaired episodic memory (*i.e.*, difficulty in learning new verbal and non-verbal material and in story recall). Temple (1997) described a 12-year-old girl who developed normally, until the age of 6, when she developed temporal lobe epilepsy. From then on, she had an impaired semantic and episodic memory, and difficulty in acquiring new verbal and nonverbal material, but her procedural memory remained intact. In a famous paper published in *Science*, Vargha-Khadem *et al.* (1997) (and later Gadian *et al.*, 2000) described the neuropsychological profile of developmental amnesia in children with bilateral early hippocampal lesions caused by hypoxic-ischaemic damage early in life. This profile was characterized by the absence of semantic memory impairments, adequate language and social capabilities, an adequate capacity to read and write, and an acquired knowledge sufficient to be rated on the medium–lower levels of the norm in cognitive assessments. There were nevertheless significant episodic memory impairments, with markedly impaired memories of the episodes of daily life (*i.e.*, disorientation in space and time, difficulty in recognizing familiar places, remembering where they had put things, saying what they had done during the day, and remembering messages, people they met, or appointments). The effect of the timing of hippocampal lesions on the neuropsychological profile of developmental amnesia is a specific feature of patients with early bilateral hippocampal damage, but for this syndrome the patients' actual age when the injury occurred can extend from birth to puberty. The extent of hippocampal volume reduction that produces this profile is in the range of 20–30 per cent on each side (Isaacs *et al.*, 2003; Vargha Khadem *et al.*, 2003).

As for the neural circuits, the perirhinal, entorhinal, and parahippocampal cortexes are capable of supporting context-free semantic memories, while the hippocampus can support context-rich episodic memory. In 2007, Vicari and colleagues described an 8-year-old who had undergone the surgical removal of an ependymoma of the left ventricle at 4 years of age, and who had mild atrophy of the left hippocampus, which was displaced downward with a twisting left fornix, and damaged posterior frontal lobe. This boy had significant difficulty in retaining daily events and information, and a severe anterograde amnesic syndrome. His performance in episodic LT memory was very poor and he was unable to recollect new verbal information a few minutes after its presentation. His ST semantic memory was normal, however. The authors came to the conclusion that the neural circuits of autobiographical and factual information do not overlap completely. In 2004, Temple and Richardson described the case of a 9-year-old boy with the classical picture of developmental amnesia, but with no apparent brain lesions, a normal intelligence, an intact episodic memory and an impaired semantic memory of facts and words. This double dissociation suggests a modularity between the episodic and semantic memory systems, and their relative independence during development.

Another question concerns the *consequences of unilateral hippocampal damage on memory*. Studies on memory in adults with hippocampal diseases have demonstrated that bilateral hippocampal lesions give rise to a clinical picture of amnesia, whereas unilateral hippocampal lesions would cause selective memory impairments for verbal and nonverbal material, depending on the hemisphere involved [though this is still debated (O'Brien *et al.*, 2003)]. Many studies in the past suggested that verbal and nonverbal memory are processed by the left or right medial temporal lobes, respectively (Milner, 1971). It has been suggested more recently that nonverbal memory comprises a series of functionally and anatomically independent subsystems; for example, memory of unknown faces is preserved in bilateral hippocampal damage. Bird *et al.* described one patient with selective hippocampal damage involving both sides and another with right hippocampal damage, who both had a preserved familiarity and recollection for faces (Cipolotti *et al.*, 2006), while topographical memory (both familiarity and recollection) was impaired. The patient with the right hippocampal lesion had no verbal memory impairment. The right hippocampus has been considered indispensable for processing the 'allocentric' space (relating to the context) rather than the egocentric space (relative to the observer) (Burgess *et al.*, 2002) in developmental amnesia as well (Burgess *et al.*, 2006; King *et al.*, 2004). Conversely, the hippocampus could not be the processor of old spatial memories (Rosenbaum *et al.*, 2005).

Does this selectivity apply to children too? Can damage to the hippocampus and the parahippocampal cortexes cause developmental amnesia, and are these impairments hemisphere-specific? To shed light on these questions, we studied nine children (five of them male) aged from 6 to 17 years at the time of testing (mean 136.1 ± 43.7 months) who had been assessed at 4 months to 15 years of age (mean 77.1 ± 62.2 months). In the seven patients with epilepsy, the symptoms were well controlled by monotherapy. The patients were matched 1:1 with normal children by gender, age, schooling, and social background. All subjects had well-articulated, fluent, syntactically correct spontaneous language skills with an adequate lexical repertoire. Their academic performance was in the normal middle range. It was impossible to predict whether their actual semantic level at the time of testing was the expected one. The patients' intelligence was in the normal range and their VIQs similar to those of the controls. For all verbal and spatial short-term semantic memory tests, the patients scored lower, though not significantly so, than controls, while in the tests assessing long-term episodic memory they differed significantly from the controls in terms of verbal episodic memory, but not in visuo-spatial episodic memory. There was also a marked difference in everyday memory by comparison with controls. Long-term semantic memory was comparable with that of controls, however. The children with lesions that also involved the perihippocampal cortexes (which are thought to process semantic memory according to the hierarchical model) scored lower, but not significantly lower than the controls. The patients also performed within normal range on the Boston Naming test and for categorical fluency, and their learning at school was normal, demonstrating that they were capable of progressing in their knowledge of the world. These patients were therefore significantly impaired in verbal (but not spatial) episodic memory and in everyday memory. Their daily life difficulties concerned remembering appointments and recalling the details of what happened the day before, people's names, etc. The relatively spared semantic memory coinciding with a more severe episodic impairment at least partially confirms Mishkin's hierarchical model. Deficiencies in verbal, but not spatial episodic memory would confirm an early hemispheric specialization of the hippocampus, as in the patients described by Milner (1971, 1980) after left or right medial temporal resections. Our results demonstrate an asymmetry, but not a complete dissociation of the two types of memory, with a weaker, but still relatively preserved semantic memory and a significantly impaired episodic memory system. These findings are more in line with the view taken by Squire and Zola that, in order to conclude for the hierarchical model, two conditions have to be satisfied: (1) there should be no residual ability to acquire new episodic information; and (2) the ability to acquire new semantic information should be completely preserved. Taking this view, these conditions apparently do not apply to our data, because episodic memory was not completely abolished and semantic memory was not completely preserved. The discrepancy between semantic and episodic memory is the same as the situation described in single cases of developmental amnesia secondary to bilateral hippocampal lesions, but less severe. In the case of unilateral left lesions, the right hippocampus could take over a proportion of the skills normally assigned to the damaged left hippocampus, triggering a reorganization of the memory system. In both models (the hierarchical and the unitary), the hippocampus is crucial to associative memory (Cohen *et al.*, 1997), while the site of semantic memory is still controversial.

To sum up, we can conclude that left hippocampal lesions (like all focal lesions) cause specific deficiencies of variable severity. Memories can be partially compensated by the intact contralateral hippocampus and parahippocampal cortexes. Unilateral left hippocampal lesions result in a limited form of anterograde amnesia, which involves both semantic and episodic memory, although the former is better preserved than the latter. The pattern is static: lesions acquired very early or in adolescence cause impairments of similar quality and severity. Children with additional damage to the parahippocampal cortexes have a slightly worse semantic memory, though not significantly worse than that of controls. The medial temporal lobe structures play a fundamental part in organizing memory through interactions with the distributed cortical regions, even at a very early age. Early and congenital hippocampal disease causes a significant loss of episodic memory, but leaves cognitive development based on semantic memory relatively intact. Since the lesions affecting the hippocampus in this study were of different types, more research is obviously needed on larger samples of children with the same disease.

Another topic of debate concerning amnesia after hippocampal damage is the possible dissociation between recognition and recall abilities. Although this type of disorder is generally uniformly identifiable in amnesia secondary to diencephalic or medial temporal lesions in adults, in developmental amnesia in children recognition abilities seem to be preserved both in experimental studies (Vargha-Khadem *et al.*, 1997) and in several clinical tasks (Baddeley *et al.*, 2001). It was Baddeley *et al.* (2001) who suggested a relationship between the observed ability to acquire semantic knowledge and the relatively spared recognition memory capacity since both require memory without context. Vargha-Khadem (1997) and Mishkin (1998) explained their findings in the context of a modular model of the medial temporal lobe derived from animal research (Gadian *et al.*, 2000; Meunier *et al.*, 1993). The dissociation between recall and recognition was also reported in some cases of adult-onset of the disorder (Barbeau *et al.*, 2005), the most salient being the patient Y.R., who had severe atrophy of the hippocampus, but normal parahippocampal gyri, and who performed very poorly in recall tests (giving 94 per cent of wrong answers), but very well in recognition tests (with 91 per cent of right answers). Several other authors have claimed that the dissociation between recall and recognition reflects the differential involvement of two memory processes. Recall robustly reflects recollection, which is defined as the mental re-establishment of previous events associated with details, sensory and emotional correlates experienced during the first occurrence of the event, and contextual cues. By contrast, recognition is mediated by both recollection and familiarity; the latter is defined as a mental awareness of having experienced an event in the past, but devoid of specific and contextual details. Recollection and familiarity are functionally distinct cognitive processes. Functional neuroimaging studies in normal and impaired subjects suggest that the two processes are dissociable in the brain (Vilberg & Rugg, 2007). Recollection has been associated with the activation of the hippocampus and, to a lesser extent, of the posterior parahippocampal gyrus (Diana *et al.*, 2007; Skinner & Fernandes, 2007). The perirhinal cortex has been found activated by a familiar component (Danckert *et al.*, 2007). Squire's group questioned this modularity after finding an impaired recollection and familiarity in adult patients with damage restricted to the hippocampus alone (Squire *et al.*, 2004) and impaired recognition memory in monkeys with selective hippocampal damage (Zola *et al.*, 2000).

This chapter has briefly discussed just a small part of the enormous mass of data relating to declarative memory and the role of the temporomedial structures in its complex processing. From studies conducted to date it is impossible to draw any final conclusions on the competencies of the hippocampus and of the adjacent cortexes in processing declarative memory, and in processing familiarity and the recall of facts and people, although it is clear that these structures' role is crucial in processing these memories.

The exact modular architecture of these functions can only be clarified by studies on individuals or groups with impairments limited to the hippocampus and/or the parahippocampal structures, and for whom we know at what age in life these impairments occurred.

References

Baddeley, A.D. & Warrington, E.K. (1970): Amnesia and the distinction between long and short term memory. *J. Verb. Learn. Verb. Behav.* **9,** 176–189.

Baddeley, A, Vargha-Khadem, F. & Mishkin, M. (2001): Preserved recognition in a case of developmental amnesia: implications for the acquisition of semantic memory? *J. Cogn. Neurosci.* **13,** 357–369.

Barbeau, E.J., Felician, O., Joubert, S., Sontheimer, A., Ceccaldi, M. & Poncet, M. (2005): Preserved visual recognition memory in an amnesic patient with hippocampal lesions. *Hippocampus* **15,** 587–596.

Basso, A., Spinnler, H., Vallar, G. & Zanobio, M.E. (1982): Left hemisphere damage and selective impairment of auditory verbal short-term memory: a case study. *Neuropsychologia* **20,** 263–274.

Brizzolara, D., Casalini, C., Montanaro, D. & Posteraro, F. (2003). A case of amnesia at an early age. *Cortex* **39,** 605–625.

Broman, M., Rose, A.L., Hotson, G. & Casey, C.M. (1997): Severe anterograde amnesia with onset in childhood as a result of anoxic encephalopathy. *Brain* **120,** 417–433.

Burgess, N., Maguire, E.A. & O'Keefe J. (2002): The human hippocampus and spatial and episodic memory. *Neuron* **35,** 625–641.

Burgess, N., Trinkler, I., King, J., Kennedy, A. & Cipolotti, L. (2006): Impaired allocentric spatial memory underlying topographical disorientation. *Rev. Neurosci.* **17,** 239–251.

Cipolotti, L., Bird, C., Good, T., Macmanus, D., Rudge, P. & Shallice, T. (2006): Recollection and familiarity in dense hippocampal amnesia: a case study. *Neuropsychologia* **44,** 489–506.

Cohen, N.J., Poldrack, R.A. & Eichenbaum, H. (1997): Memory for items and memory for relations in the procedural/ declarative memory framework. *Memory* **5,** 131–178.

Danckert, S.L., Gati, J.S., Menon, R.S. & Köhler, S. (2007): Perirhinal and hippocampal contributions to visual recognition memory can be distinguished from those of occipito-temporal structures based on conscious awareness of prior occurrence. *Hippocampus.* **17,** 1081–1092.

De Renzi, E. & Lucchelli, F. (1990): Developmental dysmnesia in a poor reader. *Brain* **113,** 1337–1345.

Diana, R.A., Yonelinas, A.P. & Ranganath, C. (2007): Imaging recollection and familiarity in the medial temporal lobe: a three-component model. *Trends Cognit. Sci.* **11,** 379–386.

Eichenbaum, H. (1997): How does the brain organize memories? *Science* **277,** 330–331.

Eichenbaum, H. (2001): The hippocampus and declarative memory: cognitive mechanisms and neural codes. *Behav. Brain Res.* **127,** 199–207.

Gabrieli, J.D., Cohen, N.J. & Corkin, S. (1988): The impaired learning of semantic knowledge following bilateral medial temporal-lobe resection. *Brain Cognit.* **7,** 157–177.

Gadian, D.G., Aicardi, J., Watkins, K.E., Porter, D.A., Mishkin, M. & Vargha-Khadem, F. (2000): Developmental amnesia associated with early hypoxic-ischaemic injury. *Brain* **123,** 499–507.

Isaacs, E.B., Vargha-Khadem, F., Watkins, K.E., Lucas, A., Mishkin, M. & Gadian, D.G. (2003): Developmental amnesia and its relationship to degree of hippocampal atrophy. *Neuroscience* **100,** 13060–13063.

King, J.A., Trinkler, I., Hartley, T., Vargha-Khadem, F. & Burgess, N. (2004): The hippocampal role in spatial memory and the familiarity–recollection distinction: a case study. *Neuropsychology* **18,** 405–417.

Kitchener, E.G., Hodges, J.R. & McCarthy, R. (1998): Acquisition of post-morbid vocabulary and semantic facts in the absence of episodic memory. *Brain* **121**, 1313–1327.

Kolb, B. & Whishaw, I.Q. (2003): *Fundamentals of Human Neuropsychology,* 5th ed., pp. 453–454, 457. New York: Freeman-Worth.

McKenna, P. & Gerhand, S. (2002): Preserved semantic learning in an amnesic patient. *Cortex* **38,** 37–58.

Meunier, M., Bachevalier, J., Mishkin, M. & Murray, E.A. (1993): Effects on visual recognition of combined and separate ablations of the entorhinal and perirhinal cortex in rhesus monkeys. *J. Neurosci.* **13,** 5418–5432.

Milner, B. (1971): Interhemispheric differences in the localization of psychological processes in man. *Br. Med. Bull.* **27,** 272–277.

Milner, B. (1980): Complementary functional specializations of the human cerebral hemispheres. In: *Nerve Cells, Transmitters and Behaviour*, ed. R. Levi Montalcini, pp. 601–625. Vatican City: Academia Scientarium.

Mishkin, M, Vargha-Khadem, F. & Gadian, D.G. (1998): Amnesia and the organization of the hippocampal system. *Hippocampus* **8,** 212–216.

O'Brien, C.E., Bowden, S.C., Bardenhagen, F.J. & Cook, M.J. (2003): Neuropsychological correlates of hippocampal and rhinal cortex volumes in patients with mesial temporal sclerosis. *Hippocampus* **13,** 892–904.

Ostergaard, A.L. (1987): Episodic, semantic and procedural memory in a case of amnesia at an early age. *Neuropsychologia* **25,** 341–357.

Reed, J.M. & Squire, L.R. (1998): Retrograde amnesia for facts and events: findings from four new cases. *J. Neurosci.* **15,** 3943–3954.

Riva, D., Saletti, V. & Nichelli, F. (2000): The organization of memory in temporo-mesial structures in developmental age. In: *Localization of Brain Lesions and Developmental Functions,* eds. D. Riva & A. Benton, pp. 15–21. Mariani Foundation Paediatric Neurology Series – IX. London: John Libbey.

Rosenbaum, R.S., Gao, F., Richards, B., Black, S.E. & Moscovitch, M.J. (2005): 'Where to?' remote memory for spatial relations and landmark identity in former taxi drivers with Alzheimer's disease and encephalitis. *Cogn. Neurosci.* **17,** 446–462.

Schacter, D.L., Peter Chiu, C.Y. & Ochsner, K.N. (1993): Implicit memory: a selective review. *Annu. Rev. Neurosci.* **16,** 159–182.

Skinner, E.I. & Fernandes, M.A. (2007): Neural correlates of recollection and familiarity: a review of neuroimaging and patient data. *Neuropsychologia* **45,** 2163–2179.

Squire, L.R. (1987): *Memory and Brain.* New York: Oxford University Press.

Squire, L.R. & Zola S.M. (1998): Episodic memory, semantic memory, and amnesia. *Hippocampus* **8,** 205–211.

Squire, L.R., Craig, E.L., Stark Craig, E.L. & Clark, R.E. (2004): The medial temporal lobe. *Annu. Rev. Neurosci.* **27,** 279–306.

Temple, C.M. (1997): Cognitive neuropsychology and its applications to children. *J. Child Psychol. Psychiatry* **38,** 27–52.

Temple, C.M. & Richardson, P. (2004): Developmental amnesia: a new pattern of dissociation with intact episodic memory. *Neuropsychologia* **42,** 764–781.

Tulving, E. & Markowitsch, H.J. (1998): Episodic and declarative memory: role of the hippocampus. *Hippocampus* **8,** 198–204.

Tulving, E., Schacter, D.L. & Stark, H.A. (1982). Priming effects in word fragment completion are independent of recognition memory. *J. Exp. Psychol. Learn. Mem. Cognit.* **8,** 336–342.

Tulving E, Hayman C.A. & MacDonald, C.A. (1991): Long lasting perceptual priming and semantic learning in amnesia: a case experiment. *J. Exp. Psychol. Learn. Mem. Cognit.* **17,** 595–617.

Vargha-Khadem, F., Gadian, D.G., Watkins, K.E., Connelly, A., Van Paesschen, W. & Mishkin, M. (1997): Differential effects of early hippocampal pathology on episodic and semantic memory. *Science* **277,** 376–380.

Vargha-Khadem, F., Salmond, C.H., Watkins, K.E., Friston, K.J., Gadian, D.G. & Mishkin, M. (2003): Developmental amnesia: effect of age at injury. *Neuroscience* **100,** 10055–10060.

Verfaellie, M., Reiss, L. & Roth, H.L. (1995): Knowledge of new English vocabulary in amnesia: an examination of premorbidly acquired semantic memory. *Int. Neuropsychol. Soc.* **1,** 443–453.

Vicari, S., Menghini, D., Di Paola, M., Serra, L., Donfrancesco, A., Fidani, P., *et al.* (2007): Acquired amnesia in childhood: a single case study. *Neuropsychologia* **45,** 704–715.

Vilberg, K.L. & Rugg, M.D. (2007): Dissociation of the neural correlates of recognition memory according to familiarity, recollection, and amount of recollected information. *Neuropsychologia* **45,** 2216–2225.

Wood, F.B., Brown, I.S. & Felton, R.H. (1989): Long-term follow-up of a childhood amnesic syndrome. *Brain Cognit.* **10,** 76–86.

Zola, S.M., Squire, L.R., Teng, E., Stefanacci, L., Buffalo, E.A. & Clark, R.E. (2000): Impaired recognition memory in monkeys after damage limited to the hippocampal region. *J. Neurosci.* **20,** 451–463.

Brain Lesion Localization and Developmental Functions, D. Riva, C. Njiokiktjien and S. Bulgheroni (eds.)

Chapter 11

Language disorders in children with morphologic abnormalities of the hippocampus

Josette Mancini*, Guillaume Agostini*, Nathalie Villeneuve°, Mathieu Milh*, Florence George*, Brigitte Chabrol* and Nadine Girard#

**Neuropaediatric Unit, Universitary Hospital La Timone, 264 rue Saint-Pierre, 13005 Marseille, France;*
°Epilepsy Center, Henri Gastaut Hospital, 300 boulevard Sainte-Marguerite, 13009 Marseille, France;
#Neuroradiologic Department, Universitary Hospital La Timone, 264 rue Saint-Pierre, 13005 Marseille, France
jmancini@ap-hm.fr

Summary

The literature provides compelling evidence that the hippocampus supports several constituents of language acquisition. Morphologic abnormalities of the hippocampal formations (HFAs) are more and more observed on magnetic resonance imaging (MRI). We wished to specify the type of clinical disorders associated with these malformations. From a retrospective case series, we planned to study the language of the children presenting with these anomalies. Our methods were as follows: From the data of all the MRI scans taken over 16 months in patients under 18 years of age, we retrospectively selected the children with an HFA, either isolated or associated with other malformations. HFAs were defined and described according to criteria of shape or orientation of defects. We studied the files of the patients with isolated HFAs. Those whose clinical presentation was compatible with language assessment were tested prospectively. Our results showed that of 2,208 MRIs from 1 January 2007 to 30 April 2008, 96 (4.3 per cent) showed an HFA; these were found in 61 boys and 35 girls aged from 2 months to 17 years. Eighty two of these 96 subjects (85 per cent) had associated anomalies. Fourteen (14 per cent) had an isolated HFA. Of these 14, nine HFAs were compatible with language assessment. Nine of the 14 children had behaviour and autism spectrum disorders, and seven of these were epileptic. Four had very serious language disorders as part of mental retardation and/or autistic disorders. Four others had language disorders prevailing in expression and phonology and manifested pathologic visual memory. We concluded that even though language disorders are often part of a larger deficiency presentation, the results we obtained suggest that isolated HFAs are not only a cause of memory disorders, but could also directly underlie language disorders, particularly in expression.

Introduction

To the degree that the hippocampus is known for playing a crucial role in memory, one might presume that this specific brain formation could interact with language. In 1988 some authors had demonstrated that the hippocampus was determinant in lexical acquisition (Gabrieli *et al.*, 1988). Currently several studies demonstrate implication of the hippocampus in syntactic elaboration. During the last several years development of such techniques as brain MRI and different functional approaches and their combination with fMRI have improved our understanding of relations between the hippocampus and language. Studies in the literature concern either normal subjects (children and adults) or those with dysfunctions that are secondary to brain lesions or pathologic disorders such as epilepsy and autism.

The hippocampus and lexicon

To memorize a new word, two strategies are possible: (1) learning of episodic type during encoding and (2) semantic storage during which the new word is related to other characteristics to give it sense. According to Ullman (2004), these strategies involve:

- the mesial temporal cortex and prefrontal cortex during episodical encoding, and
- lateral temporal cortex in semantic processing.

An fMRI experiment in adults demonstrated that hippocampal activation was observed during word encoding. Words were visually presented as triplets: Subjects were asked to undertake two types of tasks. Either they had to mentally repeat the different words or they had to classify them from the more to the less desirable (rote processing). Twenty minutes later, the subjects had to recognize previous words among different audio stimuli. The hippocampus was activated in both tasks, but it was more activated during the task that tried to establish relations between the different words (rote processing). On the other hand, item memorization was better when encoding was required to establish relations between words. So the authors (Davachi & Wagner, 2002) concluded that the hippocampus played an active role during encoding.

Another fMRI study in adults showed that the hippocampus activity differentiated good from poor learners of a novel lexicon. This acquisition of a novel lexicon generated a larger activation in the left hippocampus and left fusiform gyrus. After the first steps of learning, there was a transfer of activation from the hippocampus to the neocortical areas classically involved in language processing. These areas became more and more active, with language improving (left parietal inferior lobe: BA40) (Breitenstein *et al.*, 2005).

The hippocampus and syntaxis

Some authors have demonstrated interactions of the hippocampal system and the prefrontal cortex in learning language-like rules. The hippocampus seems to play an important role at the beginning of syntactic learning. At this stage learning is based on similarity. Later on, when syntactic learning is based on more universal rules, the activation of the prefrontal cortex becomes predominant (Opitz & Friederici, 2003, 2004). Another study using event-related potentials demonstrated the role of the hippocampus in syntactic integration by showing a P600 at the level of the hippocampus when sentences were spoken with incorrect syntaxis (Meyer *et al.*, 2005).

The hippocampus and conceptualization

According to Kumaran *et al.* (2009), the capacity to bring prior knowledge to bear in novel situations is a defining characteristic of human intelligence. To reach this goal humans use *concepts*: concepts are built through abstraction and capture the shared meaning of similar entities through an organizing principle that explains their relatedness. During an fMRI experiment, adult subjects had to be able to predict weather (sun or rain) from conceptualization from different visual components that appeared on the screen. Subjects were covertly trained to find the rules to help them make a correct answer about the future weather. There was a second part of the experiment, during which the subjects could find the correct answer only if they used such rules. When hippocampal activation occurred at the first stage, subjects were able to establish concepts that allowed them to find correct answers during the second stage. The ventromedial prefrontal cortex was activated at this second time. According to these data, the hippocampus supports conceptual learning through its unique associative-memory capacity.

The hippocampus and language lateralization

Several studies suggest that the hippocampus could play a role in language lateralization. In a morphometric study among 20 participants, those who had a right dominancy for the language had a bigger hippocampus, although the planum temporale were equivalent (Jansen *et al.*, 2010).

Does language lateralization depend on the hippocampus? This question was raised by Knecht (2004) in an editorial that appeared in *Brain* concerning the functional language reorganization after an early brain lesion. His comment was about an fMRI experiment in 10 children with early or congenital right brain lesions reported at this time by Liégeois *et al.* (2004). Transhemispheric compensation for language appeared to be more common than it was in adults. In this small population, language reorganization was not based on a shift in handedness. Neither age at onset of epilepsy nor proximity of a lesion to language areas intervened, but a critical role of the left medial temporal lobe, probably the hippocampus, was highly suspected. In these cases transhemispheric compensation for language was based on hippocampal preservation.

Another fMRI study, comparing 84 epileptic adults with different brain lesions (hippocampal sclerosis, left frontal lobe and left temporo-lateral lesions) and 45 healthy control subjects, assessed the lateralization of cerebral language representation. Patients with hippocampal sclerosis showed less left cerebral representation of language than in all other groups of subjects. Thus the hippocampus seems to play a role in the establishment of language dominance (Weber *et al.*, 2006).

Effects of hippocampal sclerosis

DeLong & Heinz (1997) reported four children with bilateral hippocampal sclerosis and severe epilepsy. They had neither motor nor sensory problems, but their language never developed. They also failed to develop social skills and complex purposive or adaptive activity. According to these authors these deficits corresponded to the cognitive deficits observed in severe infantile autism. So hippocampal function appears necessary for language learning in the infant, as well as for complex social and adaptive learning. We know that left anterior temporal lobe resection for pharmacologically intractable temporal lobe epilepsy (TLE) carries a risk for postoperative naming decline because naming is usually mediated by the perisylvian cortex in the left (language-dominant) hemisphere. Hamberger *et al.* (2007) demonstrated that this risk is lower in patients with hippocampal sclerosis (HS) relative to those without HS. This pattern might implicate direct involvement of the hippocampus in naming. On the other hand, critical naming sites have been found in anterior, lateral temporal (*i.e.*, extra-hippocampal) neocortex, the region typically removed with 'standard' TLE resection. Therefore Hamberger *et al.* speculated that the relative preservation of naming in postoperative HS patients might reflect cortical reorganization of language to areas outside this region. Using pre-resection electrical stimulation mapping, they compared the topography of auditory and visual naming sites in 12 patients with HS and 12 patients without structural brain pathology. Their results suggest that preserved naming ability in HS patients, following anterior temporal resection, might be attributable, at least in part, to intrahemispheric reorganization of language in response to the likely early development of sclerosis in the medial temporal region. These results hold theoretical implications regarding the role of the dominant hippocampus in determining the cortical representation of semantic and lexical information, and raise questions regarding the specific roles of medial and lateral temporal cortex in targeted word retrieval.

Developmental abnormalities of the hippocampus

In a recent study (Agostini *et al.*, 2010), we personally considered anomalies of shape and positioning of the hippocampal formations because they were more and more noted in the results of interpretation of miscellaneous brain MR images. We wanted to know whether these anomalies correspond to a specific clinical picture, and thus decided to look for language difficulties in this population.

Patients and methods

First we compiled brain MRI reports of children examined from January 1, 2007 to April 30, 2008 at the department of neuroradiology in our hospital under the auspices of Prof. Nadine Girard in an attempt to discover hippocampal formation abnormalities (HFAs) in this population. MRI exams were done by the same medical team. In all subjects, MRI scans were acquired on a 1.5–tesla gyroscan; at the least, axial T_2-weighted, coronal FLAIR and high-resolution T_1-weighted 3D MRI scans were obtained. We selected MRI reports that signified HFAs such as: abnormalities of shape (spherical or triangular hippocampus) or orientation (vertical orientation of the hippocampus or of the parahippocampal sulcus). Hippocampal atrophy or mesial sclerosis was excluded.

In a second round we performed some testing in children with isolated HFAs, that is, those children had no other brain anomaly. Tests were necessarily limited to children who had acquired language. They contained different batteries for French-speakers. These included evaluation of oral language (Khomsi, 2001) and tests of syntactic and semantic comprehension (Lecocq, 1996). We joined some subtests of the BREV, a screening battery for rapid evaluation of cognitive functions (Billard, 2000) concerning verbal and visual memory, and a subtest from the NEPSY that is based on phonologic segmentation (from Korkman, 2003).

Results

From January 1, 2007 to April 30, 2008, a total of 2,208 pediatric patients (less than 18 years old) underwent brain MRI. Among them, 96 presented with HFAs. These HFA patients were more often male (61 boys, 35 girls). Among diagnoses that were assigned to these patients before MRI, mental retardation was the most frequent (49 per cent). We found some chromosomal aberrations: one child with trisomy 18, one with trisomy 9p, another with partial trisomy 7, and finally a patient with an unbalanced translocation (t 1–13). There was also a patient with mucopolysaccharidosis type VII. But in these patients, as in 82 out of 96 patients with HFAs, there were also other brain anomalies; cerebral atrophy, corpus callosum anomalies, small frontal lobes, and myelinization disorders were the most frequently associated (Table 1).

Fourteen of the 96 patients (10 boys, 4 girls) presented with isolated HFAs (see Fig. 1).

Table 1. HFAs in 96 MRI brain studies (from January 2007 to April 2008)

Sex	
Male	61
Female	35
Age	2 months–17 years
Clinical context	
Mental retardation, learning disorders	47
Epilepsy	23
Psychotic, autistic, pervasive developmental disorders	22
Language disorders only	18
Hippocampal formations anomalies	
Unilateral, left	14
Prevailing on left side	5
Prevailing on right side	10
Unilateral, right	5
Associated anomalies	
Cerebral atrophy	55
Corpus callosum anomaly	18
Fontal horns with a square aspect	15
Small frontal lobes	9
Myelinization disorders	6
Periventricular heterotopias	1
Malformation Chiari type I	1
Microlissencephaly	1
Myelomeningocele	1
Syringomyelic cavity	1

Nine of these children suffered from behaviour disorders, and among them 5 were autistic and 7 were epileptic (Table 2).

We could assess nine patients of the 14 patients. One of them (patient 3) had quite normal results in all the tests. The other eight patients were divided into two groups according to their results. In the first group, language disorders were very severe and were a part of more global developmental disorders with mental retardation and/or autistic features (Table 3). In the second group, language was specifically disrupted. Disorders of expression and phonologic consciousness predominated. Visual memory was selectively impaired (Table 4)

Table 2. Patients with isolated anomalies of the hippocampal formations

Case	Sex	Age at MRI study	Brain MRI anomalies	Epilepsy	EEG	Language examination (expressive and receptive aspects)
1	F	9	Incomplete folding of the hippocampi; vertical orientation of the parahippocampal sulcus predominating on the left side	Absences	Normal	Pathologic on both sides
2	M	5	Globular shape of the anterior hippocampus	No	ND	Impossible
3	M	8	Vertical orientation and globular shape of the left hippocampus	No	Normal	Normal
4	F	10	Rounded shape of the hippocampi; atrophic parahippocampal gyrus	Temporal seizures	Left posterior focus	Impossible
5	M	5	Unusual shape of both hippocampi, parahippocampal gyri and amygdalas	Unilateral right tonic seizures	Left temporal focus	Pathologic on both sides
6	M	5	Triangular shape of left hippocampus	No	Normal	Disorders predominating on expressive items
7	M	8	Unusual folding of the hippocampi with a global round shape; vertical orientation of the parahippocampal sulcus	No	Normal	Pathologic expressive language
8	F	14	Unusual folding of the left hippocampus with vertical orientation of the left parahippocampal sulcus	Generalized seizures; myoclonias	Temporal and parietal; bilateral foci	Impossible
9	F	4	Malrotation of the anterior parts of both hippocampi (vertical orientation) especially on the right side	Loss of awareness of surroundings; sensitive hallucinations	Right temporal focus during sleep	Deficiency in verbal memory
10	M	6	Incomplete folding of the hippocampi predominating on the left side	Staring, trismus, vomiting	Left parieto-occi-pital focus	Pathologic language predominating on expressive language
11	M	14	Small right hippocampus	Staring; left clonic seizures	Right temporal focus	Pathologic on both sides
12	M	6	Rounded shape and vertical orientation of both hippocampi	No	Normal	Pathologic on both sides
13	M	15	Incomplete folding of the hippocampi predominating on the right side	No	ND	ND
14	M	6	Vertical orientation of both hippocampi	Right temporal seizures	Left temporal focus	Impossible

F, female; M, male; ND, not done; MRI, magnetic resonance imaging; EEG, electroencephalogram.

Table 3. Language evaluation for the patients with isolated HFA and global development disorder

Patient	1	5	11	12
Age	10 years, 1 month	7 years	15 years, 6 months	8 years
School	CLIS	SEES	No schooling; at home	CLIS
Receptive items				
• Lexicon				
Reception	– 1.24σ	– 2.70σ	– 7.50σ	– 1,10σ
• Syntax				
Understanding	– 3.90σ	– 1.96σ	– 4.46σ	– 0.75σ
ECOSSE	– 5.80σ	ND	– 14.47σ	– 6.71σ
Expressive items				
• Lexicon				
Production (images naming)	– 4.35σ	– 1.74σ	– 7.50σ	– 3.30σ
• Syntax				
Utterances repetition	– 2.21σ	ND	ND	ND
Utterances production	– 5.40σ	ND	ND	ND
• Phonology				
Words repetition	– 11.66σ	ND	– 55.40σ	– 8.17σ
Visual memory				
Objects locations	– 5.30σ	ND	ND	– 5.42σ
Verbal memory				
Digits	– 2.66σ	ND	ND	ND
Words	– 3.00σ	ND	ND	ND
Sentences	– 1.14σ	ND	ND	ND

CLIS, special class for children with disabilities; SEES, section for specialized teaching and education; ECOSSE, test for syntactic and semantic understanding; ND, not done

Table 4. Language evaluation for the patients with isolated HFAs and without global development disorder

Patient	3	6	7	9	10
Age	9 years, 7 months	6 years, 7 months	10 years	4 years, 1 month	8 years
School	'CM1' 4th year in primary school	'CP' 1st year in primary school	'CM1' 4th year in elementary school	Nursery school	'CE1' 2nd year in elementary school
Receptive items					
• Lexicon					
Reception	+0.19σ	−1.10σ	−0,90σ	+0.58σ	+0.95σ
• Syntax					
Understanding	+0.20σ	−1.80σ	−0,35σ	+0.17σ	+0.92σ
ECOSSE	+0,.32σ	−1.60σ	−0.44σ	NR	−0.26σ
Expressive items					
• Lexicon					
Production (images naming)	+2.12σ	−1.40σ	−1.40σ	+0.14σ	−2.20σ
• Syntax					
Utterances (repetition)	ND (acquired)	ND (acquired)	ND (acquired)	−0.50σ	ND (acquired)
Utterances (production)	+1.10σ	−2.52σ	−0.90σ	−0.24σ	−0.16σ
• Phonology					
Words repetition	+0.60σ	−4.50σ	−4.25σ	+0.15σ	+0.30σ
Visual memory					
Object location	+0.42σ	−1.50σ	−1.60σ	−1.50σ	−2.00σ
Verbal memory					
Digits	−0.66σ	−1.20σ	−0.70σ	ND	−0.33σ
Words	+0.30σ	−0.20σ	+0.33σ	−2.16σ	−0.36σ
Sentences	−0.20σ	−0.90σ	+0,.05σ	ND	+0.50σ

ECOSSE, test for syntactic and semantic understanding; ND, not done.

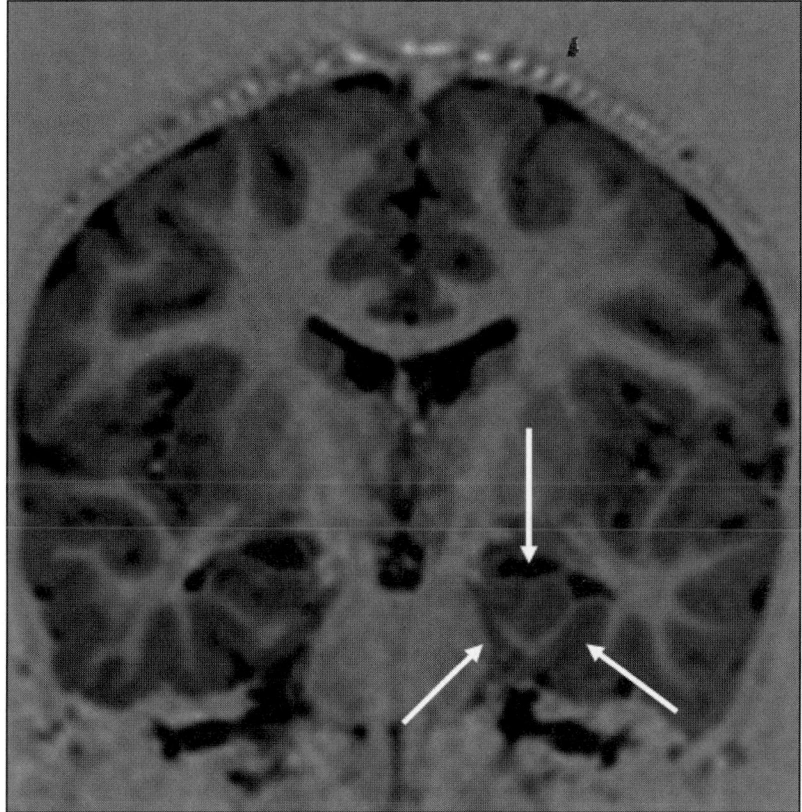

Fig. 1. Brain MRI in patient 6: coronal T_1-weighted inversion recovery sequence. White arrows point to triangular aspect of the left hippocampus with bad infolding.

Comments

HFA appeared frequently (4.3 per cent) among all MRI examinations and was often associated with developmental problems. In the literature, HFAs were reported to be associated with some syndromes, such as the Opitz syndrome (Fitoz *et al.*, 2003), Muenke syndrome (Riedl *et al.*, 2008), and septo-optic dysplasia (Grosso *et al.*, 2003); they were also sometimes associated with FGFR3 gene mutations (Tokumaru *et al.*, 1996; Hevner, 2005).

There are other circumstances of genetic pathology. Many causes, especially genetic ones, could explain the occurrence of HFA. SOX2 mutations were found in subjects with HFA and periventricular heterotopias (Sisodiya *et al.*, 2006). In another patient with DCX mutation, HFA was associated with corpus callosum agenesis (Kappeler *et al.*, 2007), allowing us to speculate that HFA could be associated with more subtle cortical dysgenesis. The co-occurrence of HFAs and malformation of cortical development (MCD) was reported recently (Kuchukhidze *et al.*, 2010). In this study, HFAs were present in 63 per cent of patients with heterotopia, in 41 per cent of those with micropolygyria, and in 38 per cent of those with cortical dysplasia, suggesting a common pathogenetic mechanism. If we consider the hippocampal formations, we know that they are the first cortical area to differentiate. With expansion of the dentate gyrus and the cornu Ammonis, infolding of the hippocampus occurs over the parahippocampal gyrus, and the hippocampal formations reach their adult stage, resulting in a nearly horizontal orientation at 18 to 20 weeks of pregnancy. Some HFAs could correspond to earlier stages of hippocampal formation.

At the molecular level, a specific protein, reelin, could play a critical role, as this protein is known to modulate neuronal migration: reelin is a secreted protein that regulates brain layer formation during embryonic development. It is secreted by Cajal–Retzius cells, which are neurons of the human embryonic marginal zone in the neocortex and hippocampus. Mutation of the human reelin gene in involved in lissencephaly, with cerebellar hypoplasia and severe cognitive deficits. Hippocampal Cajal–Retzius cells and the reelin protein are essential for neuronal positioning and formation of specific layer connections (Förster *et al.*, 2006). Reelin expression is reduced in several psychiatric disorders. During the postnatal life, reelin could play a role in synaptic plasticity (Abraham, 2003).

Language disorders

Language disorders were found in nearly all the children with isolated HFA who were tested (8 of 9). We regret that children were not evaluated for IQ. But among them, it was impossible to test the first group, and because the second group attended normal schools, we can infer that their IQ was in the normal range. In the first group (Table 3) language disorders were very severe, affecting all the components of language: lexicon, syntax and especially phonology. Pragmatic aspects were not specifically tested but were disrupted in all these four children. In the second group (Table 4) receptive language was correct; we noticed disturbances in several aspects of expressive language such as lexicon, verbal fluency, syntax and phonology. Spatial memory also appeared to be disrupted. The clinical picture of the first group could be connected with the disorders observed in bilateral hippocampal sclerosis (DeLong & Heinz, 1997). In the second group the more subtle anomalies could be connected with the different roles of the hippocampus in lexical and syntactic organization (Breitenstein *et al.*, 2005; Meyer *et al.*, 2005). In our small population with isolated HFAs, difficulties in naming did not appear to be specifically linked to left HFAs, unlike findings in other studies considering hippocampal sclerosis (Hamberger *et al.*, 2007).

Associated disorders

Among 14 patients with HFAs, 7 were epileptic; and 2 of them were in the second group. The observation of HFAs was already reported in children who were operated on for severe epilepsy (Lehéricy *et al.*, 1996). In adults, HFAs are often associated with other brain development anomalies and with TLE, and there is no relation between lateralization of the epileptic focus and lateralization of HFAs (Bernasconi *et al.*, 2005; Peltier *et al.*, 2005). Similarly, we did not find this type of correlation in our children. But, although it is difficult to draw some conclusions from our small population, epilepsy *per se* and antiepileptic treatment did not seem to play a direct role in language disorders.

Among our population with HFA some children could not be evaluated because of their severe comportment disorder. Some of them did not acquire any language. In autistic subjects, MRI has evidenced some anomalies that appear very different in each subject, such as augmentation of brain volume (Sparks *et al.*, 2002) or cerebellar hypoplasia (Pierce, 2001). Recently, in a retrospective study concerning 77 MRI scans from autistic children, Boddaert *et al.* (2009) suggested that temporal lobe anomalies were implicated in autistic disorders for 20 of them. In another study, some correlations were found between autistic or pervasive developmental disorders and the volume of HF (Hrdlicka *et al.*, 2005). More precisely, this type of disorder was correlated with a disturbance of memories, especially the episodic memory, as well as with HFA (Salmond *et al.*, 2005). Again, in a more recent study, Dager *et al.* (2007) mentioned HFA in children with autistic spectrum disorders, explaining them as resulting from functional deficits of the mesial temporal lobe.

Conclusions

We studied isolated HFAs in 14 children. Among them, we noticed the presence of some language disorders. These disorders were mostly of expressive language and seemed to be associated with visual memory disturbances. This point has to be confirmed with a more precise evaluation. These children suffered as well from impulsivity and attention deficit. Epilepsy was very frequent in this population, as were behavioural disorders. There was no correlation between language disorders and epilepsy. This first approach to the study of children with isolated HFAs has to be enhanced by further prospective studies with more evaluative tools and a greater number of subjects when possible. Functional MRI with language paradigms would be a welcome addition to such studies.

References

Abraham, H. (2003): Reelin-expressing neurons in the postnatal and adult human hippocampal formation. *Hippocampus* **13,** 715–722

Agostini, G., Mancini, J., Chabrol, B., Villeneuve, N., Milh, M., George, F., *et al.* (2010): Troubles du langage chez les enfants porteurs d'anomalies morphologiques de l'hippocampe. *Arch. Pediatr.* **17,** 1008–1016.

Bernasconi, N., Kinay, D., Andermann, F. & Bernasconi, A. (2005): Analysis of shape and positioning of the hippocampal formation: an MRI study in patients with partial epilepsy and healthy controls. *Brain* **128,** 2442–2452.

Billard, C. (2000): *BREV: Une batterie rapide d'évaluation des fonctions cognitives*. Paris: Signes.

Boddaert, N., Zilbovicius, M., Philipe, A., Robel, L., Bourgeois, M., Barthélemy, C., *et al.* (2009): MRI findings in 77 children with non-syndromic autistic disorder. *PLoS ONE* **4**(2): e4415.

Breitenstein, C. *et al.* (2005): Hippocampus activity differentiates good from poor learners of a novel lexicon, *NeuroImage* **25,** 958–968.

Dager, S.R., Wang, L., Friedman, S.D., Constantino, J.N., Artru, A.A., Dawson, G. & Csernansky J.G. (2007): Shape mapping of the hippocampus in young children with autism spectrum disorder. *AJNR Am. J. Neuroradiol.*, **28,** 672–677.

Davachi, L. & Wagner, A.D. (2002): Hippocampal contribution to episodical encoding: insights from relational and item-based learning. *J. Neurophysiol.* **88,** 982–990.

DeLong, G.R. & Heinz, E.R. (1997): The clinical syndrome of early-life bilateral hippocampal sclerosis. *Ann. Neurol.* **42,** 11–17.

Fitoz, S., Atasoy, C., Deda, G., Erden, I. & Akyar, S. (2003): Hippocampal malrotation with normal corpus callosum in a child with Opitz syndrome. *Clin. Imaging* **27,** 75–76.

Förster, E., Jossin, Y., Zhao, S., Chai, X., Frotscher, M. & Goffinet, A.M. (2006): Recent progress in understanding the role of reelin in radial neuronal migration, with specific emphasis on the dentate gyrus. *Eur. J. Neurosci.* **23,** 901–909.

Gabrieli, J.D., Cohen, N.J. & Corkin, S. (1988): The impaired learning of semantic knowledge following bilateral medial temporal-lobe resection. *Brain Cognit.* **7,** 157–177.

Grosso, S., Farnetani, M.A., Berardi, R., Bartalini, G., Carpentieri, M., Galluzzi, P., *et al.* (2003): Medial temporal lobe dysgenesis in Muenke syndrome and hypochondroplasia. *Am. J. Med. Genet.* **120A,** 88–91.

Hamberger, M.J., Seidel, W.T., Goodman, R.R., Williams, A., Perrine, K., Devinsky, O. & McKhann, G.M., 2nd (2007): Evidence for cortical reorganization of language in patients with hippocampal sclerosis. *Brain* **130,** 2942–2950.

Hevner, R.F. (2005): The cerebral cortex malformation in thanatophoric dysplasia: neuropathology and pathogenesis. *Acta Neuropathol.* **110,** 208–221.

Hrdlicka, M., Dudova, I., Beranova, I., Lisy, J., Belsan, T., Neuwirth, J., *et al.* (2005): Subtypes of autism by cluster analysis based on structural MRI data. *Eur. Child Adolesc. Psychiatry* **14,** 138–144.

Jansen, A., Liuzzi, G., Deppe, M., Kanowski, M., Olschläger, C., Albers, J.M., *et al.* (2010): Structural correlates of functional language dominance: a voxel based morphometry study. *J. Neuroimaging* **20,** 148–156.

Kappeler, C., Dhenain, M., Phan Dinh Tuy, F., Saillour, Y., Marty, S., Fallet-Bianco, C., *et al.* (2007): Magnetic resonance imaging and histological studies of corpus callosal and hippocampal abnormalities linked to doublecortin deficiency. *J. Comp. Neurol.* **500,** 239–254.

Khomsi, A. (2001): *ELO – Évaluation du langage oral.* Paris: ECPA edition.

Knecht, S. (2004): Does language lateralization depend on the hippocampus? *Brain* **127,** 1217–1218.

Korkman, M., Kirk, U. & Kemp, S. & NEPSY A (2003): *Developmental NEuroloPSYcological Assessment: version française*. Paris: ECPA edition.

Kuchukhidze, G., Koppelstaetter, F., Unterberger, I., Dobesberger, J., Walser, G., Zamarian, L., *et al.* (2010): Hippocampal abnormalities in malformations of cortical development: MRI study. *Neurology* **74,** 1575–1582.

Kumaran, D., Summerfield, J.J., Hassabis, D. & Maguire, E.A. (2009): Tracking the emergence of conceptual knowledge during human decision making, *Neuron* **63,** 889–901.

Lecocq, P. (1996): *ECOSSE, Epreuve de Compréhension Syntaxico-Sémantique*. Villeneuve d'Ascq: Presses Universitaires du Septentrion.

Lehéricy, S., Dormont, D., Sémah, F., Clémenceau, S., Granat, O., Marsault, C. & Baulac, M. (1995): Developmental abnormalities of the medial temporal lobe in patients with temporal lobe epilepsy. *AJNR Am. J. Neuroradiol.* **16,** 617–626.

Liégeois, F., Connelly, A., Cross, H., Boyd, S.G., Gadian, D.G., Vargha Khadem, F. & Baldeweg, T (2004): Language reorganization in children with early onset lesions of the left hemisphere: an fMRI study. *Brain* **127,** 1229–1236.

Meyer, P., Mecklinger, A., Grunwald, T., Fell, J., Elger, C.E. & Friederici, A.D. (2005): Language processing within the human medial temporal lobe. *Hippocampus* **15,** 451–459.

Opitz, B. & Friederici, A.D. (2003): Interactions of the hippocampal system and the prefrontal cortex in learning language-like rules. *NeuroImage* **19,** 1730–1737.

Opitz, B. & Friederici, A.D. (2004): Brain correlates of language learning: the neuronal dissociation of rule-based versus similarity-based learning. *J. Neurosci.* **24,** 8436–8440.

Peltier, B., Hurtevent, P., Trehan, G., Derambure, P., Pruvo, J.P. & Soto-Ares, G. (2005): MRI of hippocampal malformations in patients with intractable temporal lobe epilepsy. *J. Radiol.* **86,** 69–75.

Pierce, K. (2001): Evidence for a cerebellar role in reduced exploration and stereotyped behavior in autism. *Biol Psychiatry* **49,** 655–664.

Riedl, S., Vosahlo, J. & Battelino, T. (2008): Refining clinical phenotypes in septo-optic dysplasia based on MRI findings. *Eur. J. Pediatr.* **167,** 1269–1276.

Salmond, C.H., Ashburner, J., Connelly, A., Friston, K.J., Gadian, D.G. & Vargha-Khadem, F. (2005): The role of the medial temporal lobe in autistic spectrum disorders. *Eur. J. Neurosci.* **22,** 764–772.

Sisodiya, S.M., Ragge, N.K., Cavalleri, G.L., Hever, A., Lorenz, B., Schneider, A., *et al.* (2006): Role of SOX2 mutations in human hippocampal malformations and epilepsy. *Epilepsia* **47,** 534–542.

Sparks, B.F., Friedman, S.D., Shaw, D.W., Aylward, E.H., Echelard, D., Artru, A.A., *et al.* (2002): Brain structural abnormalities in young children with autism spectrum disorder. *Neurology* **59,** 184–192.

Tokumaru, A.M., Barkovich, J., Ciricillo, S.F. & Edwards, M.S. (1996): Skull base and calvarial deformities: association with intracranial changes in craniofacial syndromes. *AJNR Am. J. Neuroradiol.* **17,** 619–630.

Ullman, M.T. (2004): Contributions of memory circuits to language: the declarative/procedural model. *Cognition* **92,** 231–270.

Weber, B., Wellmer, J., Reuber, M., Mormann, F., Weis, S., Urbach, H., *et al.* (2006): Left hippocampal pathology is associated with atypical language lateralization in patients with epilepsy. *Brain* **129,** 346–351.

Brain Lesion Localization and Developmental Functions, D. Riva, C. Njiokiktjien and S. Bulgheroni (eds.)

Chapter 12

Hippocampus, neurotrophic factors and depression: possible targets for antidepressant medication

Gabriele Masi, Paola Brovedani and Angela Magazù

IRCCS Stella Maris, Scientific Institute of Child Neurology and Psychiatry, via dei Giacinti 2, 56128 Calambrone, Pisa, Italy
gabriele.masi@inpe.unipi.it

Summary

Depression is a frequent and debilitating mental disorder affecting as much as 15 per cent of the population with at least one episode during life, resulting in huge costs for society. The neurobiologic mechanisms of depression are not well known, but an interplay between genetic and environmental factors is hypothesized. Antidepressant medications are frequently used in depression, but at least 50 per cent of the patients are poor responders, clinical response occurs after weeks to months of treatment, and only chronic treatment can be effective, suggesting that the action of these agents is beyond the rapid enhancing effect on the monoaminergic systems. An impairment of synaptic plasticity (neurogenesis, axon branching, dendritogenesis, and synaptogenesis) in specific areas of the CNS, mainly the hippocampus, is related to alterations in the levels of neurotrophic factors, such as BDNF, which may be implicated in the pathophysiology of depression. Because BDNF is repressed by stress and increased by antidepressants, epigenetic regulation of the BDNF gene may play an important role in depression and its response to antidepressants. Environmental stressors triggering activation of the hypothalamic-pituitary-adrenal (HPA) axis cause the brain to be exposed to corticosteroids, affecting neurobehavioral functions with a strong down-regulation of hippocampal neurogenesis, and are thus a major risk factor for depression. Antidepressant treatment stimulates neurogenesis and reverses the inhibitory effects of stress, but this effect is evident only after 3–4 weeks of drug administration, the time course for maturation of new neurons. The ablation of hippocampal neurogenesis blocks the behavioural effects of antidepressants in animal models. These findings suggest new possible targets for pharmacotherapy.

Introduction

Depression is a highly prevalent and debilitating mental disorder, affecting up to 15 per cent of the population at least once during the lifetime, and carrying huge costs for society. Depression can begin early in life and it is estimated to affect, at any time, about 1 to 2 per cent of prepubertal children and 4 to 6 per cent of adolescents (Kessler *et al.*, 2001). Suicide accounts for about 2 per cent of the world's deaths, is among the 10 leading causes of death at all ages, and is the third largest cause of death among adolescents in the USA (Evans *et al.*, 2005). The neurobiologic mechanisms of depression are still not well known, although there is consensus about an interplay between genetic and environmental factors. The monoamine hypothesis of depression, based on a deficiency or imbalance of monoamine neurotransmitters (serotonin, norepinephrine, and dopamine), has been the leading explanation for the last 50 years, supported by the enhancing effect of all antidepressants on the monoaminergic systems (Manji *et al.*, 2000). Antidepressant medications are frequently used in depression, both in adults and in children and adolescents. However, at least 50 per cent of the patients are poor responders, even to more recently discovered medications. Furthermore, clinical response occurs only after weeks to months of treatment and often only chronic treatment can be obtained, suggesting that an adaptation of downstream events (*i.e.*, lasting changes in gene expression) is needed for greater efficacy. These events may result in long-lasting changes in the brain, beyond a simple and reductive relationship between monoamines and depression, which may be only the initiation of the antidepressant action.

Recent studies indicate that an impairment of synaptic plasticity in specific areas of the CNS, including the prefrontal cortex, amygdala, subgenual cingulate cortex, and most importantly, the hippocampus, resulting in an abnormal structural remodeling of these areas, may contribute to the pathophysiology of depression (Berton & Nestler, 2006). This abnormal neural plasticity may be related to alterations in the levels of neurotrophic factors, which play a central role in cellular proliferation (neurogenesis), migration, differentiation, and maintenance in the developing brain.

The relationship between adult hippocampal neurogenesis and depression is supported by the following findings: (1) stress inhibits hippocampal neurogenesis and is a risk factor for depression; (2) depressed patients have smaller hippocampal volumes; (3) antidepressant treatment stimulates neurogenesis and reverses the inhibitory effects of stress; (4) antidepressant effect is evident only after 3 to 4 weeks of administration, the time course for maturation of new neurons; and (5) ablation of hippocampal neurogenesis blocks the behavioural effects of antidepressants in mice.

Stress plays a major role in the precipitation or worsening of depression and other mental disorders. Environmental stressors, both internal and external, which trigger activation of the hypothalamic-pituitary-adrenal (HPA) axis, result in cortisol hypersecretion, exposing the brain to corticosteroids in the short- and long-term. These phenomena can negatively affect neurobehavioural functions of various brain structures and determine a strong downregulation of neurogenesis (Duman *et al.*, 2001). These effects are modulated by individual differences in the basal levels of the HPA axis or in the response to stressors, which are related to genetic factors or to early exposure to traumatic experiences in prenatal or neonatal life, and are possible predictors for individuals at risk (Cushing & Kramer, 2005).

However, most of the evidence of adult neurogenesis in specific areas of the CNS was found in animal models, particularly rodents. Some caveats limit extending these animal findings to humans. Possible differences in neurogenesis may reflect the different position of the animals in the evolutionary scale, as the hippocampus, amygdala, and olfactory circuits are particularly important for survival in sub-primates, whereas the cortex is pivotal in primates and humans. Considerations that should be kept in mind that may limit the implication of hippocampal neurogenesis in human depression include the following: (1) The rate of neurogenesis in the adult mammalian brain – the hippocampus as well as the olfactory bulb, neocortex, striatum, amygdala, and substantia nigra – is still uncertain (Gould, 2007). (2) The number of new neurons after antidepressant treatment in humans is low (Boldrini *et al.*, 2009). (3) Besides antidepressants, other psychotropic drugs induce neurogenesis in rodents, but they do not have an antidepressant effect in depressed patients. (4) Knock-out mice without adult brain neurogenesis do not show abnormal emotional responses or anxiety-like behaviours, compared to wild-type controls. (5) Severe bilateral hippocampal atrophy in human infants, attributable to perinatal hypoxic-ischaemic damage, is associated with later-occurring invalidating memory impairments, but no depressive symptoms are reported in these patients (Gadian *et al.*, 2000). (6) The relationship between neurotrophic factors and depression is partly controversial, as in some animal models depressogenic properties have been reported outside the hippocampus (*i.e.*, in the ventral-tegmental area) (Groves, 2007).

In this review evidence supporting a possible major role of hippocampal plasticity, particularly neurogenesis and neurotrophic factors, will be discussed in detail. Implications for pharmacotherapy of depression will be considered in the last section.

The hippocampus–depression relationship: cause or consequence?

The hippocampus is particularly sensitive to stress, given its prolonged ontogeny, postnatal neurogenesis, and high levels of glucocorticoid receptors, which are hypothesized to account for the smaller hippocampal volume in both subjects with early trauma and in those with depression (Banasr & Duman, 2007). Depression is associated with significant hippocampal atrophy, which persists after remission of depression (MacQueen *et al.*, 2003; Sheline *et al.*, 1996), with more prolonged depressions being associated with more severe atrophy (Sapolsky, 2001). However, the relation among hippocampal volume reduction, depression, and early trauma is far from clear, *i.e.*, we cannot tell whether smaller hippocampal size is a *consequence* of depression or a *pre-existing marker* for vulnerability to depression. It is well demonstrated that depressive episodes can induce further changes in hippocampal volumetry, especially in patients in whom a depressive episode failed to remit (Frodl *et al.*, 2008). However, growing evidence supports the notion of reduced hippocampal volume even before the occurrence of early-onset depressive manifestations in high-risk patients (MacMaster *et al.*, 2008; Rao *et al.*, 2010), including those with high familial risk for depression (Chen *et al.*, 2010). Smaller hippocampal volume may be a vulnerability marker for depression. However, it must be emphasized that reduction of hippocampal volume and decreased neurogenesis have been reported in other psychiatric disorders such as schizophrenia, bipolar disorder, dementia, substance addiction, and anxiety.

Pathophysiology of hippocampal morphologic changes in depression

Mechanisms implicated in hippocampal atrophy in depression have been extensively investigated in animal models, with evidence of both a reduction of hippocampal volume and a decrease of neurogenesis (Czéh *et al.*, 2001). Prenatal stress in rhesus monkeys decreases adult neurogenesis in the hippocampus and is associated with exacerbated emotional behaviour (Coe *et al.*, 2003).

Inescapable stress reduces neurogenesis and is associated with behavioural despair in a learned helplessness animal model of depression, with reversal after fluoxetine treatment (Malberg & Duman, 2003). Repeated stress can also alter the dendritic morphology of a population of hippocampal neurons, named CA3 pyramidal neurons, with decreased arborisation (McEwen, 2000).

A recent study of Hajszan and colleagues (2009) analyzed hippocampal changes in male rats after a learned helplessness paradigm, using electron microscopy, which provides sufficient resolution to visualize synaptic specializations. The study demonstrated, at the ultrastructural level, that hippocampal spine synapses undergo strong remodeling parallel to behavioural changes in this rat model of depression. Stress induced an acute and persistent loss of spine synapses in hippocampus (CA1, CA3, and dentate gyrus), associated with an acute and persistent helpless behaviour pattern. Changes in spine synapses did not occur in the motor cortex, indicating that this negative effect is not uniform in the cortical areas. Similar changes occurred after injection of corticosterone, indicating that a surge of corticosteroid levels is sufficient to induce the observed deficits. A 6-day treatment with an antidepressant (desipramine) reversed cellular and behavioural effects, while shorter treatments (1- and 3-day) were ineffective at both the cellular and behavioural levels. Similar effects of average soma size of hippocampal pyramidal neurons and of spine synapse remodeling were found in sections of hippocampal formation of patients with major depression, and these alterations could be attenuated or reversed by antidepressants (Stockmeyer *et al.*, 2004). More recent evidence indicates that the antidepressant fluoxetine can reverse the state of neuronal maturation in hippocampal granule cells in adult mice, with positive effects, by reinstating neuronal functions that were lost during development (Kobayashi *et al.*, 2010).

Hippocampal neurogenesis

Until recently, a dogmatic belief was that when the brain reached an adult level of development, the capacity for adding new neurons was lost. Although several reports of postnatal neuronal proliferation were published during the twentieth century, including neurogenesis in the rat hippocampus (Altman & Das, 1965), no consensus was reached, and these findings were forgotten for at least 20 years because of lack of definitive evidence on adult neurogenesis, as well as uncertainty about the clinical implications of this finding. During the 1990s, clear evidence of neural cell proliferation throughout the life span was available, even in humans (Eriksson *et al.*, 1998). The functional meaning of hippocampal neurogenesis in mammals is still uncertain, but it may be hypothesized that it is related to the specific functions of this brain structure, involving processing, storing, and retrieving of experience.

Multiple factors modulating hippocampal neurogenesis are increasingly defined, included exercise, hormones, neurotransmitters, and environment (hippocampus-dependent learning), suggesting a specific implication of neurogenesis in several physiologic mechanisms. Exercise can stimulate neurogenesis, increasing hippocampal volume by 2 per cent after 1 year of moderate-entity aerobic exercise even in older subjects (Erickson *et al.*, 2011) and this effect can be blocked by X-ray hippocampal irradiation (Pereira *et al.*, 2007). Glucocorticoids are associated with a marked reduction in granule cell proliferation caused by stress (Duman *et al.*, 2001).

On the contrary, several types of medications, namely antidepressants, but also mood stabilizers and some antipsychotics, are associated with a stimulation of hippocampal neurogenesis (Jope, 2003; Malberg *et al.*, 2000; Nasrallah *et al.*, 2010). Almost all antidepressants, including serotonin and/or noradrenaline reuptake inhibitors and tianeptine, and the new antidepressant agomelatine (with agonism on both melatonin and 5-$HT_{2B/C}$ receptors) increase proliferation and maturation of newborn cells and these effects, added to increased survival, may all enhance the long-term plasticity in the dentate gyrus (Li *et al.*, 2008; Wang *et al.*, 2008). The effect on hippocampal neurogenesis has been related to chronic, but not acute, antidepressant treatment (Malberg & Duman, 2003). A preferential involvement of the 5HT_{1A} receptor in serotonin effect on neuron proliferation has been proposed (Jacobs *et al.*, 2000; Santarelli *et al.*, 2003), even though 5-HT_{2A} and 5-HT_{2C} are involved as well (Banasr *et al.*, 2004). Ablation of hippocampal neurogenesis blocked the antidepressant effect (Czéh *et al.*, 2001; Santarelli *et al.*, 2003). The antidepressant effect may be mediated by hippocampal cell proliferation by antagonizing the reduction of hippocampal neurogenesis observed in animal models of depression and possibly in human patients.

The environmental effects on the function of genes are epigenetic and can operate by means of different mechanisms. A well-characterized example is the modulation of hippocampal glucocorticoid receptors by methylation of DNA and/or acetylation of DNA-associated histones (Waggoner, 2007). A chromatin modeling through methylation of DNA usually silences genes, while histone acetylation facilitates activation of transcription. The transcriptional control of gene expression through epigenetic regulation is not only a source of phenotypic variability, but it can be also related to diseases or to vulnerability for diseases. The long latency before the onset of positive effects of antidepressant treatment may be attributed to enduring changes in the state of chromatin.

A prominent locus of modification is the brain-derived neurotrophic factor (BDNF) gene, and the epigenetic control of BDNF expression has been specifically explored. Because BDNF is repressed by stress or increased by antidepressants, epigenetic regulation of the BDNF gene may play an important role in depression and in antidepressant response. Animal models of depression, such as single immobilization stress (Fuchicami *et al.*, 2009) or social defeat (Tsankova *et al.*, 2006), decrease the levels of BDNF in hippocampus on account of induction of H3-K27 dimethylation and transcriptional repression (Jenuwein & Allis, 2001). Antidepressants reverse repression of BDNF expression by H3 acetylation and H3-K4 methylation at the BDNF promoter region (Tsankova *et al.*, 2006). In this regulation, the role of histone deacetylases (HDACs) is crucial because antidepressants downregulate HDAC5, while overexpression of hippocampal HDAC5 prevents the antidepressant effects (Tsankova *et al.*, 2006). Thus, HDAC inhibitors received attention as possible treatments for depression and related mood disorders (Covington *et al.*, 2009) (see below).

Environmental stressors and the hypothalamic-pituitary-adrenal axis

A disruption of external homeostasis induced by environmental changes, but also perturbations of internal homeostasis, such as lack of food or water or excessive temperature, can activate a series of neural responses increasing the adaptation to environmental challenges. Neurons in the paraventricular nucleus (PVN) of the hypothalamus secrete the corticotrophin-releasing factor (CRF) and arginine/vasopressin (AVP), which stimulates the secretion of adrenocorticotropic hormone (ACTH) from the anterior pituitary gland. The ACTH stimulates the synthesis and release of glucocorticoids (principally cortisol in humans) from the adrenal cortex, which favours the adaptation of the organism to stress through vascular and metabolic effects. The hypothalamic-pituitary-adrenal (HPA) axis is regulated by mineralocorticoid and glucocorticoid receptor negative feedback regulation, but chronic stress can reduce the sensitivity to feedback inhibition. A feedback loop includes certain brain regions such as hippocampus and amygdala. Individual differences in basal levels or in response to stressors may affect the consequences of stress. Individual differences in vulnerability may derive from genetic processes and/or adverse events during prenatal or neonatal life (Weaver *et al.*, 2004).

An epigenetic effect resulting from an abnormal setting of the HPA axis is hypothesized to determine an atypical early neurogenesis, with consequent atypical and vulnerable neural systems. Repeated shifts of cortisol levels in hippocampus may determine a re-set of the control system as an effect of damage of glucocorticoid receptors. Although the phasic rise of cortisol under adverse circumstances may occur across the life span, it may determine different consequences in different ages, such as in the first phases of development, when early experience can more strongly modulate neurogenesis (Karl *et al.*, 2006). In different animal models, adversity and stress during pregnancy can be transmitted to the child with long-lasting effects on brain structures subserving emotion and cognition as maternal and fetal cortisol levels correlate (*e.g.*, Bhatnagar *et al.*, 2005). In rats, low maternal care has been proven to be related to increased methylation of the consensus sequence of a neurotrophic growth factor, NGFI-A, on the promoter of glucocorticoid receptor gene, resulting in a decreased expression of the glucocorticoid receptor in the brain (Weaver *et al.*, 2004). These findings suggest that the sensitive period begins in early prenatal period, and extends far beyond. Further epigenetic events may occur in this vulnerable CNS, and determine new mental illnesses when neural systems subserving cognitive processing become operative.

Stress, inflammatory cytokines, and depression

Some negative mechanisms of stress on neurogenesis can be blocked by the inhibition of the inflammatory cytokines. Pro-inflammatory cytokines, including interleukin-1β (IL-1β), IL-6, and TNF-α induced by injury or infections or psychological stress, have been implicated in depressive behaviour both in rodents and humans, and appear to be an important mediator of the anhedonic effects of stress (Koo & Duman, 2008; Miller *et al.*, 2009). The nuclear-factor κB (NF-κB) is the mediator of the signalling cascade of IL-1β and other cytokines in peripheral immune cells and in the brain (Miller *et al.*, 2009). After early life, chronic stress, social stress, and anxiety increased NF-κB signalling as documented in healthy subjects, but this effect is further enhanced in depressed patients (Pace *et al.*, 2006). Koo and colleagues (2010) have recently explored the role of NF-κB in the action of IL-1β and stress, showing that the effects of stress on hippocampal neurogenesis and the resulting depressive-like behaviours can be blocked by an inhibitor of NF-κB, and similarly with an inhibitor of IL-1β. These effects resulted in involving neural stem-like cells, but not early progenitor cells. The blockade of NF-κB may be useful in both inflammatory processes and in stress-related disorders (Koo *et al.*, 2010).

Neurotrophic factors

Neurotrophic factors play a central role in cellular proliferation, migration, and differentiation and maintenance in the developing brain (Dwivedi, 2009). Their presence is crucial during the entire life span for maintenance of neuronal functions, structural integrity of neurons, and neurogenesis. They regulate plasticity to modulate the strength and number of synaptic connections and neurotransmission. An alteration of the neurotrophic factor system may lead to alterations of neural maintenance and regeneration, structural abnormalities in the brain, and reduction of neural plasticity, resulting in an impairment of individual's ability to adapt to crisis situations.

Special attention has been given to the brain-derived neurotrophic factor (BDNF), which regulates neurogenesis, neuronal survival, maturation of connections, and plasticity (Chao, 2003). The survival rate of immature neurons in the dentate gyrus is decreased in the heterozygote BDNF knockout mice and transgenic mice with dominant negative (truncated) BDNF receptor (TrkB) (Sairanen *et al.*, 2005). It has been proposed that BDNF (and its receptor) may reactivate developmental-like cortical plasticity, with adjustment of neural networks, under appropriate environmental guidance (Castrén & Rantamaki, 2010). BDNF is a dimeric protein found throughout the brain, and is particularly abundant in the hippocampus and the cerebral cortex. The BDNF gene lies on the reverse strand of the chromosome 11p13, and encodes a precursor peptide pro-BDNF (Greenberg *et al.*, 2009). BDNF is expressed by most tissues of the body at relatively high levels (Lommatzsch *et al.*, 2005). Given the difficulty of studying BDNF levels directly in the brain, great interest is devoted to the assessment of BDNF activity peripherally from blood samples (serum, plasma, or whole blood), where BDNF is primarily stored at high levels in platelets. However, information is still lacking about the source of BDNF in the blood, which is probably platelets or, less probably, white cells (lymphocytes) (Pandey *et al.*, 2010). Little evidence is available on its regulation by stress, endocrine factors, or environmental stimuli (Sen *et al.*, 2008). In the brain, many types of stress and adrenal steroids decrease the expression of BDNF in the limbic area in rodents (Duman & Monteggia, 2006), but it is unclear whether the reduction of serum BDNF results from decreased levels of BDNF in the brain, peripheral tissues, or both (Sen *et al.*, 2008).

Given the possible bidirectional movement of BDNF (Karege *et al.*, 2005), it has been hypothesized that serum BDNF may have functional effects on the brain (Sen *et al.*, 2008). These results indicate that serum BDNF may not only be a biomarker of depression, but may also have functional effects on neurogenesis and behaviour. According to Schmidt and Duman (2010), the peripheral infusion of BDNF showed positive effects in animal models of depression and anxiety, and increased hippocampal neurogenesis after 2 weeks. These effects may result from the direct action of BDNF in the brain and/or they may be the consequence of an indirect effect of BDNF on peripheral tissues, with other growth factors, such as IGF-1, transported in the brain.

Different neurotrophic factors may share their mechanism of action and similar mitogenic effects on neural progenitor cells, but they also have complementary, different actions on cellular neuroplasticity, suggesting differential, but overlapping effects among growth factors in proliferation and survival of immature cells. A better understanding of the interactions within this system may contribute to newer insights into the antidepressant action as well as into the pathophysiology of depression and other mental disorders.

The vascular endothelial growth factor (VEGF) has been described in the hippocampus (Warner-Schmidt & Duman, 2007) as having both cytogenic and behavioural actions. The infusion of this peptide produces antidepressant responses in rodent models, while an inhibitor of VEGF receptor blocks the antidepressant neurogenic action (Warner-Schmidt & Duman, 2007). Stress downregulates VEGF in the hippocampus (Heine *et al.*, 2005), an effect that is reversed by antidepressants. Antidepressants induce a proliferation of endothelial cells in the adult hippocampus with a time course similar to that for the induction of neurogenesis. The signalling pathways involve the Flk-1 receptor and the cAMP response binding protein (CREB). VEGF may thus be another critical mediator of antidepressant action and thus a therapeutic target for antidepressant agents.

The B-cell leukaemia/lymphoma 2 (Bcl-2) protein is a member of the family of proteins involved in neuroprotective activity, as it promotes axonal growth and regeneration, protects cell from insults, and stimulates neuronal differentiation. Its activity is increased after treatment with the antidepressants amitriptyline and venlafaxine (Xu *et al.*, 2006), as well as after lithium (Manji & Chen, 2002). Elevated levels of mRNA coding for antiapoptotic protein Bcl-2 have been found in fluoxetine-treated neural stem cells derived from hippocampus (Chiou *et al.*, 2006).

Other growth factors can also operate, such as insulin-like growth factor (IGF-1) (Anderson *et al.*, 2002) and fibroblast growth factor 2 (FGF-2) (Turner *et al.*, 2008), or the glial cell–derived neurotrophic factor (GDNF) (Michel *et al.*, 2008), artemin (ARTN) and NT-3 (Otsuki *et al*, 2008), all of which are decreased in currently depressed patients.

Receptors of neurotrophic factors and intracellular cascade

Neurotrophic factors activate numerous receptors coupled with signal transduction pathways for cellular functions, including the regulation of genes involved in neural plasticity. Most functions of BDNF (and of other neurotrophic factors) are mediated by specific subtypes of the tropomycin receptor kinase (Trk) family of tyrosine kinase receptors. The TrkB is located in the synaptic sites, but further localization occurs at the synaptic sites after neuronal activity, which is critical for synthesis and intracellular targeting of TrkB receptors (Lu *et al.*, 2005). The TrkB receptor can be found in at least two isoforms, the 'full length', mediating the main biological action of BDNF, and the 'truncated' TrkB receptor (TrkB1.T1), without a large part of the intracellular domain (and without the protein tyrosine kinase activity) (Luberg *et al.*, 2010). BDNF signaling is impaired as a consequence of the formation of heterodimers (resulting from both the isoforms), suggesting that the truncated form prevents the induction of a signal transduction mechanism, and acts as a negative modulator of BDNF signaling (Eide *et al.*, 1996). Long-term antidepressant treatment can increase mRNA levels of TrkB in the rat brain (Nibuya *et al.*, 1996), as well as the signaling from TrkB in medial prefrontal cortex and hippocampus (Rantamaki *et al.*, 2007). Thus, similarly to an increase of BDNF expression, TrkB activation is associated with (and/or needed for) the behavioural effect of antidepressants. The survival rate of immature neurons in the dentate gyrus is decreased in the heterozygote BDNF knockout mice and transgenic mice with dominant negative (truncated) TrkB receptor (Sarainen *et al.*, 2005). This decreased survival is reversed by antidepressant treatment, but not in mice with TrkB-negative signaling, indicating that BDNF signaling is needed for the cellular effect of antidepressants (Sarainen *et al.*, 2005).

All neurotrophic factors can bind to the pan75 neurotrophin receptor ($P75^{NTR}$), which plays a role in neurotrophin transport, ligand binding specificity, and Trk receptor functioning, enhancing their ligand affinities (Esposito *et al.*, 2001). When TrkB is less or not activated or absent, the effect of $P75^{NTR}$ is to promote hippocampal neuronal death after neurotrophin action (Friedman, 2000) as an apoptotic mechanism. On the contrary, when TrkB receptors are active, $P75^{NTR}$ is pro-survival instead of pro-apoptotic. Thus, the ratio of TrkB and $P75^{NTR}$ is relevant in neurotrophin function. A polymorphism of the P75, which replaces a serine with a leucine residue, is associated with attempted suicide in young adults with childhood-onset depression (McGregor *et al.*, 2007).

Neurotrophic factors and depression

Increasing evidence has implicated neurotrophic factors in the pathophysiology of depression. The neurotrophic hypothesis of depression and antidepressant treatment is based on the reduction of the expression of neurotrophic factors in limbic structures, especially the hippocampus, after depression and stress (Duman & Monteggia, 2006; Schmidt & Duman, 2007). Antidepressants promote neurotrophic factor gene expression and neurogenesis, principally in the hippocampus and prefrontal cortex. Direct injection of BDNF into the hippocampus of experimental animals resulted in behavioural changes similar to those induced by antidepressant treatment (Shirayama *et al.*, 2002), while effects of antidepressant treatments are blocked in transgenic mice with a dominant negative form of BDNF receptor (TrkB). However, a depressive phenotype is not evident in BDNF deletions mutants or dominant negative TrkB (Saarelainen *et al.*, 2003; Chen *et al.*, 2006), suggesting that these are not genes for diseases, but susceptibility markers for psychologic and physiologic processing (Duman *et al.*, 2007). Although a reduction of BDNF levels in BDNF heterozygous knockout mice does not determine depressive-like symptoms (MacQueen *et al.*, 2001), an overexpression of TrkB reduces anxiety and depressive symptoms in mice (Koponen *et al.*, 2005).

The expression of neurotrophic factors is markedly reduced by stress, an important precipitant of depression, with resulting increased cellular atrophy in limbic and cortical areas of the brain. BDNF expression in animal models of depression can be dysregulated by different types of stressors, both physical and social, including early maternal separation and social defeat, with most evident changes in dentate gyrus of hippocampus (Roceri *et al.*, 2002; Pizarro *et al.*, 2004). Consistent with animal studies, experience in humans supports a role of BDNF in depression. The level of BDNF in serum or platelets of depressed subjects was decreased on account of a reduced release mechanism, and the decrease was negatively correlated with the severity of depression in female patients with lower BDNF levels (Karege *et al.*, 2005). Two meta-analyses have further supported the notion that BDNF is lower in depressed patients and that these levels significantly increase after antidepressant treatment (Brunoni *et al.*, 2008; Sen *et al.*, 2008). Another recent study found decreased levels of platelet BDNF in depressed patients, both suicidal and nonsuicidal, but not in platelet-poor plasma, indicating the importance of studying BDNF in platelets (Lee & Kim, 2009). Finally, a recent analysis including both children/adolescents and adults with depression found that levels of BDNF mRNA in the lymphocytes and protein levels in platelets were significantly lower in both paediatric and adult patients compared with matched healthy controls, without a correlation with severity of illness (Pandey *et al.*, 2010).

These effects can be reversed by antidepressants, which can reverse the downregulation of BDNF caused by stress (Alfonso *et al.*, 2006; Nibuya *et al.*, 1996; Shirayama *et al.*, 2002). Behavioural effects of two different classes of antidepressants, such as SSRIs (fluoxetine) and tricyclics (desipramine), in BDNF-deficient mice are abolished (Saarelainen *et al.*, 2003), suggesting that BDNF plays a crucial role in the antidepressant behavioural effect.

Although preclinical and clinical evidence supports a role of BDNF in the pathophysiology of depression and in mechanisms of antidepressants, some studies are inconsistent with this putative model (Groves, 2007). Mice reared in communal nests presented increased levels of BDNF and depressive-like behaviours in a forced-swim paradigm (Branchi *et al.*, 2006). Infusion of BDNF into the ventral tegmental area induced a pro-depressive effect, while suppression of the BDNF receptor TrkB delivered antidepressive-like effects (Eisch *et al.*, 2003). Social stresses in animal models are associated with increased levels of BDNF in nucleus accumbens and depressive-like behaviours, blocked by BDNF repression in the ventral tegmental area (Berton *et al.*, 2006). These authors suggest that an intact BDNF system in the ventral tegmental area–nucleus accumbens pathway is necessary for the development of depressive-like symptoms in this animal model. Functional properties in this pathway seem to be the opposite of those reported for the hippocampus, indicating that symptomatology and pathophysiology of depression may be related to diverse and regionally specific neurotrophin function (Groves, 2007).

BDNF alleles and depression

Single nucleotide polymorphisms (SNPs) in the BDNF gene may contribute to brain dysfunction and therefore to mood disorders. A single nucleotide polymorphism at nucleotide 196 encodes a variant at codon 66 (Val66-Met), with effect on the activity-dependent BDNF secretion, even when BDNF levels are unchanged (Chen *et al.*, 2004). Mice with the Met/Met or Val/Met alleles of BDNF have a smaller hippocampus, and those with Met/Met a reduced dendritic complexity, compared to that of wild-type mice (Chen *et al.*, 2004).

The role of the Val66-Met polymorphism has been explored in 152 depressed patients and 255 healthy controls (Tsai *et al.*, 2003). No significant differences were found between affected and unaffected subjects for the allele frequency of BDNF polymorphism. Similarly, Choi *et al.* (2006) failed to find differences between depressed and undepressed individuals according to Val66-Met polymorphism. Although association studies did not support a direct effect of this polymorphism on mood disorders (Groves, 2007), an association with neuroticism, a personality trait that increases the susceptibility to depression (Sen *et al.*, 2003) and with a history of childhood depression have been reported (Strauss *et al.*, 2005). Furthermore, in 100 mother–daughter pairs from a high-risk population, adolescents with Val66-Met and their mothers presented more depressive symptoms and a ruminative response style (Hilt *et al.*, 2007).

Subjects with the Met allele of BDNF and the short (s) form of the 5-HTTLPR are found to have an increased risk of depression when a prior stress (maltreatment) has occurred (three-way gene × gene × environment interaction) (Kaufman *et al.*, 2004, 2006). These studies suggest that this genetic combination (gene to gene interaction) increases the risk of the environmental event, and thus affects the vulnerability/resilience balance. A study including healthy adult individuals supported the notion that both Val66-Met polymorphism of BDNF and the 5-HTTLPR polymorphism mediated the effect of early adversity on adult depression (Aguilera *et al.*, 2009).

Hippocampus and suicidal risk

Suicidal behaviour is often seen as a complication of major depression. Altered synaptic and structural plasticity in depressed patients has been related to suicidal behaviour. The inability of the brain to make adaptive responses to environmental stimuli may result from impaired structural plasticity, as supported by studies indicating altered brain structures in suicidal subjects (cell number, neuronal and glial density, cell body size in frontal cortex and hippocampus) (Dwivedi, 2009). In post-mortem studies of suicidal individuals, levels of BDNF mRNA and circulating protein were significantly reduced in both hippocampus and prefrontal cortex, compared to healthy control subjects, and irrespective of a concurrent diagnosis of depression (Dwivedi *et al.*, 2003). This finding has been replicated by Karege *et al.* (2005), with the additional observation that suicidal patients receiving antidepressant had normal levels of BDNF. Kim *et al.* (2007) compared plasma BDNF levels in depressed persons who attempted suicide, depressed but not suicidal patients, and healthy controls, and found significantly lower BDNF levels in depressed suicidal patients. These findings suggest that low plasma BDNF levels may be related to suicidal behaviour in depression.

Also the expression of TrkB receptors is decreased in hippocampus and prefrontal cortex of individuals who committed suicide, but only in the full-length (full-functional) isoform (Dwivedi *et al.*, 2003). This decrease may influence both BDNF-induced signaling and the maintenance of neurons. The role of the impairment of TrkB receptor is supported by the finding that tyrosine phosphorylation of full-length receptor is decreased in brains of suicidal patients (Dwivedi *et al.*, 2009).

As reported above, a polymorphism of the P75, who replaces a serine with a leucine residue, has been found to be associated with attempted suicide in young adults with childhood-onset mood disorder (McGregor *et al.*, 2007). An investigation of post-mortem brain in adolescents who committed suicide showed that the protein expression of BDNF was significantly decreased in the prefrontal cortex, but not in hippocampus, while a decrease in BDNF mRNA was observed in both the brain areas (Pandey *et al.*, 2008).Whether these findings indicate developmental differences in pathophysiology of suicide is still matter of research, as these mechanisms may be more or less directly related to a greater vulnerability to suicide (or other mental or behavioural disorders).

BDNF levels in diagnosis, prognosis and treatment response

Although the relationship between BDNF levels in depressed patients before and after antidepressant treatment has been supported by empirical evidence, its implication in pathophysiology of depression must be supported by further studies. The measures of BDNF mRNA and protein may be a relevant biomarker of disease, and a possible predictor of antidepressant response. The availability of biomarkers may be helpful for the diagnosis of depression, a still unmet goal for researchers and clinicians. The simplicity of the test and the consistency of findings of reduced BDNF in depressed subjects support its utility as biomarker. The specificity of this finding needs further research, as reduced BDNF has been found in schizophrenia, bipolar disorder, eating disorders (both bulimia and anorexia nervosa), autism, and even in general medical diseases, such as lower respiratory infections or type-2 diabetes (Sen *et al.*, 2008). It is unknown whether all these disorders share a basic mechanism, which may explain some comorbidities.

Study of BDNF levels may be useful in predicting the efficacy of novel antidepressants or in predicting an individual's sensitivity to a specific antidepressant at an early time point (Pandey *et al.*, 2010). However, a similar increase of BDNF levels has been found after other conditions, including specific food intake, stress, or exercise The effect of these conditions on BDNF in depressed *versus* undepressed subjects, as well their antidepressant effect in clinical patients, is still uncertain.

These studies support the importance of determining mRNA of neurotrophic factors in depressed patients. Determining lymphocyte gene expression of BDNF and BDNF in platelets or serum may be a good peripheral biomarker for depression both in paediatric and adult patients or as a predictor of antidepressant response (Pandey *et al.*, 2010).

Whether these research findings may imply a possible window of opportunity for intervention to improve the prognosis in depressed patients, through pharmacotherapy and/or other treatments, is an important field of further research. According to the neurotrophic model of depression, improving BDNF function may be beneficial to protect hippocampal neurons after stress-induced damages. Thus, BDNF and its receptor (TrkB) may be possible targets of new antidepressant agents. Promoting neurogenesis in individuals at high risk for depression may prevent neuronal atrophy, and possibly the onset of the depressive disorder (Chen *et al.*, 2010). Furthermore, the development of new antidepressants may be facilitated by a deeper comprehension of the regulation of BDNF, VEGF, and other neurotrophins, with other specific targets on adult neurogenesis.

Conclusions

The pathophysiology of depression is still largely unknown, although preclinical and clinical observations suggest that the disorder is associated with an impaired ability of neural systems to adaptive plasticity. The neurotrophin hypothesis of depression postulates that BDNF and other neurotrophic factors play a major role in the pathophysiology of depression, through the regulation of neural structures and plasticity in the adult brain, particularly hippocampus. To date, evidence supporting a crucial role of hippocampal neurogenesis in vulnerability and/or aetiology of depression is much less stringent than data supporting a role of neurogenesis in the antidepressant effect. However, evidence for the involvement in the pathophysiology of depression is still inconclusive (Groves, 2007). The lack of a clear depressive phenotype in BDNF knockout mice, negative results from large-scale population studies, and partly inconsistent conclusions from gene polymorphisms still weaken the BDNF hypothesis of depression. A possible hypothesis is that BDNF may modulate plasticity within emotional processing networks (Castrén & Rantamaki, 2010). Changes in neural plasticity may have different behavioural effects in the hippocampus, nucleus accumbens–ventral tegmental area and amygdala, indicating the need for a dynamic role of BDNF in mood regulation.

These findings depict a new framework for understanding the pathophysiology of depression and mechanism of antidepressants, in which a restoring altered neuroplasticity and network functioning may be a primary target of the treatments. The next steps in the development of new antidepressants (and more in general new psychotropic drugs) seem to be closely related to the discovery of agents with strong neuroprotective actions. Stimulation of neurogenesis has become a potential new target for antidepressant treatment, and new candidate agents with neurogenic potential are under study, which may normalize the effects of stress on neurogenesis, including also antagonists of receptors of corticotrophin-releasing factor, vasopressin, and glucocorticoid and selective antagonists of the neurokinine-1 receptor. Novel compounds that upregulate endogenous growth factors may be more effective, faster, and more tolerable than currently available medications, and may increase remission rates. These agents may enhance neuronal plasticity, which may allow environmental inputs to modify the neuronal networks to be better fine-tuned to help individuals to deal with the the external world in a complementary way with psychotherapy, learning, and exercise, with similar action on the final common pathway of neuroplasticity (Castrén & Rantamaki, 2010). This may have implications in both prevention (protective action in vulnerable subjects with early atypical neurogenesis), and treatment (reversal of micro/macrodegenerative components of mental illnesses).

References

Aguilera, M., Arias, B., Wichers, M., *et al.* (2009): Early adversity and 5-HTT/BDNF genes: new evidence of gene environment interactions on depressive symptoms in general population. *Psychol. Med.* **39,** 1425–1432.

Alfonso, J., Frick, L.R., Silberman, D.R., *et al.* (2006): Regulation of hippocampal gene expression is conserved in two species subjected to different stressors and antidepressant treatments. *Biol. Psychiatry* **59,** 244–251.

Altman, J. & Das, G.D. (1965): Autoradiographic and histological evidence of postnatal hippocampal neurogenesis in rats. *J. Comp. Neurol.* **124,** 319–335.

Anderson, M.F., Aberg, M.A., Nilsson, M. & Erickson, P.R. (2002): Insulin-like growth factor – I and neurogenesis in the adult mammalian brain. *Brain Res. Dev. Brain Res.* **134,** 115–122.

Banasr, M. & Duman, R.S. (2007): Regulation of neurogenesis and gliogenesis by stress and antidepressant treatments. *CNS Neurol. Disord. Drug Targets* **6,** 311–320.

Banasr, M., Hery, M., Printemps, R., *et al.* (2004): Serotonin-induced increases in adult cell proliferation and neurogenesis are mediated through different and common 5-HT receptor subtypes in the dentate gyrus and the subventricular zone. *Neuropsychopharmacology* **29,** 450–460.

Berton, O. & Nestler, E.J. (2006): New approaches to antidepressant drug discoveries: beyond monoamines. *Nat. Rev. Neurosci.* **7,** 137–151.

Berton, O., McClung, C.A., Dileone, R.J., *et al.* (2006): Essential role of BDNF in the mesolimbic dopamine pathway in social defeat stress. *Science* **311,** 864–868.

Bhatnagar, S., Lee, T.M. & Vining, C. (2005): Prenatal stress differentially affects habituation of corticosterone responses to repeated stress in adult male and female rats. *Horm. Behav.* **47,** 430–438.

Boldrini, M., Underwood, M.D., Hen, R., *et al.* (2009): Antidepressants increase neural progenitor cells in the human hippocampus. *Neuropsychopharmacology* **34,** 2376–2389.

Branchi, I., D'Andrea, I., Sietzema, J., *et al.* (2006): Early social enrichment augments adult hippocampal BDNF levels and survival of BrdU-positive cells while increasing anxiety and depression-like behaviour. *J. Neurosci. Res.* **83,** 965–973.

Brunoni, A.R., Lopes, M. & Fregni, F. (2008): A systematic review and meta-analysis of clinical studies on depression and BDNF levels: implications for the role of neuroplasticity in depression. *Int. J. Neuropsychopharmacol.* **11,** 1169–1180.

Castrén, E. & Rantamaki, T. (2010): Role of brain-derived neurotrophic factor in the etiology of depression: implications for pharmacological treatment. *CNS Drugs* **24,** 1–7.

Chao, M.V. (2003): Neurotrophins and their receptors: a convergence point for many signalling pathways. *Nat. Rev. Neurosci.* **4,** 299–309.

Chen, M.C., Hamilton. J.P. & Gotlib, I.H. (2010): Decreased hippocampus volume in healthy girls at risk for depression. *Arch. Gen. Psychiatry* **67,** 270–276.

Chen, Z.Y., Patel. P.D., Sant, G., *et al.* (2004): Variant brain derived neurotrophic factor (BDNF) (Met66) alters the intracellulat trafficking and activity secretion of wild-type BDNF in neurosecretory cells and cortical neurons. *J. Neurosci.* **24,** 4401–4411.

Chen, Z.Y., Jing, D., Bath, K.G., *et al.* (2006): Genetic variant BDNF (Val66Met) polymorphism alters anxiety-related behaviour. *Science* **314,** 140–143.

Chiou, S.H., Chen, S.J., Peng, C.H., *et al.* (2006): Fluoxetine up-regulates expression of cellular FLICE-inhibitory protein and inhibits LPS-induced apoptosis in hippocampus-derived neural stem cell. *Biochem. Biophys. Res. Commun.* **343,** 391–400.

Choi, M.J., Kang, R.H., Lim, S.W., *et al.* (2006): Brain-derived neurotrophic-factor gene polymorphism (Val66Met) and citalopram response in major depressive disorder. *Brain Res.* **1118,** 176–182.

Coe, C.L., Kramer, M., Czéh, B., *et al.* (2003): Prenatal stress diminishes neurogenesis in the dentate gyrus of juvenile Rhesus monkeys. *Biol. Psychiatry* **54,** 1025–1034.

Covington, H.E., III, Maze, I., LaPlant, Q.C. *et al.* (2009): Antidepressant action of HDAC inhibitors. *J. Neurosci.* **29,** 11451–11460.

Cushing, B.S. & Kramer, K.M. (2005): Mechanism underlying epigenetic effects of early social experience: the role of neuropeptides and steroids. *Neurosci. Behav. Rev.* **29,** 1089–1105.

Czéh, B., Michaelis, T., Watanabe, T., *et al.* (2001): Stress-induced changes in cerebral metabolites, hippocampal volume, and cell proliferation are prevented by antidepressant treatment with tianeptine. *Proc. Natl. Acad. Sci. USA* **98,** 12796–12801.

Duman, R.S. & Monteggia, L.M. (2006): A neurotrophic model for stress-related mood disorders. *Biol. Psychiatry* **59,** 1116–1127.

Duman, R.S., Nagasawa, S. & Malberg, J. (2001): Regulation of adult neurogenesis by antidepressant treatment. *Neuropsychopharmacology* **25,** 836–884.

Duman, C.H., Schlesinger, L., Kodama, M., *et al.* (2007): A role for MAP kinase signalling in behavioral models of depression and antidepressant treatment. *Biol. Psychiatry* **61,** 661–670.

Dwivedi, Y. (2009): Brain derived neurotrophic factor: a role in depression and suicide. *Neuropsychiatric Dis. Treat.* **5,** 433–449.

Dwivedi, Y., Rizavi, H.S., Conley, R.R., *et al.* (2003): Altered gene expression of brain-derived neurotrophic factor and receptor tyrosine kinase B in post-mortem brain of suicide subjects. *Arch. Gen. Psychiatry* **60,** 804–815.

Dwivedi, Y., Rizavi, H., Zhang, H., *et al.* (2009): Neurotrophin receptor activation and expression in human postmortem brain: effect of suicide. *Biol. Psychiatry* **65,** 319–328.

Eide, E.F., Vioning, E.R., Eide, B.L., *et al.* (1996): Naturally occurring truncated TrkB receptors have dominant inhibitory effects on brain derived neurotrophic factor signaling. *J. Neurosci.* **16,** 3123–3129.

Eisch, A.J., Bolanos, C.A., de Witt, J., *et al.* (2003): Brain derived neurotrophic factor in the ventral midbrain-nucleus accumbens pathway: a role in depression. *Biol. Psychiatry* **54,** 994–1005.

Erickson, K.I., Voss, M.W., Prakash, R.S., *et al.* (2011): Exercise training increases size of hippocampus and improves memory. *Proc. Natl. Acad. Sci. USA* E-pub ahead of print 2011, Jan 31.

Eriksson, P.S., Perfilieva, S., Bjork-Eriksson, T., *et al.* (1998): Neurogenesis in the adult human hippocampus. *Nat. Med.* **4,** 1313–1317.

Esposito, D., Patel, P., Stephens, R.M., *et al.* (2001): The cytoplasmic and transmembrane domain of P75 and Trk A receptors regulate high affinity binding to nerve growth factor. *J. Biol. Chem.* **276,** 32687–32695.

Evans, E., Hawton, K., Rodham, K. & Deeks J (2005): The prevalence of suicidal phenomena in adolescents: a systematic review of population-based studies. *Suicide Life Threat. Behav.* **35,** 239–250.

Friedman, W. (2000): Neurotrophins induce death of hippocampal neurons via the p75 receptor. *J. Neurosci.* **28,** 6340–6346.

Frodl, T.S., Koutsouleris, N., Bottlender, R., *et al.* (2008): Depression-related variation in brain morphology over 3 years: effects of stress? *Arch. Gen. Psychiatry* **65,** 1156–1165.

Fuchikami, M., Morinobu, S., Kurata, A., *et al.* (2009): Single immobilization stress differentially alters the expression profile of transcripts of the brain-derived neurotrophic factor (BDNF) gene and histone acetylation at its promoters in the rat hippocampus. *Int. J. Neuropsychopharmacol.* **12,** 73–82.

Gadian, D.G., Aicardi, J., Watkins, K.E., *et al.* (2000): Developmental amnesia associated with early hypoxic-ischaemic injury. *Brain* **123,** 499–507.

Gould, E. (2007): How widespread is adult neurogenesis in mammals? *Nat. Rev. Neurosci.* **8,** 481–488.

Greenberg, M.E., Xu, B., Lu, B. & Hempstead, B.L. (2009): New insights in the biology of BDNF synthesis and release: implications in CNS function. *J. Neurosci.* **29,** 12764–12767.

Groves, J.O. (2007): Is it time to reassess the BDNF hypothesis of depression? *Mol. Psychiatry* **12,** 1079–1088.

Hajszan, T., Dow, A., Warner-Schmidt, J.L., *et al.* (2009): Remodeling of hippocampal spine synapses in the rat learned helplessness model of depression. *Biol. Psychiatry* **65,** 392-400.

Heine, V.M., Zareno J., Maslam, S., *et al.* (2005): Chronic stress in the adult dentate gyrus reduces cell proliferation near the vasculature and VEGF and Flk-1 protein expression. *Eur. J. Neurosci.* **21,** 1304–1314.

Hilt, L.M., Sander, L.C., Nolen-Hoeksema, S. & Simen, A.A. (2007): The BDNF Val66Met polymorphism predicts rumination and depression differently in young adolescent girls and their mothers. *Neurosci. Lett.* **429,** 12–16.

Jacobs, B.L., van Praag, H. & Gage, F.H. (2000): Adult brain neurogenesis and psychiatry: a novel theory of depression. *Mol. Psychiatry* **5,** 262–269.

Jenuwein, T. & Allis, C.D. (2001): Translating the histone code. *Science* **293,** 1074–1080.

Jope, R.S. (2003): Lithium and GSK-3: one inhibitor, two inhibitory actions, multiple outcomes. *Trends Pharmacol. Sci.* **24,** 441–443.

Karege, F., Bondolfi, G., Gervasoni, N., *et al.* (2005): Low brain derived neurotrophic factor (BDNF) levels in serum of depressed patients probably results from lowered platelet BDNF release unrelated to platelet reactivity. *Biol. Psychiatry* **57,** 1068–1072.

Karl, A., Schaefer, M., Malta, L.S., *et al.* (2006): A meta-analysis of structural brain abnormalities in PTSD. *Neurosci. Biobehav. Rev.* **30,** 1004–1031.

Kaufman, J., Yang, B.Z., Douglas-Palumberi, H., *et al.* (2004): Social supports and serotonin transporter gene moderate depression in maltreated children. *Proc. Natl. Acad. Sci. USA* **101,** 17316–17321.

Kaufman, J., Yang, B.Z., Douglas-Palumberi, H., *et al.* (2006): Brain derived neurotrophic factor – 5-HTTLPR gene interactions and environmental modifiers of depression in children. *Biol. Psychiatry* **59,** 673–680.

Kessler, R.C., Avenevoli, S. & Merikangas, K.R. (2001): Mood disorders in children and adolescents: an epidemiologic perspective. *Biol. Psychiatry* **49,** 1002–1014.

Kim, Y.K., Lee, H.P., Won, S.D., *et al.* (2007): Low plasma BDNF is associated with suicidal behaviour in depression. *Prog. Neuropsychopharmacol. Biol. Psychiatry* **31,** 578–579.

Kobayashi, K., Ikeda, Y., Sakai, A., *et al.* (2010): Reversal of hippocampal neuronal maturation by serotonergic antidepressants. *Proc. Natl. Acad. Sci. USA* **107,** 8434–8439.

Koo, J.W. & Duman. R.S. (2008): IL-1beta is an essential mediator of the antineurogenic and anhedonic effects of stress. *Proc. Natl. Acad. Sci. USA* **105,** 751–756.

Koo, J.W., Russo, S.J., Ferguson, D., *et al.* (2010): Nuclear factor-κB is critical mediator of stress-impaired neurogenesis and depressive behaviour. *Proc. Natl. Acad. Sci. USA* **107,** 2669–2674.

Koponen, E., Rantamaki, T., Voikar, V., *et al.* (2005): Enhanced BDNF signalling is associated with an antidepressant-like behavioral response and changes in brain monoamines. *Cell. Mol. Neurobiol.* **6,** 973–980.

Lee, B.H. & Kim, Y.K. (2009): Reduced platelet BDNF in patients with major depression. *Prog. Neuro-Psychopharmacol. Biol Psychiatry* **33,** 849–853.

Li, Y., Luikart, B.W., Birnbaum, S., *et al.* (2008): TrkB regulates hippocampal neurogenesis and governs sensitivity to antidepressant treatment. *Neuron* **59,** 399–412.

Lommatzsch, M., Quarcoo, D., Schulte-Herbruggen, O., *et al.* (2005): Neurotrophins in murine viscera: a dynamic pattern from birth to adulthood. *Int. J. Dev. Neurosci.* **23,** 495–500.

Lu, B., Pang, P.T. & Woo, N.H. (2005): The Yin and Yang of neurotrophin action. *Nat. Rev. Neurosci.* **6,** 603–614.

Luberg, K., Wong, J., Weickert, C.S. & Timmusk. T. (2010): Human TrkB gene: novel alternative transcripts, protein isomorphs, and expression pattern in the prefrontal cerebral cortex during postnatal development. *J. Neurochem.* **113,** 952–964.

MacMaster, F.P., Mirza, Y., Szeszko, P.R., *et al.* (2008): Amygdala and hippocampal volumes in familial early-onset major depressive disorder. *Biol. Psychiatry* **63,** 385–390.

MacQueen, G.M., Ramakrishan, K., Croll, S.D., *et al.* (2001): Performance of heterozygous brain-derived neurotrophic factor knockout mice on behavioral analogues of anxiety, nociception, and depression. *Behav. Neurosci.* **115,** 1145–1153.

MacQueen, G.M., Campbell, S., McEwen, B.S., *et al.* (2003): Course of illness, hippocampal function, and hippocampal volume in major depression. *Proc. Natl. Acad. Sci. USA* **100,** 1387–1392.

Malberg, J.E. & Duman, R.S. (2003): Cell proliferation in adult hippocampus is decreased by inescapable stress: reversal by fluoxetine treatment. *Neuropsychopharmacology* **28,** 1562–1571.

Malberg, J.E., Eisch, A.J., Nestler, E.J. & Duman, R.S. (2000): Chronic antidepressant treatment increases neurogenesis in adult rat hippocampus. *J. Neurosci.* 20, 9104–9110.

Manji, H.K. & Chen, G. (2002): PKC, MAP kinases and the Bcl-2 family of proteins as long term targets for mood stabilizers. *Mol. Psychiatry* **7,** S46–S56.

Manji, H.K., Drevets, W.C. & Charney, D.S. (2000): The cellular neurobiology of depression. *Nat. Med.* **7,** 541–547.

McEwen, B. (2000): Effects of adverse experiences for brain structure and function. *Biol. Psychiatry* **48,** 721–731.

McGregor, S., Strauss, J., Bulgin, N. *et al.* (2007): P75 (NTR) gene and suicide attempts in young adults with a history of childhood onset mood disorder. *Am. J. Med. Genet. B. Neuropsychiatr. Genet.* **144B,** 696–700.

Michel, M., Frangou, T.S., Camara, S, *et al.* (2008): Altered glial cell-line derived neurotrophic factor (GDNF) concentrations in the brain of patients with depressive disorder: a comparative post-mortem study. *Eur. Psychiatry* **23,** 413–420.

Miller, A.H., Maletic, V. & Raion, C.L. (2009): Inflammatory and its discontent: the role of cytokines in the pathophysiology of major depression. *Biol. Psychiatry* **65,** 732–741.

Nasrallah, H.A., Hopkins, T. & Pixley, S.K. (2010): Differential effects of antipsychotic and antidepressant drugs on neurogenic regions in rats. *Brain Res.* **1354,** 23–29.

Nibuya, M., Nestler, E.J. & Duman, R.S. (1996): Chronic antidepressant administration increases the expression of c-AMP response element binding protein (CREB) in rat hippocampus. *J. Neurosci.* **7,** 2365–2372.

Otsuki, K., Uchida, S., Watanuki, T., *et al.* (2008): Altered expression of neurotrophic factors in patients with major depression. *J. Psychiatr. Res.* **42,** 1145–1153.

Pace, T.W., Mletzko, T.C., Alagbe, O., *et al.* (2006): Increased stress-induced inflammatory responses in male patients with major depression and increased early life stress. *Am. J. Psychiatry* **163,** 1630–1633.

Pandey, G.N., Ren, X., Rizavi, H.S., *et al.* (2008): Brain-derived neurotrophic factor and tyrosine kinase B receptor signalling in post-mortem brain of teenage suicide victims. *Int. J. Neuropsychopharmacol.* 11, 1047–1061.

Pandey, G.N., Dwivedi, Y., Rizavi, H.S., *et al.* (2010): Brain-derived neurotrophic factor gene in pediatric and adult depressed subjects. *Prog. Neuro-Psychopharm. Biol. Psychiatry* **34,** 645–651.

Parsey, R.V., Hastings, R.V., Oquendo, M.A., *et al.* (2006): Effects of the triallelic functional polymorphism of the serotonin-transporter-linked promoter region on expression of serotonin transporter in the human brain. *Am. J. Psychiatry* **163,** 48–51.

Pereira, A.C., Huddleston, D.E., Brickman, A.M., *et al.* (2007): An in vivo correlates of exercise-induced neurogenesis in the adult dentate gyrus. *Proc. Natl. Acad. Sci. USA* **1004,** 5638–5643.

Pizarro, J.M., Lumley, L.A., Medina, W., *et al.* (2004): Acute social defeat reduces neurotrophin expression in brain cortical and subcortical areas in mice. *Brain Res.* **1025,** 10–20.

Rantamaki, T., Hendolin, P., Kankaanpaa, A., *et al.* (2007): Pharmacologically diverse antidepressants rapidly activate brain-derived neurotrophic factor receptor TrkB and induce phospholipase-C gamma signaling pathways in mouse brain. *Neuropsychopharmacology* **32,** 2152–2162.

Rao, U., Chen, L.A., Bidesi, A.S., *et al.* (2010): Hippocampal changes associated with early-life adversity and vulnerability to depression. *Biol. Psychiatry* **67,** 357–364.

Roceri, M., Hendriks, W., Racagni, G. *et al.* (2002): Early maternal deprivation reduces the expression of BDNF and NMDA receptor subunits in rat hippocampus. *Mol. Psychiatry* **7,** 609–616.

Saarelainen, T., Hendolin, P., Lucas, G. *et al.* (2003): Activation of the TrkB neurotrophin receptor is induced by antidepressant drugs and is required for anti-depressant-induced behavioral effects. *J. Neurosci.* **25,** 1089–1094.

Sairanen, M., Lucas, G., Emfors, P., *et al.* (2005): Brain-derived neurotrophic factor and antidepressant drugs have different but coordinated effects on neuronal turn-over, proliferation, and survival in the adult dentate gyrus. *J. Neurosci.* **25,** 1089–1094.

Santarelli, L., Saxe, M., Gross, C., *et al.* (2003): Requirement of hippocampal neurogenesis for the behavioral effects of antidepressants. *Science* **301,** 805–809.

Sapolsky, R.M. (2001): Depression, antidepressants and the shrinking hippocampus. *Proc. Natl. Acad. Sci. USA* **98,** 12320–12322.

Schmidt, H.D. & Duman, R.S. (2007): The role of neurotrophic factors in adult hippocampal neurogenesis, antidepressant treatment and animal models of depressive-like behaviour. *Behav. Pharmacol.* **18,** 391–418.

Schmidt, H.D. & Duman, R.S. (2011): Peripheral BDNF produces antidepressant-like effects in cellular and behavioral models. *Neuropsychopharmacology* **36,** 550.

Sen, S., Duman, R.S., Sanacora, G. (2008): Serum brain derived neurotrophic factor, depression and antidepressants: meta-analyses and implications. *Biol. Psychiatry* **64,** 527–532.

Sheline, Y.I., Wang, P.W., Gado, M.H., *et al.* (1996): Hippocampal atrophy in recurrent major depression. *Proc. Natl. Acad. Sci.* **93,** 3908–3913.

Shirayama, Y., Chen, A.C., Nakagawa, S., *et al.* (2002): Brain-derived neurotrophic factor produces antidepressant effects in behavioral models of depression. *J. Neurosci.* **22,** 3251–3261.

Stockmeyer, C.A., Mahajan, G.J., Konick, L.C., *et al.* (2004): Cellular changes in the post-mortem hippocampus in major depression. *Biol. Psychiatry* **56,** 640–650.

Strauss, J., Barr, C.L., George, C.J., *et al.* (2005): Brain-derived neurotrophic factor variants are associated with childhood-onset mood disorder: confirmation in an Hungarian sample. *Mol. Psychiatry* **10,** 861–867.

Tsai, S.J., Chen, C.Y., Yu, Y.W., *et al.* (2003): Association study of a brain-derived neurotrophic-factor genetic polymorphism and major depressive disorders, symptomatology, and antidepressant response. *Am. J. Med. Genet. B. Neuropsychiatr. Genet.* **123B,** 19–22.

Tsankova, N.M., Berton, O., Rental, W., *et al.* (2006): Sustained hippocampal chromatin regulation in a mouse model of depression and antidepressant action. *Nat. Neurosci.* **9,** 519–525.

Turner, C.A., Gula, E.L., Taylor. L.P., *et al.* (2008): Antidepressant-like effects of intra-cerebro-ventricular FGF2 in rats. *Brain Res.* **1224,** 63–68.

Waggoner, D. (2007): Mechanisms of disease: epigenesis. *Semin. Ped. Neurol.* **14,** 7–14.

Wang, J.W., David, D.J., Monckton, J.E., *et al.* (2008): Chronic fluoxetine stimulates maturation and synaptic plasticity of adult-born hippocampal granule cells. *J. Neurosci.* **28,** 1374–1384.

Warner-Schmidt, J.L. & Duman, R.S. (2007): VEGF is an essential mediator of the neurogenic and behavioral actions of antidepressants. *Proc. Natl. Acad. Sci. USA* **104,** 4647–4652.

Weaver, I.C., Cervoni, N., Champagne, F.A., *et al.* (2004): Epigenetic programming by maternal behaviour. *Nat. Neurosci.* **7,** 847–854.

Xu, J.H., Hu, H.T., Liu, Y., *et al.* (2006): Neuroprotective effects of ebselen are associated with the regulation of Bcl-2 and Bax proteins in cultured mouse cortical neurons. *Neurosci. Lett.* **399,** 210–214.

Brain Lesion Localization and Developmental Functions, D. Riva, C. Njiokiktjien and S. Bulgheroni (eds.)

Chapter 13

The role of the hippocampus in neural mechanisms of attachment and attachment disorders: a review

Charles Njiokiktjien and Catharina Anna Verschoor

Developmental Dysphasia Foundation, WG-Plein 316, NL-1054 SG, Amsterdam, the Netherlands
cn@suyi.nl

Summary

Maternal care together with the newborn's need for care – genetically driven 'instinctual' behaviours of the mother and her infant – is the start of dyadic interaction after birth, ultimately leading to attachment. This interaction is controlled by neural mechanisms in both mother and infant. In the early stages of attachment, sensory and motor mechanisms enable the infant to acquire a basic understanding of the mother's bodily behaviour, *i.e.*, her formal actions as well as her affective bodily expressions. It is thought that normal attachment creates an internal bodily experience which becomes the model for understanding and expressing social relatedness and protects humans against stressful events (or stressors) in life. The prenatal administration of corticosteroids, maternal stress, and other stress factors interfering with normal attachment may be the cause of a less than optimal basis for social relatedness in the infant and may trigger deviant stress responses in the child and adult. Research points to the hypothalamic-pituitary-adrenal (HPA) axis, with the hippocampus as the key substrate for the stress response. The hippocampus is vulnerable to adverse perinatal and postnatal events and damage, which has consequences for affect and resilience in coping with stress, as well as episodic memory functions. This article addresses the influence of stress in infancy and childhood on the hippocampus. Levels of circulating cortisol are a measurable and important biological stress index. Stress has been related in animal and clinical studies with reductions in hippocampal volume as well as with neuronal cellular and receptor damage. The implications of damage are an overly high HPA activity, deviant ways of coping with stressful emotions in general, as well as non-optimal functioning in cognitive domains such as attention and memory. While behavioural traits are largely genetically determined, an attachment disorder is a risk factor for later deviant coping with stress.

Introduction to attachment

Maternal care as well as the newborn's need for caring behaviour is the start of a dyadic interaction or bodily dialogue which begins at birth (Fonagy *et al.*, 2007). Mothers' and infants' behaviours are genetically driven 'instinctual' behaviours, modulated by the mental mechanism of the primary caregiver (Fonagy, 2001b), which result in a personal relationship. This ultimately leads to mother–infant bonding or *attachment* (a term used by Bowlby [1967, 1973]). Dyadic interaction is controlled by neural mechanisms in both infant and caretaker (the primary caregiver or attachment figure, here called mother). For example the limbic CARE system, activated by the neurohormone oxytocin, promotes maternal nurturance (mothering or parenting) and enhances feelings of care, devotion, and empathy. In the infant, a system called the PANIC system plays a key role, evoking anxiety when there is separation from the mother. This causes vocalization of distress and approach to the caretaker. In this system both oxytocin and vasopressin alleviate separation distress. Both the CARE and the PANIC systems, whose neural networks are described by Panksepp (1998), initiate, promote, and maintain attachment.

Contrary to earlier proposals, safe attachment does not come into being only through the fulfilment of vital needs (drive satisfaction), or the mere availability and physical proximity of the mother, but is instead based on *feeling safe* with the available mother. Attachment theorists have explained that 'safe' means that the caregiver is attuned to its infant's affects in an optimal way (Fonagy *et al.*, 2002). The infant's repeated proximity-seeking behaviour is answered by maternal *affect attunement* (a term used by Stern [1985]), meaning that the mother matches the infant's feelings with her own in a synchronized way. The hippocampus, as a substrate for imprinting events and their affective value, as well as the substrate that initiates the stress response, has a role during these mother–infant interactions, and may chronically be modulated towards an unfavourable balance between nice-events/no-stress and terrifying-events/much-stress. Attachment and stress-response mechanisms are connected and have neural representations in the brain that show experience-dependent plasticity.

Neural plasticity makes it possible for a normal attachment to be the basis of a life-long internal working model, a template for relatedness with others, which includes the individual's unconscious expectations and beliefs about others. This internal working model also forms the basis for theory-of-mind functions (the capacity to mentalize). Mentalizing opens a mental window to other people's thought, feelings and intentions (Fonagy, 2001a, 2002). The internal working model entails a way to cope with stress, physiologically supported by the stress-response mechanism, a hormonal and neurotransmitter mechanism.

During the early stages of attachment (the first 6 months of life) sensory and motor mechanisms enable the infant to acquire a basic understanding of the mother's bodily behaviour, which entails formal action understanding with objects, especially with the infant as object, as well as understanding the mother's affective bodily expressions towards the infant, which are part of affect attunement. Njiokiktjien *et al.* (2011) called this understanding that develops in the infant 'Theory of Body' (ToB) and found that it comes into being in the first 3–4 months of infancy. ToB, which is part of the internal working model of attachment, is thought to consist largely of memory for emotional feelings connected with the mother's bodily behaviour. After a study in adult patients, Calabrese *et al.* (1999) concluded that hippocampal formation plays a role in nonconscious, implicit emotional memory. However, the internal working model is not adult episodic memory with a notion of time, but is partly procedural – how the mother's body is handling the infant's in an affective way – processed in part by limbic structures, notably the hippocampal formation, and in part by the sensory-motor or action system (on infantile memory and amnesia; see Turnbull and Solms [2003] and Riva [this volume]).

Attachment as an internal working model which is in some ways comparable to the immune system's memory and reaction model protects humans against the stressful events that occur in everyday life, which are usually of a relational nature, and also against chronic stressors such as hunger and poverty. A secure attachment is also a relative protection against unusual acute stressors such as severe disease, aggression inflicted on the body (during war or incidentally), or the sudden loss of beloved family members or friends in accidents or natural disasters.

Prenatal maternal stress and chronic postnatal stress factors interfere with optimal attachment and may be the cause in the infant and later in life of a deviant stress response as well as a less than optimal basis for relatedness. Gunnar *et al.* (1996) hypothesized that secure attachment protects the developing brain against the potential deleterious effects of elevated cortisol (see also Feldman *et al.*, 2010 [under *Postnatal stress*]).

Within the developing brain it is the limbic system and especially the hippocampus, a part of the hypothalamic-pituitary-adrenal (HPA) axis that plays a role in coping with both pre- and postnatal stress. The HPA axis, the sympathic nervous system, and the immune system, as well as a number of neurotransmitters, are involved in the stress response. The stress response is a physiologic reaction and is present in the case of separation anxiety, when the PANIC system is active. Figure 1 provides information about the HPA axis.

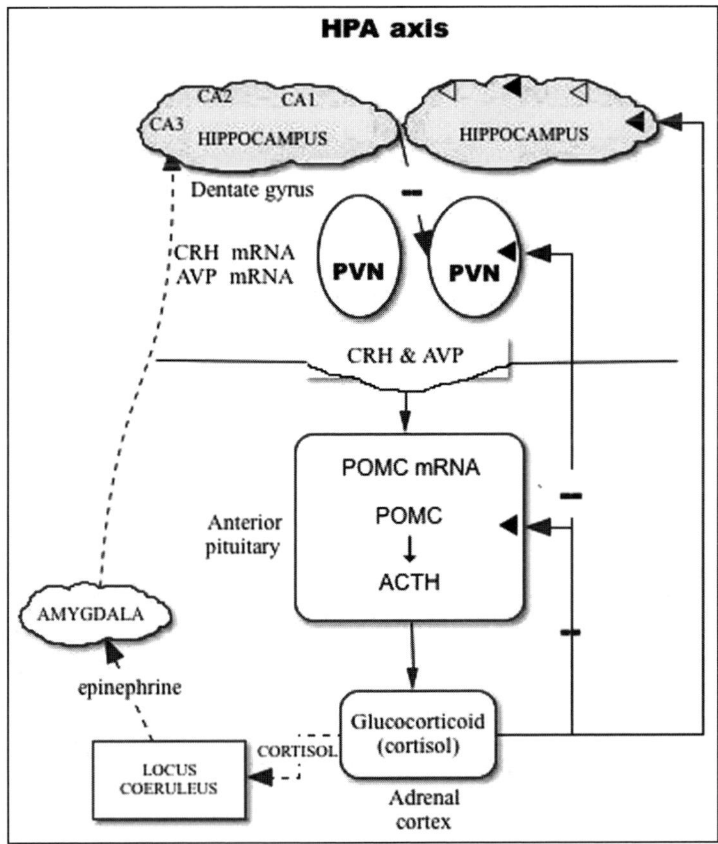

Fig. 1. Schema of the hippocampal-pituitary-adrenal axis, a connection in the brain to the adrenal cortex, which secretes cortisol. Cortisol stimulates the locus coeruleus, which activates the amygdala. Hyperstimulation of the amygdala damages hippocampal cells, which gives rise to chronic anxiety. The anterior cingulate cortex also plays a role. The hippocampus provides the major inhibitory (–) input to the hypothalamic periventricular nucleus (PVN), which controls pituitary-adrenocortical activity. Parvocellular neurons in the PVN synthesize corticotrophin-releasing hormone (CRH) and arginin-vasopressin (AVP). These are released in the hypophyseal portal circulation (downward arrow towards the anterior pituitary gland), where they promote adrenocorticotrophin (ACTH) synthesis from propriomelanocortin (POMC) and its release in the blood. ACTH initiates the synthesis of glucocorticoid (cortisol) in the adrenal cortex. Glucocorticoids have an inhibitory feedback influence (–) on the anterior pituitary, the PVN, and the hippocampus, and inhibit HPA activity. Glucocorticoid receptors are found in the hippocampal regions CA1–3. ◀ = glucocorticoid receptor; ◁ = mineralocorticoid receptor; mRNA = messenger RNA.

Neuroanatomic substrates and mechanisms of the stress system

The HPA axis and its function

The first topic we will address is the role of glucocorticoids (cortisol in humans). Glucocorticoids play an important role in brain development, influencing cellular and subcellular level (neuron-to-neuron and neuron-to-glia-cell interactions). It has been discovered, mainly though animal experiments, that excessively high or low levels of glucocorticoids may damage neuronal function.

The importance of the HPA axis for the developing infant and child is that it is involved in the early programming of the brain for coping with stress. The stress response is a learned response and plays a role later in life. Many indications point to the HPA axis with the hippocampus as a key neural substrate for the stress response.

The function of the HPA axis, described by Herman *et al.* (1996, 1997), is probably permanently programmed during development; it naturally has an impact on the individual's entire postnatal life. As shown in Fig. 1 the PVN (hypothalamic periventricular nucleus) with its neurochemical products, corticotrophin-releasing hormone (CRH) and arginin-vasopressin (AVP), controls pituitary-adrenal cortical activity, which ultimately leads to cortisol production by the adrenal cortex. CRH and AVP are accelerators of the stress axis, whereas cortisol is an inhibitor. The hippocampus supplies a major inhibitory input to the PVN, and also receives inhibitory feedback from cortisol.

The stress response

Hüther (2006) distinguishes between stressor and stress response as well as between controllable and uncontrollable stress. In the case of uncontrollable stress, the stress–response mechanism is more activated than in instances of controllable stress. When a stressor is encountered, in addition to cortisol, the brain produces other hormones and neurotransmitters, for example, noradrenaline, a stimulus which prompts immediate flight or fighting. A stressor also produces autonomous nervous system changes, such as increased heart rate and changes in physical well-being. Cortisol is connected to these changes. There is a FEAR system, described by Panksepp (1998), for fundamental forms of unconditioned fear. It is located between the lateral amygdala, hypothalamus, and peri-aquaductal gray matter (PAG) of the midbrain and can be aroused by conscious and unconscious memories of frightening past events, indirectly provided by the amygdala and hippocampus. This system can be chronically overaroused and sensitized in the case of post-traumatic stress disorders (PTSD) and the like. When a threatening stressor is encountered, the FEAR system becomes active and the bodily changes described above occur; taken together they are what is called an *emotion*, felt by the subject as an emotional feeling (Damasio, 2010) or affect (Freud), the result of enteroception. The functions of the FEAR system are not further addressed in this article.

The core system for the stress response, the HPA axis, is the cause of an increased cortisol level and leads *via* the PVN to inhibitory feedback, which brings cortisol back to a normal level. The hippocampus pyramidal neurons, with major inhibitory input to the PVN, have many receptors for cortisol, and are therefore vulnerable to high circulating cortisol caused by uncontrollable stress. Cortisol levels remaining higher than they should for extended periods of time, as they do in chronic stress, is associated with damage to the hippocampal neurons, and this changes the HPA axis function in such a way that feedback has less effect. A hyperplastic adrenal cortex and hypercortisolism have been shown.

Bremner (1997) proposed an alternative explanation, which is that some children are born with smaller hippocampal volumes which are genetically determined. This has consequences for their reaction to subsequent stressful events. Some of these reactions are classified as neuropsychiatric syndromes, such as posttraumatic stress disorder (PTSD) after traumatic brain injury (TBI), but also include syndromes such as borderline personality disorder (BPD), depression, memory problems, and unclassified physical complaints. In short, an inborn smaller hippocampus and/or previous chronic and severe stress can be the cause of subsequent deviant stress responses. The outcome is that the person is enmeshed in a vicious circle: more stress produces increasingly deviant responses, which in turn generate more stress, a phenomenon known as 'sensitization'. Possibly, the balance of CRH and AVP as accelerators of the stress axis and cortisol's inhibiting feedback become unstable or hyper-reactive in the case of PTSD. If children and adults can deal efficiently with controllable stress, it strengthens their self-confidence and increases the strategies they can use to cope with stress. This is enhanced by stable affectional relationships (attachment). Details will be discussed below.

The emotional brain

We will now describe the functioning of the Papez–MacLean–Panksepp circuit within the greater limbic system or emotional brain. Our principal reference for this section is *The Central Nervous System of Vertebrates* by Nieuwenhuys *et al.* (1998).

In 1878, six years after Darwin's book *The Expression of the Emotions in Man and Animals* was published, Broca described 'le grand lobe limbique', which possessed functions such as smell and emotions. In 1937 Papez proposed a circuit subserving functions of central emotion and their expression, and in 1952 MacLean elaborated upon this idea and used the term 'limbic system' in a functional sense (MacLean, 1990).

The limbic system consists of the hypothalamus, anterior thalamic nuclei, cingulate gyrus, and hippocampus with its interconnections (Papez, 1937), plus the prefrontal cortex and amygdalae (MacLean, 1990) and, according to Panksepp (1998), also the hypothalamus and peri-aquaeductal central gray of the mesencephalon (PAG). Neuroanatomists no longer consider the limbic system as an neuroanatomic entity – the core neural circuit is still the Papez–MacLean circuit – and the term 'greater limbic system' is now current (Nieuwenhuys, 1996, 2008).

Cortical perception, present for olfactory, gustatory, auditory and somatosensory, as well as visual stimuli – *e.g.*, the occipital-inferotemporal ventral stream to the right fusiform gyrus for perception of faces – is connected with the limbic system (notably the hippocampus *via* the perirhinal and entorhinal cortices) for processing emotions. The Papez–MacLean–Panksepp circuit contains the *hippocampus,* serving episodic memory comparison, with output in this order: → fornix → mammillary bodies → mammillothalamic tract → anterior thalamus → cingulate gyrus (the secondary paralimbic cortex for feeling emotion) → amygdala → gyrus hippocampi/ventrolateral thalamus → prefrontal cortex. The *amygdala* – which also has influence on the hippocampus after epinephrinergic input from the locus coeruleus – receives input from the PAG and neocortex and sends output *via* the dorsomedial thalamus to the prefrontal areas (orbital frontal and medial prefrontal) for cognitive evaluation and execution/expression of emotions (Korkmaz, this volume). Observed emotions ultimately lead to inhibition or expression of one's own emotions.

Panksepp (1998) wrote a comprehensive textbook entitled *Affective Neuroscience*, in which he persuasively argues that the emotional brain circuits (mainly limbic system) comprise closed and open programs. Closed programs, which are reflexive and instinctive in nature, are present in reptiles, the lower mammals, and primates, and are relatively impermeable to external influences other than a primary stimulus. In humans, evolutionary processes, including the evolution of the neocortex and emotion programs, are more open, subject to learning, memory, inner reasoning, hormones, and culture. Panksepp proposed a neurologically based taxonomy of behavioural/emotional processes (Fig. 2).

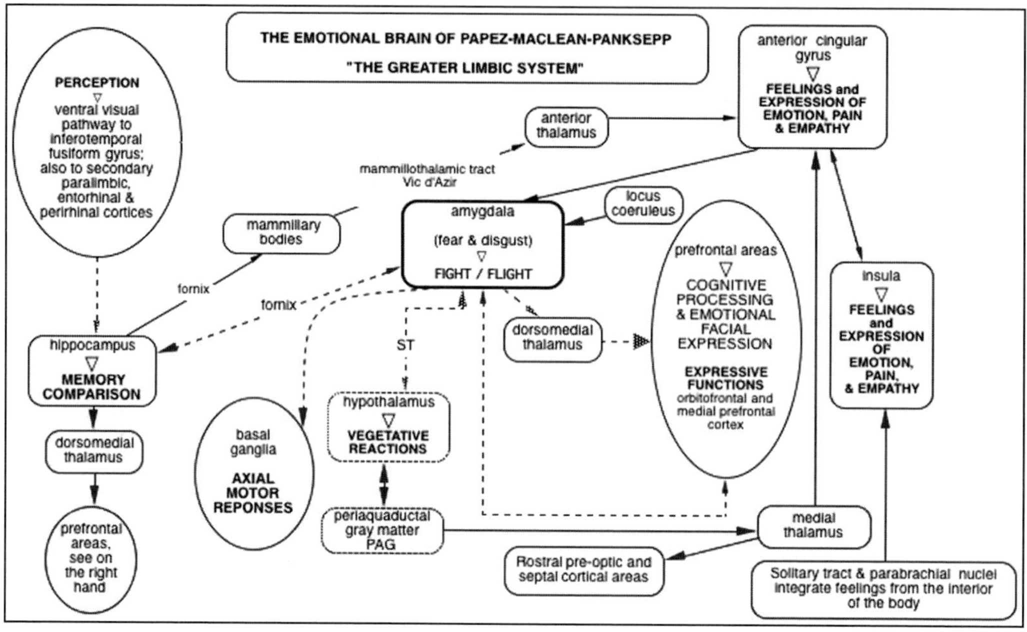

Fig. 2. Schematic figure of the Papez–MacLean–Panksepp cerebral circuits for emotion processing. It shows the main substrates and connections for emotion processing, with functions shown in boldface. The classic Papez circuit (continuous lines) is supplemented (MacLean) by the prefrontal cortex, hypothalamus, anterior thalamic nuclei, preoptic area, and amygdalae (dotted lines). The basal ganglia (below left) are part of the 'reptilian brain' and control axial or whole-body motor responses. The scheme shows how the cortical perception of emotions (top left) via *the right fusiform gyrus for the perception of facial emotion is connected with the Papez circuit, which is a memory and emotion circuit. Perception is also auditory, somatosensory, gustatory and olfactory (not shown here). The Papez circuit contains the hippocampus (for memory comparison, with input from the dorsal and ventral pathways) → fornix → mammillary bodies → mammillothalamic tract → anterior thalamus → cingulate gyrus (the secondary paralimbic cortex for feelings and emotions, basic to empathy) → hippocampal gyrus / ventrolateral thalamus (not shown) → prefrontal cortex. The amygdalae get input from the preaquaductal grey matter (PAG), cingulum, neocortex and hippocampus and send output* via *the dorsomedial thalamus to the frontal areas, including the subcortical basal ganglia for cognitive evaluation and execution/expression of emotions by face or body. Observed emotions ultimately lead to inhibition or expression of felt emotions (middle right). The diagram shows the most important connections. ST = stria terminalis, connecting the amygdalae to the hypothalamus. Reciprocal projections from the amygdalae through the stria terminalis to the medial hypothalamus and from the PAG to the medial hypothalamus and back are part of both Panksepp's* RAGE *and the* FEAR *systems. The PAG* via *the medial thalamus to the rostral preoptic and septal cortical areas, the stria terminalis, and the anterior cingulate cortex are part of the* PANIC *system. The hypothalamic and preoptic areas, medially connected to the PAG, are part of the* LUST *system. For the* RAGE, FEAR, PANIC, *and* LUST *systems, see the main text. In the system for* SHAME, GUILT, *and* DISGUST, *the hippocampus, basal ganglia, and anterior cingulate cortex play a role. Solitary tract and parabrachial nuclei integrate feelings from the interior of the body, input for the insula.*

Dealing with the difficulty of overlapping and sometimes conflicting definitions, Panksepp (1998) and Liotti and Panksepp (2004) hypothesized seven emotion systems in the brain: SEEKING, RAGE, FEAR, and PANIC (the four primitive systems which begin operating early) and LUST, CARE, and PLAY (the social emotions).

MacLean (1990), well-known for his evolutionary approach, emphasized the role of the infant–mother relationship with three behaviours that separate mammals from the lower vertebrates: nursing and maternal care, audiovocal communication to maintain contact, and play behaviour. He devoted an entire chapter to this question in his book *Participation of Thalamocingulate Division in Family-Related Behaviour*. MacLean, in fact, repeated what Bowlby (1967, 1973) had said on the deleterious effects of infant–mother separation. The PAG *via* the medial thalamus to the rostral preoptic and septal cortical areas, and the anterior cingulate cortex are part of the PANIC system, active when the infant is separated from the caretaker (discussed below).

The limbic system is involved in the perception of other people's moods and emotions and through the prefrontal cortex plays a role in the expression of moods and emotional feelings. The amygdalae ensure that cortical stimuli acquire an emotional charge and are thus better remembered. The amygdalae, as part of the FEAR system, register danger and respond, *e.g.*, to an angry facial expression. The limbic system, whose most important memory structure is the hippocampal system, is an indispensable co-processor, connected to the cortical association areas for storage. It ensures that relevant episodic biographical knowledge is imprinted and retained (long-term memory [LTM]). The limbic areas have connections with the cerebral cortex and are activated by sensory stimuli. As a result, perceptions lead to negative or positive feelings and the event is remembered with the accompanying feeling. In the case of a repetition of an event of the same kind, the limbic system becomes active again and brings the memory of the event to mind, with the feelings that accompanied the original occurrence. This means that a person will normally avoid unpleasant things and seek to gravitate towards pleasant ones. However, because the hippocampus is part of the HPA axis, very stressful events can be strongly imprinted and become the cause of a stress-response dysregulation.

The right hemisphere

Schore (2001, 2003a,b,c, 2009) wrote that the development of the right brain plays a part in early emotional life and affect regulation as well as in early attachment trauma (Schore, 2001). Attachment experiences, according to Schore and Schore (2008), shape the early organization of the right hemisphere (RH): the regulation of the infant's affect by the mother will lead to self-regulation, which is an ontogenetic network organization within the RH's arousal system, the limbic and orbitofrontal areas. As emotions and affects play a major role in infancy and as these are processed by the RH, which dominates behaviour at that age, negative moods and emotions are perceived by the RH cortices and processed by the amygdalae. Although it may seem contradictory, several MRI studies have shown more left than right hippocampus abnormalities, mostly volume reductions, in adults with PTST and previous childhood abuse (Teicher, 2002). Ito *et al.* (1998) found higher EEG coherence patterns in the left hemisphere of 15 previously abused schoolchildren, which is a reversed asymmetry. Teicher (2002) also found neuropsychological indications that abused children had a diminished left–right integration; this was supported by the finding that the middle parts of the corpus callosum were significantly smaller in abused boys. Although compensation may play a role, the left-right differences are not resolved.

Development and role of the hippocampus

Together with the adjacent subiculum, the hippocampus and the dentate gyrus make up the hippocampal formation. The medial temporal lobe (MTL) contains the hippocampal formation, as well as the parahippocampal, entorhinal, and perirhinal cortices and the amygdalae, and is important for the storage and the retrieval of episodic memory facts. The hippocampus, a subcortical structure tucked in behind the temporal lobes, together with the amygdalae, are part of what is called the limbic system (MacLean, 1990) or virtually synonymous with the 'emotional brain' (Panksepp, 1998).

The hippocampal formation is a highly complex supramodal association area, in which stimuli (including interoceptive emotional stimuli) converge from all sensory modalities, so that multimodal memory associations can come into being. These associations in the hippocampal system are thought to have connections to long-term activity with a high degree of feedback, so that reverberating activity occurs, *i.e.*, the reactivation of a memory engram (Ijima *et al.*, 1996).

Except for information from the entorhinal and perirhinal cortices (ventral stream: 'what') and parahippocampal cortices (dorsal stream: 'where'), the hippocampal formation receives little direct cortical input. Subcortical input reaches the hippocampus (CA3) *via* the fornix and diffuse systems, which link the hippocampus to the amygdalae (Fig. 1). However, its CA1 (receiving input from CA3) and subicular areas send extensive projections back to the association cortices from which they do not receive direct projections. Hippocampal output uses the fornix to reach the septum, accumbens, anterior thalamus, and mammillary body (Heimer *et al.*, 2008). The hippocampus sends output *via* the dorsomedial thalamus to the frontal areas for cognitive evaluation and execution/expression of emotions.

Payne *et al.* (2009) described normal development of the hippocampus in rhesus macaques. Their longitudinal T1-weighted MRI studies of the hippocampal formation and amygdala in *Macaca mulatta* between 1 week and 2 years of age showed that while the hippocampus increased by 117.05 per cent in males and 110.86 per cent in females, the left was significantly larger than the right, irrespective of gender, and significant age-related changes were unrelated to overall brain development. We will not address other findings here.

The hippocampus is a late-maturing structure, in which neuronal differentiation begins prenatally and is only completed after birth (Rakic & Novakowski, 1981). In addition to the slow maturation of the prefrontal cortex, this might be one reason why young children have a less efficient working memory (WM), and why they are distracted and cannot make quick decisions.

Although the hippocampus is known to be involved in LTM functions, its exact functional organization is still under debate, *i.e.*, the precise dissociation between the episodic and semantic components of declarative memory has not yet been determined. De Haan *et al.* (2006) propose that there is familiarity-based recognition memory within the first postnatal months (*e.g.*, for faces, sounds, and objects) with the ventral stream and possibly the perirhinal cortex as substrates. A semantic-like nonverbal memory (for facts such as single actions) emerges then and depends on the medial temporal lobe, possibly including the hippocampus. Episodic memory develops with progressive development of the hippocampus. Clinical observations indicate that it is likely that the hippocampus is a substrate with early hemispheric specialization and plays a crucial role in episodic implicit and context-rich LTM [Riva, (this volume)]. The following is an example of a clinical observation (present author) that demonstrates how the hippocampus functions:

T has had a phobia of elevators since early childhood, especially in the absence of other people. In infancy and early childhood she would begin to cry as soon as she had to enter an elevator. She was told by her mother that when she was three months old, her babysitter went shopping, left her alone and closed her in a wooden cabinet for over an hour. According to T's mother, this was the cause of the phobic behaviour.

Although it has been known since the 1970s which neural substrates subserve and represent memory traces, only recently have we obtained a detailed picture of how memory works at the neuronal and molecular level (Kandel, 2006). In his book *In Search of Memory* Kandel describes the influence of the hippocampal system on the multimodally excitable LTM episodic memory component. When a child perceives something, it will know whether it happened before, where it happened, and whether or not the experience was pleasant. If the child has acquired a formal notion of time, he or she may say when the episode took place. Active remembering (voluntary retrieval) is a prefrontal rather than a hippocampal function. While early hippocampal lesions cause some semantic memory disorders, they have a greater effect on episodic memory.

The LTM episodic memory component suggests long-lasting changes at the neuronal level. Bliss & Lømo (1973) found that the mechanism involved in this change is what they called long-term potentiation (LTP), considered in this context to mean lasting from a few days to throughout life. LTP underlies learning and memory formation (Setiawan *et al.*, 2007). LTP appears in different forms and is influenced by hormones and neurotransmitters, *e.g.*, glutamate. The glutamate agonist *N*-methyl-D-aspartate (NMDA) and its receptors (NMDAR) play a role in the activity-dependent maturation of synaptic connections; NMDAR also facilitates the opening of cell membrane channels for the passage of calcium. When glutamate levels are excessively high, for example, in cases of perinatal insult or when the body overproduces glucocorticoids (Stein-Behrens *et al.*, 1994), there is excessive NMDA receptor activity, which allows intracellular calcium to reach toxic levels; together this enables memory loss. In the hippocampus, two regions are important in this respect: CA1 and CA3. These regions have many glucocorticoid receptors (see the section below entitled 'Disorders of the HPA axis including the hippocampus').

Jacobson & Sapolsky (1991) described the role of the hippocampus in feedback regulation of the HPA axis and emphasized that the hippocampus is very susceptible to damage by insults such as ischaemia, hypoglycaemia, and seizures. This susceptibility to damage is linked to the maturation of its neuronal structure.

Disorders of the hippocampus

Hippocampal pathology has long been associated with memory disorders, psychoses, and epilepsy. Early hippocampal lesions cause semantic and episodic memory disorders (Riva *et al.*, 2000), while later lesions are more implicated in multimodal episodic memory disorders than in semantic ones. Like abnormalities of the hippocampus, abnormalities of the fornix (Calabrese *et al.*, 1995; Grafman *et al.*, 1985; Park *et al.*, 2000), the corpora mammillaria, and the dorsomedial thalamic nucleus, resulting from perinatal damage, cause serious imprinting problems. Memory disorders are not further addressed here as there is a separate chapter on this subject in this volume (Riva, this volume).

Disorders of the HPA axis including the hippocampus

Two lines of clinical research have advanced our knowledge of the effects of the abnormal stress mechanism mentioned above. The first is the use of synthetic glucocorticoids to treat foetuses at risk for respiratory problems if born preterm. The second focuses on the question of what happens to the HPA axis if people, especially pregnant women or infants, undergo stress.

Prenatal therapeutic use of glucocorticoids

It was in the 1970s that synthetic glucocorticoids were first used by medical research scientists to treat foetuses *via* antenatal administration to the mother (Liggins & Howie, 1972). It was demonstrated that antenatal synthetic glucocorticoid therapy (often dexamethasone) is highly effective in the prevention of severe respiratory complications. Women originally received either one dose or courses of the hormone, the latter procedure becoming common practice in the 1990s. Serious concerns about long-term side effects on neurodevelopment have since been expressed (see, for example, Barrington [2001]). These were based on animal research that demonstrated long-term effects of foetal exposure to glucocorticoids on behaviour and endocrine function. Animal studies also showed that both short-term as well as repeated treatment of mothers with synthetic glucocorticoids may permanently affect the HPA axis function in offspring. Human infants, whose mothers were treated with dexamethasone, showed reduced stress reactivity (less salivary cortisol and slowed heart rate) to a heelstick stressor (Davis *et al.*, 2004).

Long-term longitudinal research with children began recently. For example, French *et al.* (2004) suggested that repeated antenatal courses of betamethasone affects attention regulation and increases the risk of aggressive behaviour in 3- to 6-year-old children; it has also been shown to negatively influence verbal working memory in children and adolescents (Hirvikoski *et al*, 2007). As synthetic glucocorticoids bind predominantly with glucocorticoid receptors, it is likely that effects on the development of the HPA axis are mediated at the level of these receptors (De Kloet *et al.*, 1998, 2005; Herman *et al.*, 1996), and given that in primates this structure matures almost entirely before birth (Owen & Matthews, 2003), it is probable that the antenatal administration of synthetic glucocorticoids has an impact on its maturation, affecting the sense of attenuation and reducing cortisol.

Owen & Matthews (2007) found that antenatal exposure to synthetic glucocorticoids in pregnant guinea pigs led to acute downregulation of mRNA expression of the NR1 subunit of the NMDA receptor in the hippocampus of female offspring. The NMDA receptor is known to play a role in LTP, and thus in neuronal plasticity and learning.

Maternal stress

Increased maternal anxiety with elevated corticoid production may be the cause of foetal exposure to excess glucocorticoids. Prenatal stress has been found to be associated with attention deficit disorders in children (Weinstock, 1997). Elevated prenatal maternal salivary cortisol levels have been connected to both stress and behavioural problems in the child (O'Connor *et al.*, 2003).

Increased exposure to endogenous glucocorticoids has also been found to predispose to a number of neurologic, metabolic, and cardiovascular diseases, whereas reduced exposure protects against these diseases. Stress and increased cortisol can have an impact on the hippocampal structure (De Kloet *et al.*, 2005), notably a reduction in volume (Bremner *et al.*, 1995; Sapolsky, 1996; Stein *et al.*, 1997). Uno *et al.* (1990, 1994) showed a dose-dependent neuronal degeneration in rhesus monkeys in CA1–CA3, the hippocampal pyramidal neurons. In monkeys, maternal stress for 6 weeks was found to have the same effect (Coe *et al.*, 2003).

Fenoglio *et al.* (2006) showed that rats undergoing stress as a result of low maternal care, have lasting changes in the hippocampus: elevated CRH mRNA levels in the CA1 and CA3 regions. Ivry *et al.* (2008) found increased numbers of CRH-expressing neurons in both fields as well as dendritic atrophy of pyramidal cells.

What happens in the case of an attachment disorder?

Winnicott (1970) emphasized the importance of the quality of maternal handling and holding, which is a dyadic activity that provides security and is interiorized in the child, an experience that forms a hidden, indelible trace deep in autobiographic memory, not in the time-linked components of episodic memory.

During the attachment period infants can experience several types and degrees of stress:

(*a*) There are factors which make mothers unable to handle their infant in an affectively attuned way. This may be a mild problem because other caretakers can replace the mother, as has been suggested by Smeekens *et al.* (2010).

(*b*) Mothers who are autistic cannot be empathic with their child or provide adequate affect attunement. They usually do not send adequate affective signals with the face, body, voice, and by touching the infant with their hands, or they send contradictory signals, which can cause the child to misinterpret other people's signals in later life.

(*c*) Other mothers may have been raised in psychopathogenic homes, and may batter their infant, which results in the most severe form of deviant attachment.

(*d*) The bodily layer of the self is differentiated into one's own body awareness and the awareness of the bodily behaviour of others. An event perceived as aggressive touch by third persons, inflicted on the caretaker and accompanied by its caretaker's emotional signals, is "felt" by the infant and is a stressor. Such events probably resonate as empathy in the same way as actions resonate in the motor system *via* the mirror neuron system (MNS). It is still not known precisely when this component starts to be present, but it is likely that this occurs starting from the 3rd month, when infants begin to observe the world from a distance.

(*e*) Premature babies are kept in incubators and are often separated from their mothers for a long time; optimal handling is hampered because these infants sleep much of the time and are small.

(*f*) Other examples from the attachment literature include depressed mothers' behaviour towards their babies, discussed by Weinberg and Tronick (1998), by Feldman (2007), and more recently by Besser *et al.* (2008). The interactive nature of depressed infant and depressed mother and a summary of the literature are given by Golse (2004).

Attachment quality can be measured. The first psychological test was the 'strange situation test' (Ainsworth *et al.*, 1978). In this test, separation from the mother is manipulated; it provokes behaviour in the child that reflects the quality of its attachment. The stress response can also give an indication of insecure attachment as well; Smeekens *et al.* (2010) showed that cortisol reactions in 5-year-olds to an attachment story completion task are different in children with an insecure attachment than in those who are securely attached. Atypical cortisol increases were related, according to the authors, with the negativity of the caregiver (associated primarily with social signals that are threatening to the infant's social self, such as negative judgments and rejection), not with a lack of effective guidance.

It has been shown that children with a deviant or insecure attachment have abnormal stress responses, which is one of the reasons they have problems establishing and maintaining relationships.

1. *Animal models*: The consequences of postnatal stress have been shown in experiments with animals. Zhang *et al.* (1997) showed that in newborn rats even 1 day of maternal deprivation (equivalent to 6 months in humans) is sufficient for hippocampal cell death. The quality of maternal care translates in adult rats into differences in hormonal stress response: with good maternal care there is reduced CRH expression in the hypothalamus and increased hippocampus glucocorticoid receptor; with poor maternal care the reverse occurs (Meaney, 2001). Moreover, the adult offspring of rats that provide good care exhibit improved hippocampus-dependent cognitive function (Liu *et al.*, 2000), which goes along with longer dendrite branch length and increased spine density in hippocampus CA1 neurons and enhanced LTP (Champagne *et al.*, 2008).

2. *Human infants:* Studies with humans have also demonstrated the negative effects of stress. Plotsky & Meaney (1993) found that repeated periods of separation from the mother led to a stress reaction in the baby, expressed by increased glucocorticoid levels as well as by hippocampal cell death. Feldman *et al.* (2010) found that the provision of touch during moments of maternal unavailability (with the still-face paradigm) reduces infants' physiologic reactivity to stress (cortisol level). We would now like to consider a case we encountered, a story we feel exemplifies the importance of affect attunement:

N was 3 when a puppy snatched the doll she was holding. She tried to pull it from the dog's mouth but the mother dog jumped at her and bit her severely on the face, after which she had to remain in hospital. Her mother was there beside her bed for three weeks. Years later, N had no memory of the event, but her sister, who was two years older than her and told the story, remembered it clearly.

Here we can see the immediate and long-standing effects of downregulation by the affect-attuned mother on the HPA axis, expressed as a decrease in serum and salivary cortisol (not measured in this case), which results in the event becoming unimportant and forgotten. Social interaction profoundly influences activity in the stress system, called 'social buffering of the HPA axis' (DeVries *et al.*, 2003). The buffering effect of social support reduces hippocampal release of oxytocin, present in both the PANIC and CARE systems (Carter, 2003). Alternative explanations for 'forgetting' are that the episode was not encoded because an acute increase in N's cortisol level was the cause of neuronal death in the hippocampus (Markowitsch *et al.*, 1998); or severe hippocampal dysfunction uncoupled negative feedback by the hippocampus to the HPA (Solms & Turnbull, 2004); or excessive NMDA receptor activity (Stein-Behrens *et al.*, 1994), which blocked LTP for encoding.

Quirin *et al.* (2009) studied 22 adults with attachment insecurity. Using T1-weighted MRI they found bilateral hippocampal volume reduction and reduced cell concentration in the left hippocampus. Buss *et al.* (2007) found that birth weight predicts hippocampal volume in adult women reporting poor maternal care by their own mothers and concluded that maternal care as a postnatal environmental variable modulates the neurodevelopmental consequences of prenatal risk – low birth weight – in women, but not in men.

In a review article by Korosi and Baram (2009) entitled 'The pathways from mother's love to baby's future', the authors describe how early-life experiences govern the expression and functioning of stress-related genes throughout life, especially what happens in the infant's brain after early-life stress.

Stress later in life

The consequences of stress in children and adults have been clinically studied. Post-traumatic stress disorder (PTSD) is often found in people in areas where wars or natural disasters have occurred and who have suffered the sudden loss of beloved family members or friends, as well as in the victims of several kinds of personally experienced aggression.

Bremner *et al.* (1995) used MRI to demonstrate that combat veterans with PTSD have reduced right-sided hippocampal volume, accompanied by certain memory deficits. Their findings were confirmed by Kitayama *et al.* (2005). Bremner *et al.* (1997) found that adults with a history of physical abuse, including sexual/incestuous abuse, many of whom have symptoms of PTSD, have a smaller than normal hippocampus. The left hippocampus was 12 per cent smaller compared to the left hippocampus of control subjects, while the right hippocampus was 5 per cent smaller (not significant). However, the authors do not exclude the fact that some people are born with smaller hippocampal volumes, thought to be genetically determined. Female victims of childhood sexual abuse have more pronounced reduction in the volume of the left hippocampus, in addition to psychiatric disorders (Stein *et al.*, 1997).

However, a dysfunctional HPA axis is not the only explanation for deviant stress responses and ensuing neuropsychiatric disorders such as PTSD and BPD. Hippocampal damage has consequences for the stress response, learning, affect, memory and other cognitive functions. Neuronal damage in parts of the brain other than the hippocampus, which are beyond the limbic system (*e.g.*, the cerebellum and the corpus callosum), may be a contributing factor, as are abnormalities in the catecholamine system. High cortisol levels, for example, may be responsible for a deviant serotonin system. This question is not further addressed here.

Conclusions

Early attachment not only protects the infant from a hostile environment, but also creates a long-lasting, robust template, a source of resilience the individual can draw on later in life in order to cope with stress. Stress can be physical (hunger, poverty, or disease) or relational (sudden separation from loved ones, threats to or aggression inflicted on the body), and there are also milder forms of stress caused, for example, by financial loss or being deceived by friends. The relational template – secure attachment – ensures that other people's relational capacities can reduce stress in a typically attached person. A healthy stress-reduction mechanism also results from the normal development of the neural networks for physiologic stress response, which entails a number of neurochemical, hormonal, and transmitter balances, including those in the HPA axis, in which a key factor is the downregulation of cortisol, contributing to optimal functioning of the hippocampal formation. An abnormal stress mechanism in the infant – caused either by prenatal biochemical or psychological events, or severe mother–child interaction problems – ultimately leads to clinical problems in social relatedness as well as problems with learning and cognitive functions, based on inefficient coping with stress.

References

Ainsworth, M.D.S., Blehar, M.C., Waters, E. & Wall, S. (1978): *Patterns of Attachment: A Psychological Study of the Strange Situation*. Hillsdale, NJ: Erlbaum.

Barrington, K.J. (2001): The adverse neuro-developmental effects of postnatal steroids in the preterm infant: a systematic review of RCT's. *BMC Pediatrics* **1,** 1.

Besser, A., Vliegen, N., Luyten P. & Blatt, S. (2008): Investigation of vulnerability to postpartum depression from a psychodynamic perspective: systematic empirical base: commentary on issues raised by Blum (2007): *Psychoanal. Psychol.* **25,** 392–410.

Bliss, T.P.V. & Lømo, T. (1973): Long-lasting potentiation of synaptic transmission in the dentate area of the anaesthesized rabbit following stimulation of the perforant path. *J. Physiol.* **232,** 331–356.

Bowlby, J. (1967): *Attachment and Loss: Attachment* (Vol. 1). Harmondsworth: Pelican/Penguin Books.

Bowlby, J. (1973): *Attachment and Loss: Separation, Anxiety and Anger* (Vol. 2). New York: Basic Books.

Bremner, J.D., Randall, P., Scott, T. M., Bronen, R.A., Selbyl, J.P., Southwick, S.M., *et al.* (1995): MRI-based measurement of hippocampus volume in patients with combat-related posttraumatic stress disorder. *Am. J. Psychiatry* **152,** 973–981.

Bremner, J.D., Randall, P., Vermetten, E. Staib, L., Bronen, R.A., Mazure, C., *et al.* (1997): MRI-based measurement of hippocampus volume posttraumatic stress disorder related to childhood physical and sexual abuse: a preliminary report. *Biol. Psychiatry* **41,** 23–32.

Buss, C., Lord, C., Wadiwalla, M., Hellhammer, D.H., Lupien, S.J., Meaney, M.J. & Pruessner, J.C. (2007): Maternal care modulates the relationship between prenatal risk and hippocampus volume in women but not in men. *J. Neurosci.* **27,** 2592–2595.

Calabrese, P., Markowitsch, H.J., Harders, A.G., Scholz, M. & Gehlen, W. (1995): Fornix damage and memory. A case report. *Cortex* **31,** 555–564.

Calabrese, P., Markowitsch, H.J., Durwen, H.F., Falk, A., Heuser, L., Gehlen, W. & Harders, A.G. (1999): The role of limbic and basal forebrain structures in the processing of nonconscious, emotional information. In: *Neuronal Bases and Psychological Aspects of Consciousness*, eds. C. Taddei-Feretti & C. Musio, pp. 100–104. Singapore: World Scientific.

Carter, S. (2003): Developmental consequences of oxytocin. *Physiol. Behav.* **79,** 383–397.

Champagne, D.L., Bagot, R.C., van Hasselt, F., Ramakers, G., Meaney, M.J., de Kloet, E.R., *et al.* (2008): Maternal care and hippocampus plasticity: evidence for experience-dependent structural plasticity, altered synaptic functioning, and differential responsiveness to glucocorticoids and stress. *J. Neurosci.* **28,** 6037–6045.

Coe, C., Kramer, M., Czéh, B., Gould, E., Reeves, A.J., Kirschbaum, C. & Fuchs, E. (2003): Prenatal stress diminishes neurogenesis in the dentate gyrus of juvenile rhesus monkeys. *Biol. Psychiat.* **54,** 1025–1034.

Damasio, A. (2010): *Self Comes to Mind*. New York: Pantheon Books.

Davis, E.P., Snidman, N., Wadhwa, P.D., Glynn, L.M., Schetter, C.D. & Sandman, C.A. (2004): Prenatal maternal anxiety and depression predict negative behavioral reactivity in infancy. *Infancy* **6,** 319–331.

De Haan, M., Mishkin, M., Baldeweg, T. & Vargha-Khadem, F. (2006): Human memory development and its function after early hipppocampal injury. *Trends Neurosci.* **29**: 374–381.

De Kloet, E.R., Vreugdenhil, E., Oitzl, M.S. & Joëls, M. (1998): Brain corticosteroid receptor balance in health and disease. *Endocr. Rev.* **19,** 269–301.

De Kloet, E.R., Joëls, M. & Holsboer, F. (2005): Stress and the brain: from adaptation to the brain. *Nature Rev. Neurosci.* **6,** 463–475.

DeVries, A.C., Glasper, E.R. & Detillion, C.E. (2003): Social modulation of stress responses. *Physiol. Behav.* **79,** 399–407.

Feldman, R. (2007): Parent-infant synchrony and the construction of shared timing: physiological precursors, developmental outcomes, and risk conditions. *J. Child Psychol. Psychiat.* **48,** 329–354.

Feldman, R., Singer, M. & Zagoory, O. (2010): Touch attenuates infants' physiological reactivity to stress. *Dev. Sci.* **13,** 271–278.

Fenoglio, K.A., Brunson, K.L. & Baram, T.Z. (2006): Hippocampus neuroplasticity induced by early-life stress: functional and molecular aspects. *Front. Neuroendocrinol.* **27,** 180–192.

Fonagy, P. (2001a): *Attachment Theory and Psychoanalysis*. New York: Other Press.

Fonagy, P. (2001b): The human genome and the representational world: the role of early mother–infant interaction in creating an interpersonal interpretive mechanism. *Bull. Menninger Clin.* **65,** 427–448.

Fonagy, P., Gergely, G., Jurist, E.L. & Target, M. (2002): *Affect Regulation, Mentalization and the Development of the Self.* New York: Other Press.

Fonagy, P., Gergely, G. & Target, M. (2007): The parent–infant dyad and the construction of the subjective self. *J. Child Psychol. Psychiatry* **48,** 288–328.

French, N.P., Hagan, R., Evans, S.F. Mullan, A. & Newnham, J.P. (2004): Repeated antenatal corticosteroids: effects on cerebral palsy and childhood behavior. *Am. J. Obstet. Gynecol.* **190,** 588–595.

Golse, B. (2004): *Du corps à la pensée.* Paris: Presses Universitaires de France.

Grafman, J., Salazar, A.M., Weingartner, H., Vance, S.C. & Ludlow, C.L. (1985): Isolated impairment of memory following a penetrating lesion of the fornix cerebri. *Arch. Neurol.* **42,** 1162–1168.

Gunnar, M.R., Brodersen, L., Nachmias, M., Buss, K. & Rigatuso, J. (1996): Stress reactivity and attachment security. *Dev. Psychobiol.* **29,** 191-204.

Heimer, L., Van Hoesen, G.W., Trimble, M. & Zahm, D.S. (2008): *Anatomy of Neuropsychiatry. The New Anatomy of the Basal Forebrain and Its Implications for Neuropsychiatric Illness.* Amsterdam: Elsevier.

Herman, J.P. & Cullinan, W.E. (1997): Neurocircuitry of stress: central control of the hypothalamic-pituitary-adrenocortical axis. *Trends Neurosci.* **20,** 78–84.

Herman, J.P., Prewitt, C.M. & Cullinan, W.E. (1996): Neuronal circuit regulation of the hypothalamo-pituitary-adrenocortical stress axis. *Crit. Rev. Neurobiol.* **10,** 371–394.

Hirvikoski, T., Nordenström, A., Lindholm, T., Lindblad, F, Ritzén, E.M., Wedell, A. & Lajic, S. (2007): Cognitive functions in children at risk for congenital adrenal hyperplasia treated prenatally with dexamethasone. *J. Clin. Endrocrinol. Metab.* **92,** 542–548.

Hüther, G. (2006): *The Compassionate Brain.* Boston: Shambhala.

Ijima, T., Witter, M.P., Ichikawa, M., Tominaga, T., Kajiwaga, R. & Matsumoto, G. (1996): Entorhinal-hippocampus interactions revealed by real time imaging. *Science* **272,** 1176–1179.

Ito, Y., Teicher, M.H. & Glod, C.A. (1998): Preliminary evidence for aberrant cortical development in abused children: a quantitative EEG study. *J. Neuropsychiat. Clin. Neurosci.* **10,** 298–307.

Ivry, A.S., Brunson, K.L., Sansman, C. & Baram, T.Z. (2008): Dysfunctional nurturing behavior in rat dams with limited access to nesting material: a clinically relevant model for early-life stress. *Neuroscience.* **154,** 1132–1142.

Jacobson, L. & Sapolsky, R. (1991): The role of the hippocampus in feedback regulation of the hypothalamic-pituitary-adrenocortical axis. *Endocrine Rev.* **12,** 118–140.

Kandel, E.R. (2006): *In Search of Memory. The Emergence of a New Science of Mind.* New York: W.W. Norton.

Kitayama, N., Vaccarino, V., Kutner, M., Weiss, P. & Bremner, J.D. (2005): Magnetic resonance imaging of hippocampal volume in PTSD: a meta-analysis. *J. Affect. Disord.* **88,** 79–86.

Korosi, A. & Baram T. Z. (2009): The pathways from mother's love to baby's future. *Frontiers Behav. Neurosci.* **3,** 1–8.

Liggins, G.C. & Howie, R.N. (1972): A controlled trial of antepartum glucocorticoid treatment for prevention of the respiratory distress syndrome in premature infants. *Pediatrics* **50,** 515–525.

Liotti, M. & Panksepp, J. (2004): Imaging human emotions and affective feelings: implications for biological psychiatry. In: *Textbook of Biological Psychiatry*, ed J. Panksepp. Hoboken, NJ: Wiley–Liss.

Liu, D., Diorio, J., Day, J., Francis, D.D. & Meaney, M.J. (2000): Maternal care, hippocampus synaptogenesis and cognitive development in rats. *Nat. Neurosci.* **3,** 799–806.

MacLean, P. (1990): *The Triune Brain in Evolution.* New York: Plenum Press.

Markowitsch, H.J., Kessler, J., Van der Ven, C., Weber-Luxenburger, G, Albers M. & Heiss, W.D. (1998): Psychic trauma causing grossly reduced brain metabolism and cognitive deterioration. *Neuropsychology* **36,** 77–82.

Meaney, M.J. (2001): Maternal care, gene expression and the transmission of individual differences in stress reactivity across generations. *Annu. Rev. Neurosci.* **24,** 1161–1192.

Nieuwenhuys, R. (1996): The greater limbic system, the emotional motor system and the brain. In: *The Emotional Motor System,* eds. G. Holstege, R. Bandler & C.B. Saper. *Prog. Brain Res.* **107,** 551–580.

Nieuwenhuys, R., ten Donkelaar, H.J. & Nicholson, C. (1998): *The Central Nervous System of Vertebrates.* Berlin: Springer.

Nieuwenhuys, R., Voogd, J. & van Huijzen, Chr. (2008): *The Human Central Nervous System* (4th ed.). Berlin: Springer.

Njiokiktjien, C., de Sonneville, L. & Verschoor, C.A. (2011): Understanding of its caretaker's affective gestures by the young infant is the basis of a theory of body. *Neuropsychoanalysis.* In press.

O'Connor, T.G., Heron, J., Golding, J., Gover, V., and the AL SPAC Study Team (2003): Maternal antenatal anxiety and behavioural/emotional problems in children: a test of a programming hypothesis. *J. Child Psychol. Psychiatry* **44,** 1025–1036.

Owen, D. & Matthews, S.G. (2003): Glucocorticoids and sex dependent development of brain glucocorticoid and mineralocorticoid repeptors. *Endocrinology* **144,** 2775–2784.

Owen, D. & Matthews, S.G. (2007): Repeated maternal glucocorticoid treatment affects activity and hippocampus NMDA receptor expression in juvenile guinea pigs. *J. Physiol.* **578,** 249–257.

Panksepp, J. (1998): *Affective Neuroscience. The Foundations of Human and Animal Emotions.* Oxford: Oxford University Press.

Papez, J.W. (1937): A proposed mechanism of emotion. *Arch. Neurol. Psychiatry* **38,** 725–43.

Park, S.A., Hahn, J.H., Kim, J.I., Na, D.L. & Huh, K. (2000): Memory deficits after bilateral anterior fornix infarction. *Neurology* **54,** 1379–1382.

Payne, C., Machado, C.J., Bliwise, N.G. & Bachevalier, J. (2009): Maturation of the hippocampus formation and amygdala in *Macaca mulata*: a volumetric magnetic resonance study. *Hippocampus* **3,** 183–192.

Plotsky, P.M. & Meaney, M.J. (1993): Early postnatal experience alters hypothalamic corticotrophin-releasing factor (CRF): mRNA, median eminence CRF content and stress-induced release in adult rats. *Mol. Brain Res.* **18,** 195–200.

Quirin, M., Gillath, O., Pruessner, J.C. & Eggert, L.D. (2009): Adult attachment insecurity and hippocampus cell density. *Soc. Cogn. Affect. Neurosci.* **5,** 39–47.

Rakic, P. & Novakowski, R. (1981): The time and origin of neurons in the hippocampus region of the rhesus monkey. *J. Comp. Neurol.* **196,** 99–128.

Riva, D., Saletti, V. & Nichelli, F. (2000): The organization of memory in temporo-mesial structures in developmental age. In: *Localization of Brain Lesions and Developmental Functions*, eds. D. Riva & A. Benton, pp. 15–21. Mariani Foundation Paediatric Neurology Series-IX. London: John Libbey.

Sapolsky, R.M. (1996): Why stress is bad for your brain. *Science* **273,** 749–750.

Schore, A.N. (2001): The effects of early relational trauma on right brain development, affect regulation, and infant mental health. *Inf. Men. Health J.* **22,** 201–269.

Schore, A.N. (2003a): The human unconscious: the development of the right brain and its role in early emotional life. In: *Emotional Development in Psychoanalysis, Attachment Theory and Neuroscience*, ed. V. Green, pp. 23–55. New York: Brunner-Routledge.

Schore, A.N. (2003b): *Affect Regulation and the Repair of the Self*, pp. 205–278. New York: W.W. Norton.

Schore, A.N. (2003c): *Affect Regulation and Disorders of the Self*, pp. 54–70, 89–265. New York: W.W Norton.

Schore, A.N. (2009): Relational trauma and the developing right brain: an interface of psychoanalytic self psychology and neuroscience. *Ann, N.Y. Acad. Sci.* **1159,** 189–203.

Schore, J.R. & Schore, A.N. (2008): Modern attachment: the central role of affect regulation in development and treatment. *Clin. Soc. Work* **36,** 9–20.

Setiawan, E., Jackson, M.F., Macdonald, J.F. & Matthews, S.G. (2007): Effects of repeated prenatal glucocorticoid exposure on LTP in the juvenile guinea pig hippocampus. *J. Physiol.* **581,** 1033–1042.

Smeekens, S., Riksen-Walraven, J.M., van Bakel, H.J.A. & de Weerth, C. (2010): Five-year-olds' cortisol reactions to an attachment story completion task. *Psychoneuroendocrinology* **35,** 858–865.

Solms, M. & Turnbull, O. (2004): *The Brain and the Inner World.* London: Karnac.

Stein, M.B., Koverola, C., Hanna, C., Torchia, M.G. & McClarty, B. (1997): Hippocampus volume in women victimized by childhood sexual abuse. *Psychol. Med.* **27,** 951–959.

Stein-Behrens, B.A., Lin, W.J. & Sapolsky, R.M. (1994): Physiological elevations of glucocorticoids potentiate glutamate accumulation in the hippocampus. *J. Neurochem.* **63,** 596–602.

Stern, D. (1985): *The Interpersonal World of the Infant: A View from Psychoanalysis and Developmental Psychology.* New York: Basic Books.

Teicher, M.H. (2002): Scars that won't heal: the neurobiology of child abuse. *Sci. Am.* (March), 54–61; and *Cerebrum* **2,** 50–67.

Turnbull, O. & Solms, M. (2003): Memory, amnesia and intuition: a neuro-psychoanalytic perspective. In: *Emotional Development in Psychoanalysis, Attachment Theory and Neuroscience*, ed. V. Green, pp. 55–85. New York: Brunner-Routledge.

Uno, H., Lohmiller, L., Thieme, C., Kemnitz, J.W., Engle, M.J., Roecker, E.B. & Farrell, P.M. (1990): Brain damage induced by prenatal exposure to dexamethasone in fetal rhesus macaques. I. Hippocampus. *Dev. Brain Res.* **53,** 157–67.

Uno, H., Eisele, S., Sakai, A., Shelton, S., Baker, E., DeJesus, O. & Holden, J. (1994): Neurotoxicity of glucocorticoids in the primate brain. *Horm. Behav.* **28,** 336–48.

Weinberg, M.K. & Tronick, E.Z. (1998): Emotional care of the at-risk infant: emotional characteristics of infants associated with maternal depression and anxiety. *Pediatrics* **102,** 1298–1304.

Weinstock, M. (1997): Does prenatal stress impair coping and regulation of hypothalamic, pituitary-adrenal axis? *Neurosci. Biobehav. Rev.* **21,** 1–10.

Winnicott, D.W. (1970): The mother–infant experience of mutuality. In: *Parenthood, its Psychology and Psychopathology*, eds. E. Antony & T Beneder. Boston: Little, Brown.

Zhang, L., Xing, G., Levine, S., Post, R. & Smith, M. (1997): Maternal deprivation introduces neuronal death. *Soc. Neurosci. Abstr.* **23,** 1113.

Brain Lesion Localization and Developmental Functions, D. Riva, C. Njiokiktjien and S. Bulgheroni (eds.)

Chapter 14

Music, emotions and the limbic system

Maria Cristina Saccuman*,§, Guido Andreolli^ and Danilo Spada°

**Faculty of Psychology, Università Vita-Salute San Raffaele, via Olgettina 58, 20132 Milan, Italy;*
§Division of Neurosciences, Istituto Scientifico San Raffaele, via Olgettina 58, 20132 Milan, Italy;
^Faculty of Philosophy, Università Vita-Salute San Raffaele, via Olgettina 58, 20132 Milan, Italy;
°Centro di Eccellenza per la Risonanza Magnetica ad Alto Campo (CERMAC), Istituto Scientifico San Raffaele, via Olgettina 60, 20132 Milano
cristina.saccuman@gmail.com

Summary

Music has the ability to evoke profound emotions, and yet it is unique among the stimuli that induce emotional responses, in that it does not appear to have any obvious role in promoting the survival of our species. But even though its biologic function remains unspecified, the human brain is exquisitely sensitive to the emotional language of musical communication. In this chapter, we review the literature that suggests that music induces emotions directly, causing measurable physiologic changes and cortical and subcortical activation similar to that of other emotional stimuli. We then consider how music is perceived in infancy, and whether infants, who have no experience with cultural conventions, experience musical emotions. We report studies showing that infants show an emotional reaction to music, and recent neuroimaging data suggesting that the newborn brain responds to music specifically and shows activation of limbic structures. There appears to be a basic, instinctual emotional response to music, and in infancy music modulates affect, promotes the growth of emotional attachment, and might get infants tuned to language and communication.

Introduction

As a human experience, music goes back to ancient times, probably to more than 35,000 years ago. There is evidence that individuals played flutes in diverse social and cultural contexts. The instruments were later found together with many other forms of occupational debris (Conard *et al.*, 2009). Such an ancestral and apparently simple experience constitutes an extraordinary complex object of study. Musical activity covers an extremely wide spectrum, going from apparently effortless everyday appreciation of music to the highly specialized competence of expert performers and composers. In recent years, music has become a fruitful research field for cognitive neuroscience because of the possibility it offers to address brain functional specialization, integration, and plasticity. On the other hand, neuroscience has become a means to address questions about music perception, production, and appreciation. In the neuroscientific literature, we simplify such a complex object of study, leaving aside many fundamental aspects pertaining to ethnomusicological, aesthetic, historical, and social issues, and focus on some general features common to all music forms. Even the common distinction between musicians and nonmusicians (people with or without formal musical training) is only useful as a starting point on account of the profound differences between musicians in terms of age of onset of training, proficiency level (amateur to outstanding), and specialization (instrument, genre, style, *etc.*).

Very generally speaking, beside timbre (*e.g.*, the particular instrument or voice performing music) and loudness (*i.e.*, the perceived intensity of sound), music is produced by combining sounds of defined pitch (tones) and duration. Pitch is the psychological quality of the perceived frequency of a sound, and has two dimensions: *height*, monotonically related to frequency, and *chroma*, which is the quality of tones that are in the 2:1, or octave ratio, and are perceived as highly similar. These two features of pitch make the existence of musical scales possible. Different musical scales are the basis of the world's various musical systems, including the Western tonal system.

In music, both pitch and duration are in particular ratios – usually expressed by integer numbers – with each other, leading to the formation of structures characterized by properties that in the current literature are often defined as 'syntactic', in analogy with language. From such a perspective, the idea is that beyond the linear order of sounds, principles of hierarchic organization are working at various levels, both in production and in perception. Most human beings have a tacit 'competence', as they do for their native language, for the musical idiom of their native culture. Despite the profound differences between musicians and nonmusicians in terms of performance and perception abilities, it seems that other abilities, like the competence for one's native musical idiom or the emotional response to certain features of music, are quite similar irrespective of expertise (Jackendoff & Lerdahl, 2006; Lerdahl & Jackendoff, 1996).

A musical feature in the pitch domain, namely consonance/dissonance, is particularly relevant for some experiments reviewed in the chapter, and it might be worth defining it here. Consonance and dissonance are basic perceptual properties of tones occurring simultaneously. Consonant tone combinations (in the Western-theory terminology: harmonic *intervals*, when two tones are combined, or *chords*, when three or more tones in particular ratios sound together) are generally perceived as more pleasant and calm than are dissonant ones, particularly by Western listeners (Blood & Zatorre, 2001; Koelsch *et al.*, 2006). Since antiquity, it has been recognized that consonance tends to be generated by tones whose fundamental frequencies are related to each other by simple (small-integer) ratios, while combinations of tones related to each other by complex (large-integer) ratios are perceived as unpleasant and 'rough.' The available evidence indicates that the perception of sensory dissonance is a function of physical properties of auditory stimuli as well as of basic physiologic and anatomic constraints, independent of specific cultural experience (Fritz *et al.*, 2009). According to one leading hypothesis, when the upper harmonic components of a complex sound are separated from one another in frequency by less than the width of a critical bandwidth (Zwicker, 1982), they remain unresolved by the basilar membrane within the cochlea. Unresolved excitation patterns overlap and produce fluctuations that are perceived as unpleasant beats or 'roughness' (Fishman *et al.*, 2001; Tramo *et al.*, 2001). The ability to discriminate isolated consonant and dissonant intervals and chords has been observed across species, including song birds (Hulse *et al.*, 1995), rodents (Fannin & Braud, 1971), and monkeys (Izumi, 2000), pointing to a perceptual mechanism that is not specific for music processing, and that is only a prerequisite for the complex experience of music listening and appreciation in humans. It is worth saying that a variable amount of dissonance in a musical piece is not only tolerable but desirable. In the Western tradition, all polyphonic music contains dissonances interspersed between consonances. In jazz, dissonance is important for giving chords particular nuances. Music is characterized by patterns in which consonances and dissonances alternate, leading to the perception of patterns of tension and resolution which are fundamental for the aesthetic and emotional experience of music.

In this chapter we will focus on one important feature of music: the way sound structures developing through time affect our emotional responses.

Music and emotions

Music has the unique ability to evoke profound emotions, trigger memories, and intensify our social experiences. We do not need to be trained in music performance or appreciation to be moved by music. We seem to relate to it spontaneously and effortlessly (Molnar-Szakacs & Overy, 2006). All humans, in all known cultures, are attracted to music, and yet music is unique among the stimuli that induce emotions (and by emotional responses we indicate a wide range of reactions, going from autonomic behaviours to the evocation of complex and rich feelings, imagination, and memories), in that it seems to have no apparent role in promoting the survival of our species. But even though music's biologic role remains unspecified, the human brain is exquisitely sensitive to the emotional language of musical communication.

This form of communication based on emotion appears to be largely independent of exposure to a specific musical culture. Fritz and colleagues (2009) recently investigated the recognition of basic musical emotions, as expressed in Western music, in a population never previously exposed to such music. The individuals tested belonged to the Mafa ethnic group of Cameroon, who live in isolated villages with no source of electricity. When presented with instrumental pieces chosen by Western listeners to express basic emotions (happy, sad, scared), Mafa listeners recognized all three emotional expressions beyond chance. This study suggests that at least these basic emotions conveyed by Western music can be universally recognized, similar to the recognition of facial expressions and language prosody.

Basic emotions expressed through music appear to be recognizable independently of cultural experience, and even in populations who have difficulties with pitch processing (Peretz *et al.*, 2001) or interpersonal relationships (Heaton, 2009). This raises questions about the relation between musical structure and emotional content processing. There does not seem to exist a univocal mapping between musical features and emotions, and at least some basic emotions can be recognized without the need to discriminate the structural details of a piece of music. This is partly because affective responses are driven by relatively superficial characteristics of music. In particular, tempo and pitch range account for a large proportion of the variance in people's judgement of happy *vs.* sad music (Thompson *et al.*, 2001). Some emotions are expressed with more precision than others. In general, listeners readily agree that an example of music is sad – with its quiet, slow, *legato* articulation and large deviation from metrical timing, or happy – with high-pitched, fast, *staccato* features and small variations from metrical timing – but they might not agree on whether a music expresses a more nuanced emotion, such as *tenderness* as opposed to *sadness* (Trainor & Schmidt, 2003).

There is another aspect that sets music apart from other stimuli that evoke emotional reactions. Music, even sad or scary music, does not induce withdrawal behaviours. In fact, people feel attracted to music with different emotional colouring, and find it rewarding regardless of whether it is marked as sad or happy (Menon & Levitin, 2005). Because of the seemingly complex relation between music and approach/withdrawal behaviours, it would be possible to think that music describes emotions we *recognize*, without leading us to *feel* the emotions.

There is still debate in the field of neuroscience as to the nature of emotional experiences and the relationship between cognitive and emotional states. How do conscious cognitive processes and unconscious automatic processes interplay in assigning emotional value to a specific stimulus? In the case of music, how does a basic perceptual judgement (of consonance or dissonance, for example) lead to an emotional reaction, or the qualification of a piece of music as 'pleasant' or 'unpleasant'?

The first issue we address in this chapter is whether music engages autonomic and neocortical systems in a way similar to other emotion-inducing stimuli. We then consider how music is perceived in infancy, and whether infants, who have no experience with cultural conventions, experience musical emotions.

Physiologic response

The experience of emotion is linked to physiologic events, such as changes in breathing and heart rate, muscle contraction, salivation and sweating, skin conductance, and immune responses. These peripheral, autonomic, endocrine and skeletomotor responses are regulated by subcortical structures: the amygdala, the hypothalamus, and the brain stem (Phillips *et al.*, 2003). The first step in studying the emotional reactions to music is the search for these basic, physiologic effects in response to music, which could set the ground for more complex emotional responses.

Measure of skin conductance, known to be sensitive to variations in emotional arousal, have been taken in response to music of different valence (positive or negative) and arousal level (high or low), showing that music induces changes in skin conductance response that vary with underlying dimensions of emotions, in particular arousal. In fact, fear and happiness, both highly arousing emotions, were associated with higher skin conductance response than were sadness and peacefulness (Khalfa *et al.*, 2002).

Other studies considered cardiovascular and respiratory parameters, showing that when musicians and nonmusicians were exposed to different musical styles, faster tempo, and simpler rhythmic structures there was an increase in breathing rate, heart rate, and blood pressure, with musicians being more sensitive to the music tempo than were nonmusicians. The effect seemed to be independent of a person's musical preferences and of habituation (Bernardi *et al.*, 2006). In another study, cardiovascular and respiratory fluctuations appeared to mirror the music profile, particularly if it contained a 'crescendo', that is, a gradual increase in loudness. In this case, the physiological changes were independent of musical training, musical preference, and subjects' conscious reaction to music (Bernardi *et al.*, 2009). Exposure to music also seems to affect the immune system through a reduction of stress levels, as shown in rats suffering from asthma (Lu *et al.*, 2010).

We can tentatively conclude that music induces emotions directly, leading to measurable physiologic changes. In particular, these physiologic parameters seem to capture the dimension of the emotional experience of 'arousal'. It is worth noting that some of these effects vary with the subject's musical training, while others do not, and that effects have been observed not only in humans, but also in other vertebrates, like rats, and are thus presumably independent of an explicit understanding and enjoyment of music (Lu *et al.*, 2010; Nakamura *et al.*, 2007). More research is needed to explore how the autonomic response is affected by personal preference and musical training, and whether there are specific physiological reactions in response to emotional dimensions other than arousal.

Central nervous system response to music

Evidence from neurophysiologic, electrophysiologic, neuropsychological, and imaging studies has shown a consistent network for music processing in adults, involving the superior temporal gyrus, and inferior frontal and parietal areas (Parsons, 2003). Right hemispheric dominance is generally observed for tasks with a focus on pitch processing, but laterality is sensitive to strategy (analytic *vs.* holistic processing) and degree of musical training (Peretz & Morais, 1987; Peretz *et al.*, 1987). However, less is known about the neural correlates of emotional response to music, their relation to music perception and to other forms of emotion (Trainor & Schmidt, 2003). This is because of difficulties in isolating and measuring something elusive like emotion and correlating it in a quantitative fashion with variations in haemodynamic or neural activity.

In the previous section we have discussed basic physiologic responses to music, showing that they can be elicited by superficial features, such as loudness or tempo. Another perceptual feature, consonance/dissonance, has been used to explore the neural response to musical emotions. The perception of dissonance, which is known to correlate with subjective judgements of pleasantness and unpleasantness, relies mostly on peripheral structures of the auditory system, and appears to be consistent and stable, independent of musical preference and musical training. Blood *et al.* (1999) used positron emission tomography (PET) to identify brain structures where regional cerebral blood flow (rCBF) correlates with increasing dissonance and consonance of musical stimuli. These authors found that the activity in paralimbic and neocortical areas known to be involved in the processing of emotion correlated with varying levels of dissonance or consonance. The areas were the right parahippocampal gyrus, right precuneus, bilateral orbitofrontal, medial subcallosal cingulate and right frontal polar regions, with different patterns of activation associated with consonance as opposed to dissonance. In particular, the activity in the parahippocampal gyrus and precuneus correlated with increasing dissonance.

It is worth remarking that this first study does not address a valence distinction *per se*, as dissonant stimuli are likely to be perceived as irritating (negative valence, high intensity) rather than sad (negative valence, low intensity), in opposition to neutral or mildly pleasant consonant stimuli (positive valence, low intensity) (Trainor & Schmidt, 2003).

A further step has been the identification of an indicator that besides physiologic arousal included clearly describable subjective feelings, such as a highly rewarding experience of pleasure. In a second study, Blood and Zatorre (2001) investigated the neural correlates of intensely pleasurable response to music, the so called 'chills' or 'shivers-down-the-spine' that some people feel in response to their favourite music. Each of the musically-trained subjects selected a piece of music that consistently elicited 'chills', and listened to it while PET was used to measure their brain response. Music selected by other subjects was used as control condition. Physiological responses, such as heart rate and respiration depth, were also recorded during PET scans. Compared to control conditions, chills were associated with increases in physiologic parameters, and changes in rCBF: increases were measured in left ventral striatum and dorsomedial midbrain, paralimbic regions, and thalamus, whereas decreases were measured in right amygdala, left hippocampus, and ventromedial prefrontal cortex. These responses are similar to those observed in association with feelings of euphoria and pleasant emotion, for example, during cocaine administration in cocaine-dependent subjects, and in response to rewarding stimuli such as food and sex. Remarkably, an abstract stimulus like music recruited neural systems known to respond to biologically relevant stimuli or pharmacologic substances.

The fact that the subjects were musicians, and were selected because of their consistent and intense response to music, could limit the generalization of these results, as other subjects might respond less intensely.

More recently, Koelsch *et al.* (2006) addressed a similar question as Blood *et al.* (1999) using fMRI and pleasant, naturalistic music, as opposed to the digitized music used by Blood (Blood *et al.*, 1999). The hypothesis was that the naturalistic music would evoke more positive emotions than its digitalized version. Nonmusician subjects heard a set of pleasant stimuli, and permanently dissonant versions of the same stimuli qualified as unpleasant. In the left hemisphere, the amygdala, hippocampus, and parahippocampal gyrus, and the temporal pole in the right hemisphere, were more active for unpleasant compared to pleasant music. These structures are involved in affective state regulation, and in the processing of emotions with unpleasant valence. The hippocampus, parahippocampal gyrus and temporal poles are interconnected with the amygdala, and both the parahippocampal gyrus and temporal poles receive input from auditory association areas, and appear to be part of a paralimbic circuit involved in processing of complex auditory information with emotional valence.

The areas more active for pleasant music were the left inferior frontal gyrus, and insula, ventral striatum, Heschl's gyrus, and the rolandic operculum bilaterally. According to the authors, this pattern suggests that pleasant music activates a motor-related circuit that serves the formation of premotor representation for vocal sound production. The rolandic operculum, also involved in overt and covert singing, possibly contains a representation of the larynx, as if subjects coded vocal sound production when they heard the pleasant music, with the activation of a perception–execution matching mechanism similar to that of mirror neurons. Also possible, as suggested by studies on sentence processing, is an involvement of the rolandic operculum in the processing of music syntactic information. The superior insula is involved in articulatory planning, whereas the ventral striatum, as in Blood (2001), is implicated in the processing of stimuli with positive valence. It receives input from limbic structures (amygdala, hippocampus), and sends output to structures involved in behaviour expression, forming a 'limbic–motor interface'.

In another study, Menon and Levitin (2005) expanded on Blood and Zatorre's (2001) study, making the results more generalizable with nonmusician subjects, and using fMRI with functional and effective connectivity techniques to characterize the dynamics of the activations observed. Stimuli were classical music excerpts, *not* selected by the subjects and rated for pleasantness, while control stimuli were the same pieces cut up and scrambled.

Like Blood and Zatorre (2001), the authors focused on reward processing, known to involve the nucleus accumbens (NAc) and the ventral tegmental area (VTA). Previous studies had found activation for NAc in tasks involving monetary rewards and recreational and addictive drugs. The hypothesis to be tested was that the NAc would be strongly activated when subjects listened to classical music, though in the case of music no explicit reward was present, and that its response would correlate with activation in the hypothalamus. Note that PET, used by Blood and Zatorre (2001), lacks the spatial resolution to image the NAc, even though the ventral striatum was found to be active in correlation with the pleasurable response to music.

The results confirmed the hypothesis: activation for music was observed in the NAc, VTA, and hypothalamus activation also occurred in frontal areas, the anterior cingulate, cerebellar vermis, and brainstem. It is worth noting that activation in response to music in the hypothalamus, which modulates the autonomic responses described above, was here observed for the first time. Functional connectivity showed correlation between responses in the NAc and VTA, and between responses in NAc and the hypothalamus. Effective connectivity, testing for regions co-activated with both the NAc and the VTA, showed VTA-dependent NAc interactions with the hypothalamus, insula, and OFC, allowing inferences to be drawn about regions affected by the dopaminergic reward pathway.

The VTA is in fact the site of mesolimbic dopamine neurons that project to the NAc, and there is an association between dopamine release and the NAc response to pleasant music. The rewarding aspect of music seems to be related to increased levels of dopamine in NAc and VTA.

This set of studies confirms that listening to music activates neural resources involved in the processing of emotional responses. The overall picture shows an integration of the reward and affective systems with the cognitive and autonomic systems during the experience of listening to pleasant music.

Development of the emotional response to music

Despite the complexity of the cognitive operations implied by music perception, mounting evidence indicates that newborns and young infants are already highly sensitive to musical information. From the first days of life, music appears to play an important role for emotional, cognitive, and social development, and infants are surprisingly skilled at processing subtle aspects of musical stimuli. In fact, their music perception skills are very similar to those of adult untrained listeners. Infants possess the abilities for relational processing of pitch and tempo, for the differentiation of consonant versus dissonant intervals, and for the detection of variations in meter, timbre, and tempo as well as duration of tones and musical phrases (Trehub, 2001).

This musical competence of infants plays a crucial role in early language learning, since the processing of speech prosody (that is, of the musical features of speech such as speech melody and rhythm) provides important cues for the identification of syllables, words, and phrases (Jusczyk, 1999; Jusczyk *et al.*, 1999; Thiessen & Saffran, 2003). The available evidence indicates that infants are predisposed to perceive music, but only a handful of studies have focused on whether infants experience emotions through music.

In all cultures, caretakers provide some form of musical input to young babies, usually in the form of singing performed in a distinctive style, some aspects of which are recognizable across cultures and musical systems (Trehub *et al.*, 1997). Mothers have a small repertoire of soothing lullabies and rhythmic playsongs that they perform in a highly ritualized manner, with each song rendered in pitch and tempo that remain very consistent from one performance to the next (Trehub *et al.*, 1997).

Infants respond to such music, showing a clear preference for songs delivered with the rich emotional intonations that characterize maternal style (Masataka, 1999) and responding with focused attention and a reduction in movements to performances where they are allowed to hear and see the singer (Masataka, 1999; Trainor, 1996). Shenfield and colleagues have shown that after their mother sang to them for 10 minutes, 6-month-old infants showed a change in the cortisol level in their saliva. In particular, salivary cortisol levels decreased in infants with initially high cortisol levels, and increased in infants with initially low levels of cortisol (Shenfield *et al.*, 2003).

A number of studies on premature infants has shown that, as in adults, music has a direct impact on physiological parameters, leading to decreases in heart rate, salivary cortisol, and distress behaviour, and increases in oxygen saturation and non-nutritive sucking rate (Arnon *et al.*, 2006; Standley, 2002, 1998; Standley & Moore, 1995). In preterm infants, exposure to music promotes weight gain, possibly through a reduction of resting energy expenditure, resulting in a shorter hospital stay (Lubetzky *et al.*, 2009).

Thus, it appears that music has a measurable effect on infant physiology, but the bases for infants' emotional reaction to music remains mostly unclear, although it is probable that, as in adults, they depend on specific characteristics of pitch, tempo, and timbre of musical pieces. One aspect that has received considerable attention is the difference in infants' response to consonance and dissonance. Studies have shown that already at 4 months infants show preference for consonant melodies over dissonant ones (Zentner & Kagan, 1998), and at 2 months they prefer to listen to consonant intervals (Trainor & Desjardins, 2002). In a recent study, Masataka tested 2-day-old newborns, showing that newborns looked longer at a visual display when the original version of a Mozart minuet was played during their looking time, rather than a version modified to contain dissonant intervals. Remarkably, this effect was also measured on hearing infants born to deaf parents who did not use vocal language. The results in the babies who had been exposed to considerably less prenatal auditory input did not differ from those of infants born to hearing parents (Masataka, 2006). The specific weighting of genetic and cultural factors in shaping early sensitivity to consonance and dissonance remains to be specified. In principle, it is possible that the auditory system is tuned by pre- and perinatal exposure to speech and musical sounds, which tend to be consonant, but data like Masataka's (2006) suggest that the preference for consonant sounds might be somewhat independent of extensive exposure to auditory stimuli *in utero*. The existence of an early bias towards consonance in infants also suggests that there might be a link between ease of processing and the judgment of pleasantness, as if the former would be the only available experiential correlate of consciously inaccessible neurophysiologic events.

The observation that singing is part of infant care in all cultures and the evidence that music can modulate infants' attention, arousal level, and physiologic state raise the possibility that maternal singing, and the biological predisposition to enjoy music, results in important biologic adaptations. Maternal singing could enhance reciprocal emotional attachment and sustain parental commitment, promoting the infant's well-being, sleep induction, a reduction in crying and displays of positive affect (Trehub, 2001). In addition, the emotional response induced by musical input could support infants' early interest in speech and social interaction. These social and emotional abilities, combined with computational skills, appear to form the basis for humans' capacity for language and communication (Meltzoff *et al.*, 2009).

Despite significant evidence for the importance of auditorily-induced emotional response from the first days of life, its neural basis in infancy and the neural basis of music processing in general have remained largely unexplored. Recently, a number of noninvasive brain imaging and electrophysiologic techniques have proved to be both reliable and comfortable for use with infants, providing informative data on auditory processing from the first hours after birth. Sambeth and colleagues used magnetoencephalography (MEG) to explore the response to emotional speech prosody in young infants (Sambeth *et al.*, 2008). They reported a sensitivity of the newborn brain to prosodic cues in language, as shown by a decrease of brain response when the speech prosody was impoverished (compared to prosodically rich conditions). Another study used event-related brain potentials to measure the response of 7-month-olds to emotional prosody: babies heard words pronounced with neutral, happy, or angry intonations (Grossmann *et al.*, 2005). A positive slow wave (700–1,000 ms) over temporal sites was elicited by happy or angry prosody compared to the neutral intonation, indicating a difference in processing based on the emotional content of speech stimuli.

In a recent study, our group used functional magnetic resonance imaging (fMRI) to investigate the neural correlates of music processing, including the processing of dissonant music, in neonates (Perani *et al.*, 2010). The goal of the study was to examine how the brain processes musical stimuli at a point where exposure to music has been minimal and presumably not sufficient to induce major shaping of the processing networks, providing information on the biologic constraints that lead, with normal experience, to the typical trajectory of brain development. We also aimed at exploring the early sensitivity of the core structures of emotional processing, and the specificity of their responses, to original and altered music stimuli.

Eighteen healthy, full-term, nonsedated newborns within the first 3 days of life heard excerpts of classical music pieces (Original Music), and counterparts of these excerpts that varied in their structural properties, and in their degree of consonance and dissonance (two sets of Altered Music). For one set of Altered Music (key shifts), all voices were infrequently shifted one semitone up or down, thus infrequently shifting the tonal centre to a tonal key that was harmonically only distantly related to the preceding harmonic context (*e.g.*, from C major to C$^{\#}$ major). For the other set (dissonance), the upper voice (*i.e.*, melody) of the musical excerpts was permanently shifted one semitone upward, rendering the excerpts permanently dissonant. The control conditions were chosen so as to be acoustically closely matched to the original stimuli, and still containing similar structural musical elements. While the Original Music condition addressed a basic question about the neural substrate of music processing in newborns, the Altered Music conditions tested the specificity of the newborn brain's response to music. In other words, the experiment explored whether the brain would be sensitive to subtle variations of the musical stimuli, or respond indifferently to any generically music-like stimulus. The Altered Music condition would also provide information on the involvement of brain structures known to be active in correlation with emotional responses.

For original music perception, results showed an extended activation cluster focused in the right superior temporal gyrus, with its peak activation being located in the primary auditory cortex (transverse temporal gyrus), extending into the secondary auditory cortex, and anteriorly into the planum polare, as well as posteriorly into the planum temporale, temporoparietal junction, and inferior parietal lobule. A smaller, weaker cluster of activation was observed in the left primary and secondary auditory cortices (Fig. 1A). Thus, hemispheric functional asymmetry for music perception in the primary, secondary, and higher-order auditory cortices is present at birth. This is in accordance with the right-dominant asymmetric activation pattern observed in adults during music processing (Peretz & Zatorre, 2005). In adult brains, the asymmetry has been attributed to specialization of the left and right auditory cortices for the processing of temporal and spectral aspects of acoustic stimuli, with the left hemisphere having better temporal resolution (crucial for speech analysis) and the right hemisphere having a better frequency resolution (required for pitch processing) (Zatorre & Belin, 2001). The lateralized specialization of brain structures has been observed very early in development, in studies of both anatomy (Chi *et al.*, 1977) and of gene-expression (Sun & Walsh, 2006; Sun *et al.*, 2005, 2006). Early hemispheric asymmetries, observed before the beginning of auditory capabilities, may contribute to the early functional asymmetries reported in this study.

The study also showed that the hemodynamic response was modulated by alterations of the musical stimuli, with less activation in the right primary and secondary auditory cortex as well as surrounding regions, and left-hemispheric activations in associative temporal and inferior frontal cortex when Altered Music was presented (the two altered conditions elicited a similar response, and the data were pooled for increased statistical power) (Fig 1B). These findings indicate that newborns' neural responses to music can be modulated by structural variations of

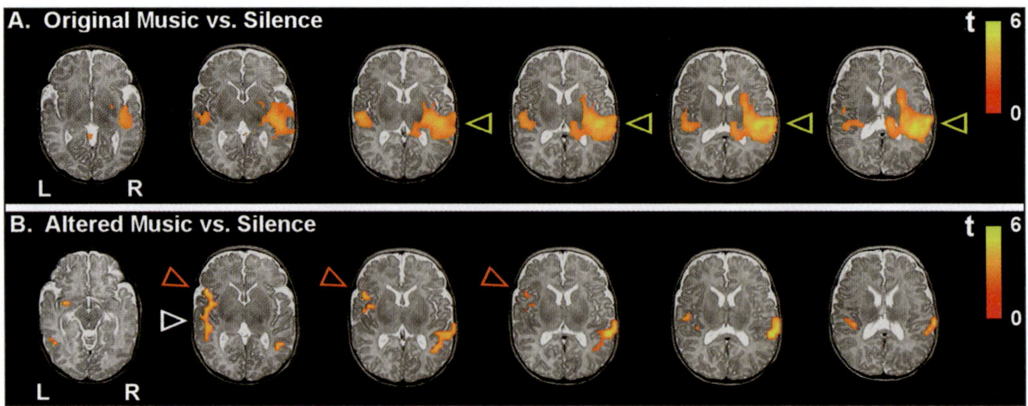

Fig. 1. Functional MRI activations elicited by musical stimuli in 18 newborns in a study showing random effects group analyses, false discovery rate corrected; $p < 0.0002$ *at the voxel level and* $p < 0.05$ *at the cluster level. (**A**) Mean activations for original music* vs. *silence are shown for six axial slices, showing right-hemispheric predominance of temporal activation (yellow arrowheads). (**B**) Mean activations for music with altered structure* vs. *silence. Note the left-hemispheric activation in the inferior frontal gyrus (orange arrowheads) and the reduced activation in the right temporal lobe (compared with the contrast of original music* vs. *silence; white arrowhead). (From Perani* et al.*, 2010; reproduced by permission from the* Proceedings of the National Academy of Sciences of the United States of America).

the stimuli, even when they remain fully musical. As both altered sets contained a higher degree of sensory dissonance compared to the original set, the pattern of activation observed for the Altered Music condition presumably reflects a sensitivity of auditory cortex to dissonance already at birth, as implied by previous studies (Masataka, 2006).

The engagement of neural resources in the inferior frontolateral cortex of the left hemisphere in response to the Altered Music might be attributed to the frequent changes of key during the *Key Shifts* condition and the tonal ambiguity of the chords in the *Dissonance* condition, requiring more left hemispheric neural capacities for the processing of acoustic relations between chords.

Finally, our data from newborns also suggest effects of music on activity of cerebral core structures for emotional music processing, as shown in adults (Phillips *et al.*, 2003). Even though these results demand to be interpreted with caution, the BOLD [blood oxygenation level-dependent] signal increase was observed in response to the original music in the right amygdala hippocampal complex and during perception of altered music in the left hippocampal/entorhinal cortex, possibly including the amygdala. As mentioned above, previous behavioural studies in infants showed a clear preference for consonant sounds in comparison to dissonant sounds (Trainor *et al.*, 2002; Masataka, 2006). Our experimental technique does not allow us to conclude that newborns were experiencing any particular emotion in response to music, but the activation of limbic structures suggests that newborns activate brain structures known to be involved in emotion processing while hearing musical stimuli. The observed hemispheric differences in activation of limbic structures remain to be specified.

It needs to be noted that these findings do not imply that the specific response observed when the newborn brain is exposed to musical information evolved for, and is exclusively involved in, instrumental music processing. It is likely that similar responses would be elicited by song and by the melodic aspects of speech.

Together these data point to an early neural predisposition for the emotional response to music, independent of extensive exposure to music or speech sounds. They also support the hypothesis that the emotional language of music might be a crucial ingredient for human development.

Conclusions

The existing literature appears to confirm that music elicits emotions directly. The fact that music affects physiologic parameters such as heart rate and skin conductance indicates that music is not simply describing emotions we recognize, in the same way it describes a running stream in the second movement of Beethoven's Symphony No. 6, but rather leading us to *feel* specific emotions. Music also activates the central nervous system, involving those networks associated with affective and reward systems. Even though much work remains to be done to explore the dynamics of music processing in real time, it is quite remarkable that abstract patterns of sound, with no obvious survival value, recruit neural systems known to respond to biologically relevant stimuli. Perhaps what is really adaptive, and could partly explain the involvement of the reward system, is the fact that auditory stimuli, especially the ones that, like music, more closely resemble our conspecifics' vocalizations, are always weighed for their emotional content. In fact, speech prosody, like facial expression, conveys relevant information about the emotional state of the speaker, which is fundamental for regulating our social behaviour, and is described using the same parameters that characterize music: pitch contour, rhythm and pauses, loudness, and timbre.

Another part of the answer may lie in the role musical communication plays in early infancy. We have reported studies revealing that infants show an emotional reaction to music, and recent neuroimaging data suggesting that the newborn brain responds to music specifically, and shows activation of limbic structures. The literature on infants suggests that our emotional response to music, at least at some level, does not require specific experience or culture. There appears to be a basic, instinctual response to music, or to at least some aspects of music. In infancy, music and singing modulate affect, promote the growth of emotional attachment, and possibly get infants 'turned on' to language and communication. It is still unknown whether the infants' reward system is involved in music processing, but behavioural observation suggests it might.

The pleasure induced by music does not seem to derive from the pleasant emotions it induces, but simply from the fact that it does induce emotions. People find sad music profoundly rewarding, just as they find sad films or stories rewarding. Music might allow listeners to 'move their affects' (*muovere gli affetti*), as stated by the Italian musicians Monteverdi and Frescobaldi, and music theorists in the 16th and 17th century. This 'practice' of feeling might be what humans mostly enjoy about music (Trainor & Schmidt, 2003).

References

Arnon, S., Shapsa, A., Forman, L., Regev, R., Bauer, S., Litmanovitz, I. & Dolfin, T. (2006): Live music is beneficial to preterm infants in the neonatal intensive care unit environment. *Birth* **33,** 131–136.

Bernardi, L., Porta, C. & Sleight, P. (2006): Cardiovascular, cerebrovascular, and respiratory changes induced by different types of music in musicians and nonmusicians: the importance of silence. *Heart* 445–452.

Bernardi, L., Porta, C., Casucci, G., Balsamo, R., Bernardi, N. F., Fogari, R. & Sleight, P. (2009): Dynamic interactions between musical, cardiovascular, and cerebral rhythms in humans. *Circulation* **119,** 3171–3180.

Blood, A.J., Zatorre, R.J., Bermudez, P. & Evans, A.C. (1999): Emotional responses to pleasant and unpleasant music correlate with activity in paralimbic brain regions. *Nat. Neurosci.* **2,** 382–387.

Blood, A.J. & Zatorre, R.J. (2001): Intensely pleasurable responses to music correlate with activity in brain regions implicated in reward and emotion. *Proc. Natl. Acad. Sci. USA* **98,** 11818–11823.

Chi, J.G., Dooling, E.C. & Gilles, F.H. (1977): Left-right asymmetries of the temporal speech areas of the human fetus. *Arch. Neurol.* **34,** 346–348.

Conard, N.J., Malina, M. & Munzel, S.C. (2009): New flutes document the earliest musical tradition in southwestern Germany. *Nature* **460,** 737–740.

Fannin, H.A. & Braud, W.G. (1971): Preference for consonant over dissonant tones in the albino rat. *Percept. Motor Skills* **32,** 191–193.

Fishman, Y.I., Volkov, I.O., Noh, M.D., Garell, P.C., Bakken, H., Arezzo, J.C., *et al.* (2001): Consonance and dissonance of musical chords: neural correlates in auditory cortex of monkeys and humans. *J. Neurophysiol.* **86,** 2761–2788.

Fritz, T., Jentschke, S., Gosselin, N., Sammler, D., Peretz, I., Turner, R., *et al.* (2009): Universal recognition of three basic emotions in music. *Curr. Biol.* **19,** 573–576.

Grossmann, T., Striano, T. & Friederici, A.D. (2005): Infants' electric brain responses to emotional prosody. *NeuroReport* **16,** 1825–1828.

Heaton, P. (2009): Assessing musical skills in autistic children who are not savants. *Phil. Trans. R. Soc. Lond. B Biol. Sci.* **364,** 1443–1447.

Hulse, S.H., Bernard, D.J. & Braaten, R.F. (1995): Auditory discrimination of chord-based spectral structures by European starlings (*Sturnus vulgaris*). *J. Exp. Psychol. Genl.* **124,** 409–423.

Izumi, A. (2000) Japanese monkeys perceive sensory consonance of chords. *J. Acoust. Soc. Amer.* **108,** 3073–3078.

Jackendoff, R. & Lerdahl, F. (2006): The capacity for music: what is it, and what's special about it? *Cognition* **100,** 33–72.

Jusczyk, P.W. (1999) How infants begin to extract words from speech. *Trends Cogn. Sci.* **3,** 323–328.

Jusczyk, P.W., Houston, D.M. & Newsome, M. (1999): The beginnings of word segmentation in English-learning infants. *Cogn. Psychol.* **39,** 159–207.

Khalfa, S., Isabelle, P., Jean-Pierre, B. & Manon, R. (2002): Event-related skin conductance responses to musical emotions in humans. *Neurosci. Lett.* **328,** 145–149.

Koelsch, S., Fritz, T., von Cramon, D.Y., Muller, K. & Friederici, A.D. (2006): Investigating emotion with music: an fMRI study. *Hum. Brain Mapp.* **27,** 239–250.

Lerdahl, F. & Jackendoff, R. (1996): *A Generative Theory of Tonal Music.* Cambridge, MA: MIT Press.

Lu, Y., Liu, M., Shi, S., Jiang, H., Yang, L., Liu, X., Zhang, Q. & Pan, F. (2010): Effects of stress in early life on immune functions in rats with asthma and the effects of music therapy. *J Asthma* **47,** 526–531.

Lubetzky, R., Mimouni, F.B., Dollberg, S., Reifen, R., Ashbel, G. & Mandel, D. (2009): Effect of music by Mozart on energy expenditure in growing preterm infants. *Pediatrics* **125,** e24–28.

Masataka, N. (1999): Preference for infant-directed singing in 2-day-old hearing infants of deaf parents. *Dev. Psychol.* **35,** 1001–1005.

Masataka, N. (2006): Preference for consonance over dissonance by hearing newborns of deaf parents and of hearing parents. *Dev. Sci.* **9,** 46–50.

Meltzoff, A.N., Kuhl, P.K., Movellan, J. & Sejnowski, T.J. (2009): Foundations for a new science of learning. *Science* **325,** 284–288.

Menon, V. & Levitin, D. J. (2005): The rewards of music listening: response and physiological connectivity of the mesolimbic system. *NeuroImage* **28,** 175–184.

Molnar-Szakacs, I. & Overy, K. (2006) Music and mirror neurons: from motion to 'e'motion. *Soc. Cogn. Affect. Neurosci.* **1,** 235–241.

Nakamura, T., Tanida, M., Niijima, A., Hibino, H., Shen, J. & Nagai, K. (2007): Auditory stimulation affects renal sympathetic nerve activity and blood pressure in rats. *Neurosci. Lett.* **416,** 107–112.

Parsons, L.M. (2003) Exploring the functional neuroanatomy of music performance, perception, and comprehension. In: *The Cognitive Neuroscience of Music,* eds. I. Peretz & R. Zatorre. New York: Oxford University Press.

Perani, D., Saccuman, M.C., Scifo, P., Spada, D., Andreolli, G., Rovelli, R., Baldoli, C. & Koelsch, S. (2010): Functional specializations for music processing in the human newborn brain. *Proc. Natl. Acad. Sci. USA* **107,** 4758–4763.

Peretz, I. & Morais, J. (1987): Analytic processing in the classification of melodies as same or different. *Neuropsychologia* **25,** 645–652.

Peretz, I. & Zatorre, R.J. (2005): Brain organization for music processing. *Annu. Rev. Psychol.* **56,** 89–114.

Peretz, I., Morais, J. & Bertelson, P. (1987) Shifting ear differences in melody recognition through strategy inducement. *Brain Cognit.* **6,** 202–215.

Peretz, I., Blood, A.J., Penhune, V. & Zatorre, R. (2001): Cortical deafness to dissonance. *Brain* **124,** 928–940.

Phillips, M.L., Drevets, W.C., Rauch, S.L. & Lane, R. (2003): Neurobiology of emotion perception. I: The neural basis of normal emotion perception. *Biol. Psychiatry* **54,** 504–514.

Sambeth, A., Ruohio, K., Alku, P., Fellman, V. & Huotilainen, M. (2008): Sleeping newborns extract prosody from continuous speech. *Clin. Neurophysiol.* **119,** 332–341.

Shenfield, T., Trehub, S. & Nakata, T. (2003): Maternal singing modulates infant arousal. *Psychol. Music* 365–375.

Standley, J.M. (1998): The effect of music and multimodal stimulation on responses of premature infants in neonatal intensive care. *J. Pediatr. Nurs.* **24,** 532–538.

Standley, J.M. (2002): A meta-analysis of the efficacy of music therapy for premature infants. *J. Pediatr. Nurs.* **17,** 107–113.

Standley, J.M. & Moore, R.S. (1995): Therapeutic effects of music and mother's voice on premature infants. *Pediatr. Nurs.* **21,** 509–512, 574.

Sun, T. & Walsh, C.A. (2006): Molecular approaches to brain asymmetry and handedness. *Nat. Rev. Neurosci.* **7,** 655–662.

Sun, T., Patoine, C., Abu-Khalil, A., Visvader, J., Sum, E., Cherry, T.J., *et al.* (2005): Early asymmetry of gene transcription in embryonic human left and right cerebral cortex. *Science* **308,** 1794–1798.

Sun, T., Collura, R.V., Ruvolo, M. & Walsh, C.A. (2006): Genomic and evolutionary analyses of asymmetrically expressed genes in human fetal left and right cerebral cortex. *Cereb. Cortex* **16** (Suppl. 1), i18–25.

Thiessen, E.D. & Saffran, J.R. (2003): When cues collide: use of stress and statistical cues to word boundaries by 7- to 9-month-old infants. *Dev. Psychol.* **39,** 706–716.

Thompson, W.F., Schellenberg, E.G. & Husain, G. (2001): Arousal, mood, and the Mozart effect. *Psychol. Sci.* **12,** 248–251.

Trainor, L.J. (1996): Infant preference for infant-directed versus noninfant-directed playsongs and lullabies. *Infant Behav. Dev.* **19,** 83–92.

Trainor, L.J. & Desjardins, R.N. (2002): Pitch characteristics of infant-directed speech affect infants' ability to discriminate vowels. *Psychon. Bull. Rev.* **9,** 335–340.

Trainor, L. & Schmidt, L.A. (2003): Processing emotion induced by music. In: *The Cognitive Neuroscience of Music.* eds. I. Peretz & R. Zatorre. New York: Oxford University Press.

Trainor, L.J., Tsang, C.D. & Cheung, V.H. (2002): Preference for sensory consonance in 2- and 4-month-old infants. *Music Percept.* **20,** 187–194.

Tramo, M.J., Cariani, P.A., Delgutte, B. & Braida, L.D. (2001): Neurobiological foundations for the theory of harmony in western tonal music. *Ann. N.Y. Acad. Sci.* **930,** 92–116.

Trehub, S.E. (2001): Musical predispositions in infancy. *Ann. N.Y. Acad. Sci.* **930,** 1–16.

Trehub, S.E., Unyk, A.M., Kamenetsky, S.B., Hill, D.S., Trainor, L.J., Henderson, J.L. & Saraza, M. (1997): Mothers' and fathers' singing to infants. *Dev. Psychol.* **33,** 500–507.

Zatorre, R.J. & Belin, P. (2001): Spectral and temporal processing in human auditory cortex. *Cereb. Cortex* **11,** 946–953.

Zentner, M.R. & Kagan, J. (1998): Infants' perception of consonance and dissonance in music. *Infant Behav. Dev.* **21,** 483–492.

Zwicker, E. (1982): *Psychoacoustics.* Berlin: Springer.

Brain Lesion Localization and Developmental Functions, D. Riva, C. Njiokiktjien and S. Bulgheroni (eds.)

Chapter 15

The amygdala and the pathophysiology of autism

Baris Korkmaz

Istanbul University, CERRAHPASA Medical Faculty, Department of Neurology, Division of Child Neurology, P.K. 18 Cerrahpasa, 34301 Istanbul, Turkey
bkorkmaz@istanbul.edu.tr

Summary

The amygdala is involved in a wide range of normal and abnormal behaviours associated with emotions such as fear and anger, and in numerous neuropsychiatric and neurodevelopmental disorders including anxiety, depression, and autism. Autism, a neurodevelopmental disorder characterized by impairments in verbal and nonverbal communication and sociability, includes various behavioural problems such as avoidance of eye contact and failure to recognize emotion on faces, all of which are associated with pathologic disorders and dysfunctions in the amygdala. Stimulation and lesion studies in animals have shown that the amygdala is at the centre of several behavioural systems, including those involved in avoidance and approach behaviour. Studies in nonhuman primates indicate that pure bilateral lesions in the amygdala in neonates cause loss of object fear, but increase social fear, thereby resembling some features of autism. Techniques including neuropathologic, neuroimaging, and neuropsychological investigations as well as clinical studies and combinations of all these methods have provided important insights into the relations between the functions of the amygdala and the pathophysiology of autism. Pathologically, the most consistent finding is the decreased number of cells found in the amygdala. Structural imaging studies indicate precocious enlargement of the amygdala, while functional MRI findings show abnormal activation (usually hyper) in response to fearful stimuli, interpreted as amygdala hyperarousal. It is therefore likely that the amygdala's involvement in autism is connected to prevailing comorbid anxiety disorders, unusual fears, and stereotypies, rather than being the cause of core social deficits.

Introduction

The amygdala, first described as a separate brain region by Burdach in 1819, is located deep within the ventral temporal lobe of the brain in mammals (Heimer *et al.*, 2008) and is part of the limbic system. Amygdala means 'almond' in Greek, a name that derives from the shape of one of its major nuclei. Perhaps more than any other brain region, it has been implicated in a wide range of normal and abnormal behaviours associated with emotions, such as fear and anger, and in the implicit emotional memory system, as well as in numerous neuropsychiatric and neurodevelopmental disorders including anxiety, depression, childhood bipolar disorder, childhood schizophrenia, posttraumatic stress disorder, antisocial personality disorder, fragile X syndrome, Williams syndrome, and autism (Schumann *et al.*, 2010).

Autism is a neurodevelopmental disorder characterized by impairments in verbal and nonverbal communication, sociability, imagination, and learning ability (Wing & Gould, 1979). Various socioemotional problems, such as avoidance of eye contact, difficulties in recognizing emotion on faces, failures in judging a person's trustworthiness, and generating a deviant sense of personal space, which are frequently included among the symptoms of autism, are found to be associated with pathologic disorders and dysfunctions of the amygdala (Adolphs, 2009, 2010; Kennedy *et al.*, 2009).

The functional neuroanatomy and neurophysiology of the amygdala

Although the molecular mechanisms guiding migration, positioning, and connectivity for the immense variety of amygdaloid nuclei are still far from being fully understood, the amygdala is known to be part of the developing telencephalon (Hirata *et al.*, 2009; Medina *et al.*, 2004). In primitive chordates the telencephalon is the site of the processing of olfactory stimuli and the amygdala is a small, undifferentiated cell mass within it, which merges with primordial piriform gray matter (Deussing & Wurst, 2007). Hence the amygdala has an important role in moving organisms away from harmful substances and towards food and is involved in sexual mating behaviour. Primates, however, rely more on visual input than smell and, compared to other orders of animals, have greatly expanded visual association areas in their brains (Blinkov & Glezer, 1968). In primates the major input to the perirhinal cortex, a smell-related area in rodents with which the amygdala has strong connections, is from the visual-association areas (Suzuki & Amaral, 1994). Hence the perirhinal areas in primates subserve as centres for complex visual analysis and phylogenetically the olfactory regions of the amygdala tend to diminish in size, while the deep nuclei (*e.g.*, basolateral complex) are relatively larger (Stephan *et al.*, 1987). Figure 1 gives an overview of the connections between the nuclei of the amygdaloid complex, their input and output, and how these are related (Heimer *et al.*, 2008; LeDoux, 2007; Sah *et al.*, 2003; Davis, 1997).

The amygdaloid nuclear complex

The amygdaloid nuclear complex is composed of 13 subnuclei, each of which has different functions, different projection systems, different thresholds of activation, and even a different morphologic ultrastructure (Davis, 1997; Heimer *et al.*, 2008; LeDoux, 2007; Sah *et al.*, 2003) and different timetable of synaptogenesis (Ulfig *et al.*, 1999, 2003). Swanson and Petrovich (1998) therefore questioned the existence of the amygdala as a structural unit. Unfortunately there is hardly any consensus on the naming and groupings of nuclei in the amygdala, which makes the literature on the subject notoriously difficult to understand. Nevertheless the amygdaloid nuclear complex has been shown to have a powerful, dense intrinsic circuitry which links its componential structures so that the same neuron may innervate several amygdaloid nuclear divisions or nuclei and extra-amygdaloid regions and also modulate other brain areas (Pitkänen *et al.*, 2003). Physiologically, the amygdala, because of its strong inhibitory network, is a relatively silent region of the brain. Hence only repetition of a novel stimulus in association with a significant event leads to potentiation (LeDoux, 2007). On the other hand, it is also one of the regions principally responsible for seizure generation (Gloor, 1990).

All the diverse functions of the amygdala, such as its modulation of the cortical circuits of perception and of attention, and regulation of visceral and somatic activity, involve the dense, reciprocal, varying connections of its subnuclei, in connection with central nervous system

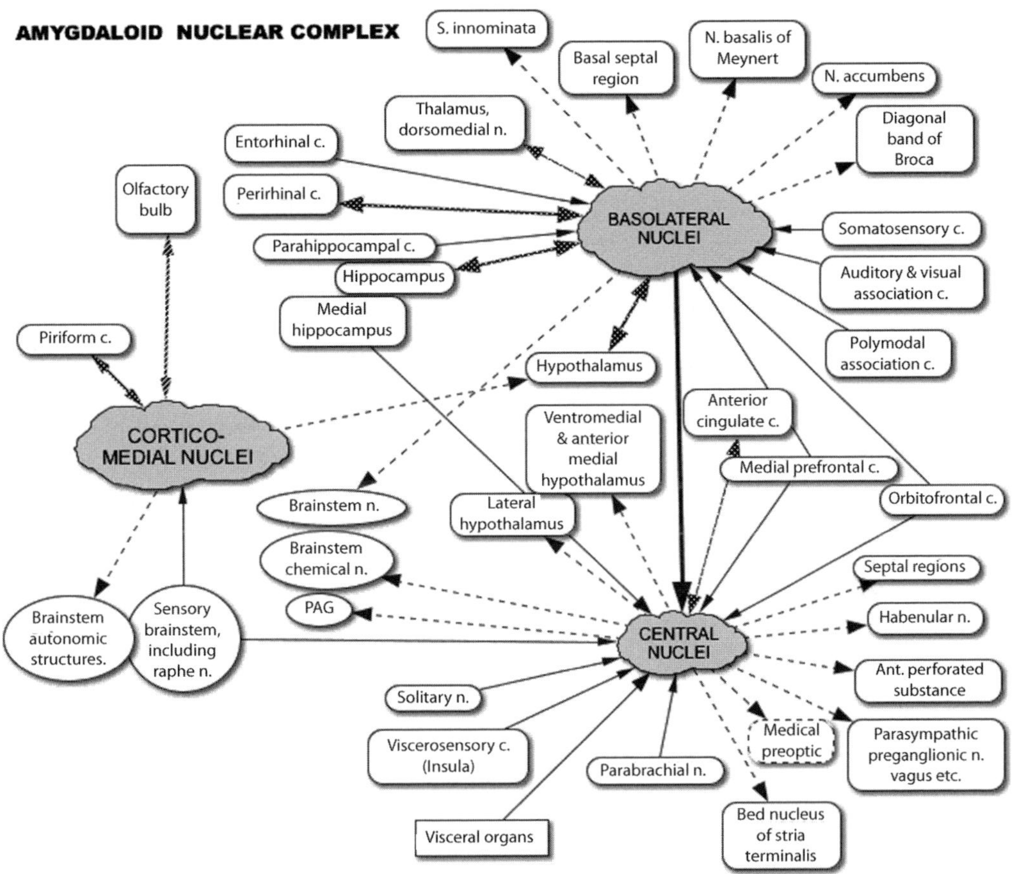

Figure 1. Major amygdala nuclei and their connections. Dashed lines = output connections; solid lines = input connections; c. = cortex, n. = nucleus or nuclei; PAG = periaqueductal gray (matter); s. = substantia.

structures, including the prefrontal lobe (orbitofrontal, piriform, and medial prefrontal), the primary and polymodal sensory cortices, parts of the limbic system (cingulate, septum, hypothalamus, hippocampus, entorhinal cortex, and ventral striatum), the brain stem, and thalamus (Heimer *et al.*, 2008; Morgane *et al.*, 2005; Sah *et al.*, 2003), as well as the peptide (opioid peptides, oxytocin, vasopressin, *etc.*) and hormone (glucocorticoid, androgen, and oestrogen) receptors they contain.

The basolateral complex

The basolateral complex includes the lateral, basal, and accessory basal nuclei (LeDoux, 2007). It identifies the positive and negative emotional aspects of various external stimuli, analyzing all incoming sensory information and charging it with an affect, either through brief and rapid evaluation or access to an inherited or past experience, so that an appropriate behavioural response can be generated. The projections to the accumbens, dorsomedial thalamus, and orbitofrontal cortex are important in assessing the gratifying or aversive nature of a stimulus (Ambroggi *et al.*, 2008; Baxter *et al.*, 2000). This circuitry provides the link by which the responses are associated with appetitive and aversive consequences. Hence the functions of the basolateral amygdala in human beings are interpreted in relation to motivation (including social motivation) and to the representation of the values and processes involved in decision making (Pessoa, 2010). The amygdala is involved in providing the emotional aspects of apperception (gnosis); the organism evaluates the affect-related cues in another's gaze, determines gaze direction, recognizes facial expressions (including the significance of the other's gaze), and makes trustworthiness judgments *via* the amygdala's multiple reciprocal connections with the sensory association cortices, particularly with the superior temporal gyrus, superior temporal sulcus, perirhinal area, and inferior temporal gyrus/facial fusiform area (Adolphs *et al.*, 1998). The role of the amygdala in the recognition of emotions (particularly fear) is well known (Baird *et al.*, 1999; Killgore *et al.*, 2001; Thomas *et al.*, 2001). The polymodal sensory association cortex (superior temporal gyrus and sulcus), which has been shown to involve mirror neurons, participates in some components of Theory of Mind functions (Emery, 2000). Projections from the basal amygdala to multiple levels across the visual cortex are interpreted to provide affective attention related to visual processing (Pessoa, 2010). The amygdala may coordinate the functioning of cortical networks during evaluation of the biological significance of affective visual stimuli (Pessoa & Adolphs, 2010). Recent evidence shows the contribution of a subcortical path to the cortical face–processing specialisation (Kleinhans *et al.*, 2009).

The central nucleus

The central nucleus is important in the development of adaptive and appropriate responses (active or passive strategies) to the conditions surrounding the organism. The central nucleus of the amygdala produces autonomic components of emotion (*e.g.*, changes in heart rate, blood pressure, and respiration) primarily through output pathways to the lateral hypothalamus and brain stem. The central nucleus of the amygdala also produces conscious interoception of emotional feelings (Damasio, 2010), primarily through the ventral amygdalofugal output pathway to the anterior cingulate cortex, orbitofrontal cortex, and prefrontal cortex. Consequently this region of the amygdala is involved principally in the expression of emotions and related physiologic reactions. It regulates the autonomic nervous system and endocrine system *via* modulatory systems localized in the brainstem.

The central nucleus, *via* the extensive connections that the amygdala has with brain stem, striatal, and hypothalamic centres (LeDoux, 2007), is basic to developing avoidance to frightening or harmful stimuli and mobilizing and regulating appropriate behavioural responses. One important related function is the regulation of cortical tone and vigilance mechanisms. Cortical activation, increased vigilance and behavioural arousal occur through the stimulation of modulatory systems including norepinephrine, dopamine, and 5-hydroxytryptamine neurotransmitters and adrenocorticotropic hormone. It also plays an important role in the modulation of visceral activities, acting on the autonomic nervous system and endocrine system. Hence the amygdala becomes one of the major structures in the synthesis of the peripheral and central elements of fear and fear-related behaviours (see also Njiokiktjien and Verschoor [this volume] for a discussion of stress-related mechanisms).

The corticomedial nucleus

The smallest portion of the amygdaloid complex – the corticomedial nucleus – which fuses with the cortex in the medial temporal lobe, is also known as the olfactory amygdala, because, *via* the piriform cortex, it has reciprocal direct and indirect connections with the olfactory bulb (Heimer *et al.*, 2008). These connections are important for the behaviour triggered by smells and are also involved in sexual responses.

Most experimental neurophysiologic studies indicate that the amygdala is necessary for the acquisition of certain types of conditioned reflexes, such as Pavlovian fear conditioning (Barot *et al.*, 2009; Bechara *et al.* 1995), aversive conditioning (Davis, 2000; Everitt *et al.*, 2003), startle reflex, and instrumental or appetitive conditioning, through which new rewards are learned and acquire motivational salience (Everitt *et al.*, 2003; Martin-Soelch *et al.*, 2007). The subnuclei of the amygdala are involved in different stages of various types of conditioning paradigms (Everitt *et al.*, 2003; Gabriel *et al.*, 2003). It was recently reported that the amygdala in the nonhuman primate is necessary for the initial acquisition, but not the retention and expression, of fear-potentiated startle and fear conditioning (Antoniadis *et al.*, 2007, 2009). Findings show that the amygdala plays a crucial role during the initial period of learning how to interpret emotions (*e.g.*, in childhood), when the stimuli may be ambiguous or neutral, and it has also been found that the amygdala is more active in response to neutral facial expressions than to those depicting fear (LaBar *et al.*, 1998; Monk *et al.*, 2003; Thomas *et al.*, 2001).

Clinical lesions of the amygdala

Damage to the amygdala can occur in several clinical disorders. Herpes simplex encephalitis may affect both amygdalae as a result of its predilection for both temporal lobes, but almost always causes some extra-amygdalar damage (Adolphs, 1999). Surgical intervention for intractable epilepsies may include pure amygdalectomies, but these are rarely bilateral (Daniel & Chandy, 1999). As the seizure activity propagates and involves other brain areas, the symptoms of amygdalar epilepsies may be difficult to distinguish with respect to their precise relationship to amygdala functions. Isolated bilateral amygdala damage occurs in a rare disorder, congenital Urbach–Wiethe disease, with many symptoms resembling autism. It may cause impaired recognition of emotion and other social cues from faces (Adolphs *et al.*, 1998; Adolphs *et al.*, 1999), impaired Theory-of-Mind abilities (Stone *et al.*, 2003), and impaired regulation of social distance (Kennedy *et al.*, 2009) as well as a high incidence of failure to make use of information from the eye region of faces (Adolphs *et al.*, 2005, 2008; Spezio *et al.*, 2007a), an impairment related to the failure to fixate eyes in faces (Pelphrey *et al.*, 2002; Spezio *et al.*, 2007b).

Experimental lesions of the amygdala

Behavioural observations of nonhuman primates with experimental lesions in neonates and in adults (bilateral temporal lobe and isolated amygdala lesions) in general confirm an important role for the amygdala in detecting threats and mobilizing an appropriate behavioural response, part of which is fear (Amaral *et al.*, 2003; Bachevalier *et al.*, 2001; Barot *et al.*, 2009; Kalin, 2001; LeDoux, 2007; Machado *et al.*, 2009; Prather *et al.*, 2001; Thompson, 1981; Thompson *et al.*, 1969). Infant macaques that lack an amygdala demonstrate impaired ability to correctly evaluate dangerous *vs.* benign stimuli, as indicated by a lack of fear response when exposed to normally fear-inducing objects, such as a rubber snake, or the diminished fear of novel objects, which normal macaques typically reveal (Bachevalier *et al.*, 2001; Bauman *et al.*, 2004a; Prather *et al.*, 2001). They readily retrieve food rewards placed near these objects and physically explore all objects without differentiating between levels of object complexity (Bliss-Moreau *et al.*, 2010); and these problems persist during adulthood and permanently compromise emotional processing (Bliss-Moreau *et al.*, 2011).

Damage to the amygdala in nonhuman primates has been associated with diminished avoidance of unfamiliar, distasteful, or potentially tainted foods, as well as inedible items that intact animals typically reject. These results confirm a general role for the amygdala in the detection of danger and prevention of harm in the presence of novel or noxious stimuli, regardless of whether such stimuli are conspecifics, predators, or foods (Machado *et al.*, 2010).

Many researchers found heightened social fear (Thompson *et al.*, 1969; Thompson, 1981); reduced eye contact; avoidance of social encounters; inexpressive faces; lack of normal play behaviours; less overall activity, exploration of the testing environment and initiation of social behaviour; and presence of locomotor stereotypies in neonatal amygdala-lesioned animals as compared to age-matched controls (Bachevalier, 1994; Bachevalier *et al.*, 2001), which inevitably caused an absence of the social interactions that resembled those of 'autistic' symptomatology. It is possible that the behavioural changes in these monkeys appeared because of unintended collateral damage to neural tissue surrounding the amygdala and/or to the restrictive rearing practices that were employed (Schumann *et al.*, 2010). Macaque monkeys that were reared by their mothers in a social environment and received discrete amygdala lesions at 2 weeks of age did not demonstrate profound impairments in social development within the first year of life (Bauman *et al.*, 2004a,b; Prather *et al.*, 2001). In a recent study, it was noted that lesioned animals displayed autistic-like behaviour due to their abnormal social-fear response, although they were very vigilant and very attentive to the other monkey in the cage (Prather *et al.*, 2001). In contrast to the increased social approach behaviour that occurred in adult animals, neonatal lesions caused reduced social approach and increased social anxiety in animals as well as an exaggerated expression of fear behaviours, particularly when monkeys were paired with an unthreatening conspecific (Bauman *et al.*, 2006; Prather *et al.*, 2001). Some recent evidence indicates that the fear behaviour may change as the monkeys age (Toscano *et al.*, 2009), but the significance of the dissociation between fear of conspecifics and fear of other species/objects calls for detailed social psychological analysis.

In one study, adult monkeys with bilateral amygdala lesions were observed to display more approach behaviour towards unfamiliar humans and other normal monkeys, with decreased anxiety and increased confidence compared with control monkeys. The lesioned monkeys were reported to have abandoned their normal caution and tendency to withdraw when confronted by a strange monkey, particularly during early encounters in dyadic social interactions. In turn they were approached and groomed more by normal monkeys with an increased social affiliation (Emery *et al.*, 2001). Interestingly, in more complex groups (the lesioned monkey together with three healthy monkeys in a tetrad), these effects were not seen. Instead other monkeys displayed subtly increased avoidance and stress behaviour towards the amygdalectomized monkey (Machado & Bachevalier, 2006). The increased exploration and sexual behaviour recorded for amygdala-lesioned monkeys in pairs was not found in the four-member groups (Machado *et al.*, 2008b).

In early studies on nonhuman primates with lesions of the temporal lobe structures, amygdalectomized female monkeys were described as exhibiting maladaptive maternal behaviours toward their infants, including physical abuse and neglect (Kling & Brothers, 1972; Steklis & Kling, 1985). Female rhesus monkeys that received lesions to the amygdala in early infancy displayed significantly less species-typical interest in infants of other mothers later in life, as compared to monkeys that received lesions to the hippocampus or a control sham surgical procedure. Nevertheless female monkeys with bilateral lesions of the amygdala may preserve the ability to display proper maternal behaviour to their offspring, probably because of parturition and its associated hormones (Toscano *et al.*, 2009).

Neonatal lesions of the amygdala caused locomotor stereotypies (Bachevalier *et al.*, 2001) and ritualistic behaviour such as rocking (Bauman *et al.*, 2008). These behaviours remained when the monkeys became adults. Early lesions of the amygdala (and ventral hippocampus) were found to cause stereotypy in rats (Daenen *et al.*, 2002) and smaller amygdala volume is associated with higher levels of restricted-repetitive behaviour in people with Asperger's syndrome (Dziobek *et al.*, 2006).

An early study reported that in monkeys with nonselective lesions, severe impairments in social relations occurred, with the consequence that the monkeys lost social status (Rosvold *et al.*, 1954), whereas more recent research found that this condition causes monkeys to be ostracized by the group, resulting in death in the wild (Kling & Brothers, 1992). In a recent study, it was found that juvenile monkeys with neonatal neurotoxic amygdala lesions had less frequent initial access to the group's preferred food, had longer latencies to obtain the food, and demonstrated fewer species-typical aggressive behaviours compared to intact monkeys. The outcome was reduced aggression and increased avoidance, as a result of which the monkeys ranked lower on indices of social dominance (Bauman *et al.*, 2006). However, in another study, selective amygdala damage in adolescent monkeys did not alter presurgical social status (Machado & Bachevalier, 2006).

Structural and functional abnormalities of the amygdala in autism: some behavioural correlations

Several types of abnormalities of the amygdala have been reported in persons with autism (Amaral *et al.*, 2008). Histopathologic changes were found in six postmortem examinations of autistic persons aged between 9 and 29 years (five of the six had mental retardation and four had a seizure disorder). These findings included unusually small and more densely packed neurons (an increased number of neurons per unit volume) and simplified dendritic patterns bilaterally in certain nuclei of the amygdala of the autistic persons compared to age-matched controls (Kemper & Bauman, 1993). The most significant increase in cell-packing density was noted in the medially-placed nuclei (the only exception was in the one individual of normal intelligence), and the lateral nucleus appeared to be uninvolved. The histopathologic features, such as reduced cell size and a simplified dendritic pattern, seen together with the volumetric findings, suggested the presence of 'excessive inessential synapses', which corresponded to the early phase of brain development (Bauman & Kemper, 1994).

In another study, significantly fewer neurons in the total amygdala and in the lateral nucleus were found in nine autistic persons 10–44 years of age without seizure disorder than in controls (Schumann & Amaral, 2006). The authors showed reduced cell size and simplified dendritic pattern, without dysmorphic features, a pattern they felt indicated the curtailment of maturation (stunted dendritic arbours), in line with the conclusions of an earlier study (Kemper & Bauman, 1993). However, to date, the only consistent finding in autism in relation to amygdala pathology has been a decreased number of neurons in the amygdala.

Despite the fact that there is a decreased number of neurons in the amygdala, volumetric MRI findings show that the amygdala is larger relative to total cerebral volume in early childhood in autism at about the time symptoms become clinically evident (Mosconi *et al.*, 2009; Schumann *et al.*, 2004; Sparks *et al.*, 2002). Sparks *et al.* (2002) reported a 13–16 per cent abnormal enlargement of the amygdala in 36- to 56-month-old children with autism; in other studies enlargement was shown using structural MRI in children between 2 and 4 years of age (Mosconi *et al.* 2009; Nacewicz *et al.*, 2006; Schumann *et al.*, 2004, 2009). This developmental trajectory of amygdala volume is abnormal, occurring far earlier than the 40 per cent increase in volume seen from 4 to 30 years of age in typically developing males (Giedd *et al*, 1996, 1997; Ostby *et al.*, 2009). The findings of a recent study differed from previous ones in that amygdala enlargement was found to be more pronounced in females with autism, compared to age- and gender-matched typically developing counterparts, than in males with autism (Schumann *et al.*, 2009). This suggests considerable heterogeneity in amygdala growth in children with autism and the possible presence of subgroups (Nordahl *et al.*, 2009).

Bilateral enlargement of a specific subnucleus (laterobasal) of the amygdala in 6- to 7-year-old children with autism has also been reported (Kim *et al.*, 2010). Although the amygdala appears to undergo an abnormal pattern of postnatal development in children with autism, the ultimate size of the amygdala is usually the same as in typically developing children, as in autistics the amygdala does not undergo the same preadolescent increase in volume that takes place in typically developing children. Studies on a wide age range of subjects, including older adolescents and adults have found no difference in size (Haznedar *et al.*, 2000) or even smaller amygdala volumes (Aylward *et al.*, 1999; Dziobek *et al.*, 2006) in individuals with autism relative to age-matched controls. It is likely that a decreased number of neurons in autistic individuals may contribute to the reduction in amygdala volume in adulthood (Schumann & Amaral, 2006). It is possible that the excessive number of neurons that are generated initially is partly consistent with the hypothesis of early brain overgrowth (Courchesne *et al.*, 2001, 2007), and, while the aberrant growth trajectory of the amygdala may extend to a later age (Schumann *et al.*, 2004), some neurons will have subsequently been eliminated during adulthood, either as part of the evolving disease process or as a repercussion of earlier stages of abnormal development. There is, however, currently no evidence to confirm or disprove this hypothesis (Schumann *et al.*, 2010).

It is not only in the amygdala that abnormal developmental changes occur. Such changes have been observed in all areas of the brain (Herbert *et al.*, 2003; Ostby *et al.*, 2009) and in different structures and regions (Bailey *et al.*, 1998; Courchesne, 2004; Hashimoto *et al.*, 1995; Herbert *et al.*, 2003; Leinhart *et al.*, 1997), including the fusiform gyrus (van Kooten *et al.*, 2008), the septal diagonal band of Broca (Kemper & Bauman, 1993), and the dentate gyrus and hippocampus field CA4 (Saitoh *et al.*, 2001).

Many studies (Paul *et al.*, 2010; Schumann *et al.*, 2010) have indicated anatomic and functional abnormalities of the amygdala in association with corresponding behavioural dysfunction in autism, although the precise significance of these abnormalities is still debatable. In male, but not female toddlers who were later diagnosed with autism, the degree of amygdala enlargement at 3 years of age was associated with the severity of the child's social and communicative impairments at final clinical evaluation at around 4 years of age and poorer outcome at 6 years of age (Munson *et al.*, 2006; Schumann *et al.*, 2009). The amygdala is thought to play a major role in the recognition of fearful expressions from faces (Adolphs, 2002) and it is activated even by masked presentation of emotional faces (Critchley *et al.*, 2000a; Monk *et al.*, 2008; Suslow *et al.*, 2006). One of the consequences of amygdala damage is impairment in recognizing fear from facial expressions (Adolphs *et al.*, 1995). In one study, autistic adolescents with small amygdalae were found to be the slowest to distinguish emotional from neutral expressions, to display more gaze avoidance, and to have been the most socially impaired subjects in early childhood (Nacewicz *et al.*, 2006). Other studies demonstrated the opposite pattern in younger children: larger amygdala volume was found to be associated with a more severe clinical course and worse outcome (Munson *et al.*, 2006; Schumann *et al.*, 2009).

Several studies have reported reduced amygdala responses in individuals with autism spectrum disorders when viewing emotional expressions (Ashwin *et al.*, 2007; Critchley *et al.*, 2000a,b). Persons with autism, the broad autism phenotype, and patients with bilateral amygdala lesions display a strikingly similar specific failure to make use of information from the eye region of faces (Adolphs *et al.*, 2005, 2008; Spezio *et al.*, 2007a), an impairment related to their failure to fixate eyes in faces (Adolphs *et al.*, 2005; Pelphrey *et al.*, 2002; Spezio *et al.*, 2007b). Individuals with autism (8–25 years of age) who had a smaller amygdala have been shown to spend the least amount of time fixating on the eye region of the face (Nacewicz *et al.*, 2006; Spezio *et al.*, 2007). In a study of 17 adult individuals with Asperger's syndrome and 17 well-matched controls, smaller amygdala volumes were associated with higher levels of restricted-repetitive behaviour domains (Dziobek *et al.*, 2006).

A functional MRI study done in the late 1990s found hypoactivation of the amygdala in autistic people while they were attempting to make social inferences about a broad range of mental states from the face and especially the eyes (Baron-Cohen *et al.*, 1999). A more recent study revealed that in individuals with autism the diminished amount of time spent looking at the eye region correlated with hypoactivation of the fusiform gyrus, which occurred as a result of amygdala hyperactivity when responding to faces (not to the affects on the face) (Dalton *et al.*, 2005). A recent study confirmed reduced amygdala habituation to faces in an autism spectrum disorder group (amygdala hyperactivity to social stimuli), with the degree of reduction related to the severity of the individual's social impairment (Kleinhans *et al.*, 2009). A number of other neuroimaging studies have noted abnormal amygdala activation when people with autism process faces (Pelphrey *et al.*, 2007; Pierce *et al.*, 2004). Reduced activation in the amygdala, fusiform gyrus, inferior occipital gyrus, and superior temporal sulcus is reported when individuals with autism viewed faces depicting fear (Pierce *et al.*, 2001). Individuals with autism were consistently shown to have reduced responses within the fusiform (occipitotemporal) gyrus to face stimuli (Critchley *et al.*, 2000a,b; Pierce *et al.*, 2001; Schultz *et al.*, 2000; Wang *et al.*, 2004). This area is of importance for the recognition of facial expressions (Adolphs, 2002; Kanwisher *et al.*, 1997). It is possible that in autism any reduction in amgydala activity may cause face-processing deficits within the fusiform gyrus, given the fact that the amygdala modulates the neural activity in the fusiform gyrus (Dziobek *et al.*, 2010) *via* reciprocal projections (Freese & Amaral, 2005). Autistic subjects were, however, able to appropriately activate the amygdala in response to familiar faces (Pierce *et al.*, 2004), suggesting that familiar faces enhanced motivation and prompted amygdala function.

Both congenital and early pathologies of the amygdala in autism cause hypoactivation of the facial fusiform area (Schultz, 2005); it is also possible that the reduction in amygdala activity in response to faces that is typical of autism may reflect problems in the representation of these faces within the fusiform gyrus (Blair, 2008). When exposed to a series of pictures of human faces, the amygdala activation in adults with autism remained elevated long after the activation of that of control subjects, who showed less activation to repeated exposures to faces (hyperarousal reactions in the amygdala cause an individual to miss important information during learning). Those individuals with autism who had the most prominent social impairment exhibited the highest levels of amygdala arousal. The fusiform gyrus, which helps people to determine what kind of object they are looking at – a face or a house, for example – also showed no habituation in either group (Kleinhans *et al.*, 2009).

As confirmed by both neuropsychological (Adolphs *et al.*, 2002) and neuroimaging studies (Baron-Cohen *et al.*, 1999), the amygdala has been implicated in the ability to judge complex social emotions based only on the information coming from the eye region (Baron-Cohen *et al.*, 1997), and the ability to make affect-related judgments is based on facial stimuli (Adolphs, 2003; Baron-Cohen *et al.*, 2000). Individuals with autism have been shown to have deficits in this task (Baron-Cohen *et al.*, 1997), while individuals with psychopathy do not (Richell *et al.*, 2003). Individuals with autism were reported to display deficits in making trustworthiness judgments (Adolphs *et al.*, 2001; Winston *et al.*, 2002), although these findings are still questioned (White *et al.*, 2006).

The structural and functional abnormalities of amygdalar nuclei may explain the difficulties people with autism have in face recognition and in appreciating/understanding the affective states of another person on the basis of their facial expression (Schultz, 2005). Although there is an inconsistency in the direction of abnormality, there is definitely an amygdala dysfunction and pathology associated with certain mental functions. The correlation between the size of the amygdala and increased activation is not entirely clear: although both enlargement and reduction in the size of the amygdala can be associated with increased anxiety, hyperactivity of the amygdala is generally associated with increased anxiety (Schumann *et al.*, 2010).

Discussion

Across a variety of species (mammals and birds), the amygdala appears to play a key role in the rapid evaluation of whether a stimulus is positive (good /rewarding) or negative (bad/threatening/dangerous), possibly in reference to imprinted/inherited information and/or traces of early experience (Davis, 1997; LeDoux, 2007). All of these processes, which are involved in the emergence of the tendency to 'avoid or approach', depending on the situation or object being confronted, are incorporated in the structure of most forms of elementary and higher (*e.g.*, social) behaviour. Approach behaviour includes reward detection, maternal attraction, sexual attraction, and appetitive (eating and drinking) behaviours. Avoiding danger and coping behaviour comprises alarm, defence, flight or attack, and the related emotions of fear, anger, *etc.* in response to physical and psychological threat (stress), including noxious stimuli or potential dangers, regardless of whether such stimuli are conspecifics, unfamiliar social partners, potential predators, novel objects or foods, contexts, *etc.* (Machado *et al.*, 2010). Hence the amygdala primarily appears to be a relay centre for the coordination of neural circuits that give rise to the emergence of species-specific innate fears in response to certain stimuli (Davis, 1997; Prather *et al.*, 2001). The amygdala may also be taking part in the transference of this type of reaction to other situations that are not intrinsically threatening (Davidson, 2002).

The precise mechanisms of amygdala dysfunction in the symptomatology of autism is not yet entirely clear, although experimental and clinical studies have consistently indicated a role for the amygdala in at least some aspects of social cognition, especially social fear and face/gaze recognition. However, even complete lesions of both amygdalae in maternally reared monkeys do not preclude the development of species-typical social behaviour such producing and responding to their species' social signals and interacting with conspecifics in a social context (Amaral *et al.*, 2003; Bauman *et al.*, 2004a,b; Emery *et al.*, 2001; Machado *et al.*, 2009; Prather *et al.*, 2001). On the basis of this evidence it was concluded that the amygdala is not essential for the early development of fundamental components of social cognition (Amaral *et al.*, 2003; Paul *et al.*, 2010), and the validity of the amygdala theory of autism (Baron-Cohen *et al.*, 2000) was questioned (Amaral *et al.*, 2003; Dziobek *et al.*, 2006). It is nonetheless possible that the amygdala is responsible for some symptoms of autism that are present in other neurodevelopmental and neuropsychiatric disorders (Schumann *et al.*, 2010). In terms of experimental science, one of the main symptoms is *fear*, as in the anticipation of a condition or an object that would be physiologically and psychologically painful and could damage the body and mental integrity; however, in terms of more complex human behaviour it is *anxiety* as in the anticipation of a realistic or nonrealistic (imaginary) fear. The amygdala is strongly implicated in the formation of anxiety (Muris *et al.*, 1998; Roozendaal, 2009).

Another slightly different but related mechanism may involve the amygdala's function in mediating or directing visual attention and visual processing based on motivation (Adolphs *et al.*, 2005; Grelotti *et al.*, 2002; Pierce *et al.*, 2004; Schultz, 2005). In social interaction, the normal function of the amygdala is to direct attention to the eye region of the face. Autistic individuals fail to look at the eyes, as has been shown by their reduced amygdala activation when viewing faces depicting emotion (fear) (Pierce *et al.*, 2001). However, they may respond appropriately when looking at a familiar face (Pierce *et al.*, 2004). The explanation may be that people with autism are indifferent to social relations and therefore are simply less motivated to look at faces. Alternatively, it may be that since they perceive social interaction *per se* as threatening, they avoid any behaviour, such as looking at another person's eyes (regardless of whether the person is someone they know or a stranger), that would place them in a situation that might involve physical or psychological danger and in autistic individuals could ultimately give rise to a heightened emotional or even fearful response (Dalton *et al.*, 2005; Nacewicz *et al.*, 2006; Spezio, *et al.*, 2007). A recent study (Kleinhans *et al.*, 2009) supports the theory that in people with autism affective hyperarousal due to amygdala hyperactivity occurs particularly in response to socially relevant stimuli, which are likely to be related to their high levels of anxiety.

Autism frequently overlaps and even coexists with social phobia and avoidant or schizoid personality features. Clinically, autism is characterized by a number of behavioural problems related to high and /or inappropriate anxiety and unusual fears. Amygdala function is associated with increased social anxiety (anticipation of a threat) (Davidson, 2002). Hence, amygdala pathology (enlargement) in subjects with autism may contribute to their abnormal fears and increased anxiety (Juranek *et al.*, 2006), causing secondary problems in their social and communication skills (Munson *et al.*, 2006). Human society largely depends on regulations, customs, and laws conceived to prevent people from harming one another. Because the amygdala is at the centre of a system that evolved principally to detect dangers in the environment and modulate subsequent responses, its functioning can ultimately profoundly influence human behaviour. If the threshold of amygdala functioning in an individual is set too low either for genetic reasons or because of early traumatic experiences, normally benign aspects of the environment and human relations will be perceived as dangers and this will cause anxiety and limit social interaction, while risk-taking behaviour and inappropriate sociality may occur if the threshold is set too high (Schumann *et al.*, 2010). Considering that many neurodevelopmental disorders are comorbid with anxiety disorders, it is not surprising that the amygdala has been implicated in many of them. The socioemotional changes found in monkeys with amygdala lesions may be interpreted as a trait change in personality (Mason *et al.*, 2006), giving rise to secondary and permanent changes in some components of the animal's social behaviour (Amaral *et al.*, 2003) rather than a change in mood (Kalin *et al.*, 2001). This means that it is likely that bilateral amygdala lesions impede the formation and maintenance of an appropriate hierarchy of social dominance because of their impact on affiliation and aggression behaviours (Bauman *et al.*, 2004b, 2006; Prather *et al.*, 2001), although no status change was observed in a recent study done with adult animals (Machado & Bachevalier, 2006).

Lastly, it should be noted that human and animal studies consistently indicate the amygdala as a mediator for the third criterion for the diagnosis of autism (American Psychiatric Association, 1994), that is, stereotypies and the imposition of routines and rituals (Bachevalier *et al.*, 2001; Bauman *et al.*, 2008; Daenen *et al.*, 2002; Dziobek *et al.*, 2006).

It is possible that several different functions of the amygdala are connected to autism in humans. These include affective analysis of social stimuli, the emergence of social fear and related harm-avoiding behaviour (*e.g.*, anxiety) involved in regulating social relations, and instrumental learning, which has a significant effect on motivation (Adolphs, 2003). While there is a great deal of evidence that implicates abnormal amygdala development in autism, to date it has not been possible to establish the causal correlations between amygdala pathologies/ dysfunctions and the symptoms of autism. There are a number of reasons for this.

(1) Animal models may not correspond to autism in humans and using them for study may give rise to misinterpretations of the behaviours observed. There is a major social difference between nonhuman primates and humans with respect to the higher aspects of consciousness. Humans have a camera view of themselves in their social relations, which significantly affects their social cognition (Laming, 2004). The amygdala nuclei may have acquired different functions in human beings because of the overall changes in the human brain, its connections and human-specific tasks that have taken place during evolution.

(2) Most nonhuman primate studies are done on macaques, which are not the primates most proximal to humans on the evolutionary scale in terms of brain structure and behavioural features (particularly sociability).

(3) Experimental studies on animals differentiate isolated nuclei and focus on the functions of different nuclei in the amygdala, whereas human studies involve the whole of the amygdala. Experimental studies on animals benefit from being able to directly record responses from neurons in awake, behaving animals. However, the experimental lesions are not truly neonatal or prenatal.

(4) Another potential problem is that lesions and stimulation, hypo- and hyperactivation of the amygdala, may be associated with both with fear and rage as well as with the suppression of these emotions (Davidson, 2002). This interesting phenomenon is probably due to the different effects the involvement of different nuclei and their connections have in response to different contexts. Furthermore, the relationship between the objective behavioural findings of studies of conditioned reflexes and the interpretive behavioural findings of human studies, including research on human consciousness, has never (starting with Pavlov) been entirely clear.

(5) Studies of lesioned monkeys reveal that rather than being rigid and universal, the amygdala's effect on social behaviour is context-dependent and susceptible to individual differences (Babineau *et al.*, 2011; Machado & Bachevalier, 2006). It is clear that the amygdala functions together with other structures within an interconnected system for social cognition (Adolphs, 2010) and these functions cannot be interpreted in isolation from their connections. For example, the amygdala plays an important role in context-dependent modulation of social behaviour through its connections to the orbitofrontal cortex (Babineau *et al.*, 2011).

(6) The chronology of events is important (Courchesne & Pierce, 2005). Early lesion onset may either affect the formation of subsequently developing structures and/or give rise to alterations in their connectivity (hypo- and hyper-) (Jou *et al.*, 2011), or may alter development of

later developing complex intellectual functions that are dependent on the presence of previously developed elementary intellectual processes (Mosconi *et al.*, 2009). Both of these factors eventually bias an individual toward different life experiences. Early permanent neural injury may also induce morphologic and neurochemical reorganization elsewhere in the brain and this may lead either to functional compensation or to exacerbation of behavioural alterations (Machado *et al.*, 2008a).

(7) There are several variables of amygdala functioning, which should be in taken into consideration. These include anatomic, developmental, and functional differences between the right and left amygdalae (Dalton *et al.*, 2007) and male and female sex (Cahill *et al.*, 2001; Giedd *et al.*, 1997), as well as age and individual and genetic differences, which may be relevant to the amygdala's role in autism. For example, the fact that in males the amygdala increases in size at the same time the neocortex decreases, whereas in females hippocampal formation increases with age (Giedd *et al.*, 1997), remains to be understood.

(8) It is hoped that the discovery of polymorphisms of genes such as stathmin, which are preferentially expressed in the amygdala (Brocke *et al.*, 2010; Shumyatsky *et al.*, 2005), and other genes (Zirlinger *et al.*, 2001), in relation to various chemical systems such as oxytocin (Furman *et al.*, 2011; Hurlemann *et al.*, 2010), serotonin (Gibboni *et al.* 2009; Munafo *et al.* 2008), and structural and functional connectivity between the amygdala and medial parts of the prefrontal cortex (Heinz *et al.*, 2005; Pacheco *et al.*, 2009; Pezawas *et al.*, 2005) will shed light on the relations between the amygdala and susceptibility to neuropsychiatric illnesses (Mayberg *et al.*, 1999; Pezawas *et al.*, 2005), trait anxiety (Kim & Whalen, 2009), and some aspects of decision-making (Roiser *et al.*, 2009).

(9) It is possible that the amygdala is not directly responsible for the generation of specific emotional responses, but instead functions to provide the formation of appropriate links between emotional and visceral responses and external stimuli (Bachevalier & Málková, 2006) by modulating the function of cortical networks during evaluation of the biologic significance of affective visual stimuli (Pessoa & Adolphs, 2010). Hence congenital or early amygdala dysfunction may be the factor triggering events that disrupt the harmonious development of the affective and cognitive functions and give rise to the developmental associative agnosia (Schulz, 2005) as the whole relationship between perception and apperception becomes altered as a result of the separation of the emotional expressions from the concepts with which they are closely associated (Vygotsky, 1934).

Acknowledgments: I am grateful to Dr. Gülçin Benbir for her editorial help with the references.

References

Adolphs, R. (1999): The human amygdala and emotion. *Neuroscientist* **5,** 125–137.

Adolphs, R. (2002): Recognizing emotion from facial expressions: psychological and neurological mechanisms. *Behav. Cogn. Neurosci. Rev.* **1,** 21–62.

Adolphs, R. (2003): Is the human amygdala specialized for processing social information? *Ann. N.Y. Acad. Sci.* **985,** 326–340.

Adolphs, R. (2009): The social brain: neural basis of social knowledge. *Ann. Rev. Psychol.* **60,** 693–716.

Adolphs, R. (2010): What does the amygdala contribute to social cognition? *Ann. N.Y. Acad. Sci.* **1191,** 42–61.

Adolphs, R., Tranel, D., Damasio, H. & Damasio, A.R. (1995): Fear and the human amygdala. *J. Neurosci.* **15,** 5879–5891.

Adolphs, R., Tranel, D. & Damasio, A.R. (1998): The human amygdala in social judgment. *Nature* **393,** 470–474.

Adolphs, R., Tranel, D., Hamann, S., Young, A., Calder, A., Phelps, E.A., *et al.* (1999): Recognition of facial emotion in nine subjects with bilateral amygdala damage. *Neuropsychologia* **37,** 1111–1117.

Adolphs, R., Sears, L. & Piven, J. (2001): Abnormal processing of social information from faces in autism. *J. Cogn. Neurosci.* **13,** 232–240.

Adolphs, R., Baron-Cohen, S. & Tranel, D. (2002): Impaired recognition of social emotions following amygdala damage. *J. Cogn. Neurosci.* **14,** 1264–1274.

Adolphs, R., Gosselin, F., Buchanan, T.W., Tranel, D., Schyns, P.G. & Damasio, A.R. (2005): A mechanism for impaired fear recognition after amygdala damage. *Nature* **433,** 68–72.

Adolphs, R., Spezio, M.L., Parlier, M. & Piven, J. (2008): Distinct face-processing strategies in parents of autistic children. *Curr. Biol.* **18,** 1090–1093.

Amaral, D.G., Bauman, M.D. & Schumann, C.M. (2003): The amygdala and autism: implications from non-human primate studies. *Genes. Brain Behav.* **2,** 295–302.

Amaral, D.G., Schumann, C.M. & Nordahl, C.W. (2008): Neuroanatomy of autism. *Trends Neurosci.* **31,** 137–145.

Ambroggi, F., Ishikawa, A., Fields, H.L. & Nicola, S.M. (2008): Basolateral amygdala neurons facilitate reward-seeking behavior by exciting nucleus accumbens neurons. *Neuron* **59,** 648–661.

American Psychiatric Association (1994): *Diagnostic and Statistical Manual of Mental Disorders*, fourth edition, pp. 65–78. Washington, D.C.: American Psychiatric Association.

Antoniadis, E.A., Winslow, J.T., Davis, M. & Amaral, D.G. (2007): Role of the primate amygdala in fear-potentiated startle: effects of chronic lesions in the rhesus monkey. *J. Neurosci.* **27,** 7386–7396.

Antoniadis, E.A., Winslow, J.T., Davis, M. & Amaral, D.G. (2009): The nonhuman primate amygdala is necessary for the acquisition but not the retention of fear-potentiated startle. *Biol. Psychiatry* **65,** 241–248.

Ashwin, C., Baron-Cohen, S., Wheelwright, S., O'Riordan, M., Bullmore, E.T. (2007): Differential activation of the amygdala and the 'social brain' during fearful face-processing in adults with and without autism. *Neuropsychologia* **45,** 2–14.

Aylward, E.H., Minshew, N.J., Goldstein, G., Honeycutt, N.A., Augustine, A.M., Yates, K.O., *et al.* (1999): MRI volumes of amygdala and hippocampus in non mentally retarded autistic adolescents and adults. *Neurology* **53,** 2145–2150.

Babineau, B.A., Bliss-Moreau, E., Machado, C.J., Toscano, J.E., Mason, W.A. & Amaral, D.G. (2011): Context-specific social behavior is altered by orbitofrontal cortex lesions in adult rhesus macaques. *Neuroscience* **14,** 80-93.

Bachevalier, J. (1994): Medial temporal lobe structures and autism: a review of clinical and experimental findings. *Neuropsychologia* **32,** 627–648.

Bachevalier, J. & Málková, L. (2006): The amygdala and development of social cognition: theoretical comment on Bauman, Toscano, Mason, Lavenex, and Amaral (2006). *Behav. Neurosci.* **120,** 989–991.

Bachevalier, J., Málková, L. & Mishkin, M. (2001): Effects of selective neonatal temporal lobe lesions on socioemotional behavior in infant rhesus monkeys *(Macaca mulatta). Behav. Neurosci.* **115,** 545–559.

Bailey, A., Luthert, P., Dean, A., Harding, B., Janota, I., Montgomery, M., *et al.* (1998): A clinicopathological study of autism. *Brain* **121,** 889–905.

Baird, A.A., Gruber, S.A., Fein, D.A., Maas, L.C., Steingard, R.J., *et al.* (1999): Functional magnetic resonance imaging of facial affect recognition in children and adolescents. *J. Am. Acad. Child Adolesc. Psychiatry* **38,** 195–199.

Baron-Cohen, S., Wheelwright, S. & Jolliffe, T. (1997): Is there a 'language of the eyes'? Evidence from normal adults and adults with autism or Asperger syndrome. *Visual Cognition* **4,** 311–331.

Baron-Cohen, S., Ring, H.A., Wheelwright, S., Bullmore, E.T., Brammer, M.J., Simmons, A. & Williams, S.C. (1999): Social intelligence in the normal and autistic brain: an fMRI study. *Eur. J. Neurosci.* **11,** 1891–1898.

Baron-Cohen, S., Ring, H.A., Bullmore, E.T., Wheelwright, S., Ashwin, C. & Williams, S.C. (2000): The amygdala theory of autism. *Neurosci. Biobehav. Rev.* **24,** 355–364.

Barot, S.K., Chung, A., Kim, J.J. & Bernstein, I.L. (2009): Functional imaging of stimulus convergence in amygdalar neurons during Pavlovian fear conditioning. *PloS ONE* **4,** e6156.

Bauman, M.L. & Kemper, T.L. (1994): Neuroanatomic observations of the brain in autism. In: *The Neurobiology of Autism*, eds. M.L. Bauman & T.L. Kemper, pp. 119–145. Baltimore, MD: The Johns Hopkins University Press.

Bauman, M.D., Lavenex, P., Mason, W.A., Capitanio, J.P. & Amaral, D.G. (2004a): The development of mother-infant interactions after neonatal amygdala lesions in rhesus monkeys. *J. Neurosci.* **24,** 711–721.

Bauman, M.D., Lavenex, P., Mason, W.A., Capitanio, J.P. & Amaral, D.G. (2004b): The development of social behavior following neonatal amygdala lesions in rhesus monkeys. *J. Cogn. Neurosci.* **16,** 1388–1411.

Bauman, M.D., Toscano, J.E., Mason, W.A., Lavenex, P. & Amaral, D.G. (2006): The expression of social dominance following neonatal lesions of the amygdala or hippocampus in rhesus monkeys *(Macaca mulatta). Behav. Neurosci.* **120,** 749–760.

Bauman, M.D., Toscano, J.E., Babineau, B.A., Mason, W.A. & Amaral, D.G. (2008): Emergence of stereotypies in juvenile monkeys *(Macaca mulatta)* with neonatal amygdala or hippocampus lesions. *Behav. Neurosci.* **122,** 1005–1015.

Baxter, M.G., Parker, A., Lindner, C.C., Izquierdo, A.D. & Murray, E.A. (2000): Control of response selection by reinforcer value requires interaction of amygdala and orbital prefrontal cortex. *J. Neurosci.* **20,** 4311–4319.

Bechara, A., Tranel, D., Damasio, H., Adolphs, R., Rockland, C. & Damasio, A.R. (1995): Double dissociation of conditioning and declarative knowledge relative to the amygdala and hippocampus in humans. *Science* **269,** 1115–1118.

Blair, R.J.R. (2008): Fine cuts of empathy and the amygdala: dissociable deficits in psychopathy and autism. *Q. J. Exp. Psychol.* **61,** 157–170.

Blinkov, S.M. & Glezer, I.I. (1968): *The Human Brain in Figures and Tables: A Quantitative Handbook.* New York: Basic Books.

Bliss-Moreau, E., Toscano, J.E., Bauman, M.D., Mason, W.A. & Amaral, D.G. (2010): Neonatal amygdala or hippocampus lesions influence responsiveness to objects. *Dev. Psychobiol.* **52,** 487–503.

Bliss-Moreau, E., Toscano, J.E., Bauman, M., Mason, W.A. & Amaral, D.G. (2011): Neonatal amygdala lesions alter responsiveness to objects in juvenile macaques. *Neuroscience* **178,** 123–132.

Brocke, B., Lesch, K.P., Armbruster, D., Moser, D.A., Müller, A., Strobel, A. & Kirschbaum, C. (2010): Stathmin, a gene regulating neural plasticity, affects fear and anxiety processing in humans. *Am. J. Med. Genet. B. Neuropsychiatr. Genet.* **153B,** 243–251.

Cahill, L., Haier, R.J., White, N.S., Fallon, J., Kilpatrick, L., Lawrence, C., *et al.* (2001): Sex related difference in amygdala activity during emotionally influenced memory storage. *Neurobiol. Learning & Memory* **75,** 1–9.

Courchesne, E. (2004): Brain development in autism: early overgrowth followed by premature arrest of growth. *Ment. Retard. Dev. Disabil. Res. Rev.* **10,** 106–111.

Courchesne, E. & Pierce, K. (2005): Brain overgrowth in autism during a critical time in development: implications for frontal pyramidal neuron and interneuron development and connectivity. *Int. J. Dev. Neurosci.* **23,** 153–170.

Courchesne, E., Karns, C.M., Davis, H.R., Ziccardi, R., Carper, R.A., Tigue, Z.D., *et al.* (2001): Unusual brain growth patterns in early life in patients with autistic disorder: an MRI study. *Neurology* **57,** 245–254.

Courchesne, E., Pierce, K., Schumann, C.M., Redcay, E., Buckwalter, J.A., Kennedy, D.P. & Morgan, J. (2007): Mapping early brain development in autism. *Neuron* **56,** 399–413.

Critchley, H.D., Daly, E., Phillips, M., Brammer, M., Bullmore, E., Williams, S., *et al.* (2000a): Explicit and implicit neural mechanisms for processing of social information from facial expressions: a functional magnetic resonance imaging study. *Hum. Brain Mapp.* **9,** 93–105.

Critchley, H.D., Daly, E.M., Bullmore, E.T., Williams, S.C., Van Amelsvoort, T., Robertson, D.M., *et al.* (2000b): The functional neuroanatomy of social behaviour: changes in cerebral blood flow when people with autistic disorder process facial expressions. *Brain* **123,** 2203–2212.

Daenen, E.W., Wolterink, G., Gerrits, M.A. & van Ree J.M. (2002): The effects of neonatal lesions in the amygdala or ventral hippocampus on social behaviour later in life. *Behav. Brain Res.* **136,** 571–582.

Dalton, K.M., Nacewicz, B.M., Johnstone, T., Schaefer, H.S., Gernsbacher, M.A., *et al.* (2005): Gaze fixation and the neural circuitry of face processing in autism. *Nat. Neurosci.* **8,** 519–526.

Dalton, K.M., Nacewicz, B.M., Alexander, A.L. & Davidson, R.J. (2007): Gaze-fixation, brain activation, and amygdala volume in unaffected siblings of individuals with autism. *Biol. Psychiatry* **61,** 512–520.

Damasio, A. (2010): *Self Comes to Mind.* New York: Pantheon Books.

Daniel, R.T. & Chandy, M.J. (1999): Epilepsy surgery: overview of forty years experience. *Neurol. India.* **47,** 98–103.

Davidson, R. (2002): Anxiety and affective style: role of prefrontal cortex and amygdala. *Biol. Psychiatry* **51,** 68–80.

Davis, M. (1992a): Major output of central nucleus of amygdala. *Trends Pharmacol Sci.* **13,** 35–41.

Davis, M. (1992b): The role of the amygdala in fear-potentiated startle: implications for animal models of anxiety. *Trends Pharmacol Sci.* **13,** 35–41.

Davis, M. (1992c): The role of the amygdala in fear and anxiety. *Annu. Rev Neurosci.* **15,** 353–375.

Davis, M. (1997): Neurobiology of fear responses: the role of the amygdala. *J. Neuropsych. Clin. Neurosci.* **9,** 382–402.

Davis, M. (2000): The role of the amygdala in conditioned and unconditioned fear and anxiety. In: *The Amygdala,* (2nd edition), ed. J.P. Aggleton, pp. 213–288. Oxford: Oxford University Press.

Deussing, J.M. & Wurst, W. (2007): Amygdala and neocortex: common origins and shared mechanisms. *Nat. Neurosci.* **9,** 1001–1002.

Dziobek, I., Fleck, S., Rogers, K., Wolf, O.T. & Convit, A. (2006): The 'amygdala theory of autism' revisited: linking structure to behavior. *Neuropsychologia* **44,** 1891–1899.

Dziobek, I., Bahnemann, M., Convit, A. & Heekeren, H.R. (2010): The role of the fusiform-amygdala system in the pathophysiology of autism. *Arch. Gen. Psychiatry* **67,** 397–405.

Emery, N.J. (2000): The eyes have it: the neuroethology, function and evolution of social gaze. *Neurosci. Biobehav. Rev.* **24,** 581–604.

Emery, N.J., Capitanio, J.P., Mason, W.A., Machado, C.J., Mendoza, S.P. & Amaral, D.G. (2001): The effects of bilateral lesions of the amygdala on dyadic social interactions in rhesus monkeys *(Macaca mulatta). Behav. Neurosci.* **115,** 515–544.

Everitt, B.J., Cardinal, R.N., Parkinson, J.A. & Robbins, T.W. (2003): Appetitive behavior: impact of amygdala-dependent mechanisms of emotional learning. *Ann. N.Y. Acad. Sci.* **985,** 233–250.

Freese, J.L. & Amaral, D.G. (2005): The organization of projections from the amygdala to visual cortical areas TE and V1 in the macaque monkey. *J. Comp. Neurol.* **486,** 295–317.

Furman, D.J., Chen, M.C. & Gotlib, I.H. (2011): Variant in oxytocin receptor gene is associated with amygdala volume. *Psychoneuroendocrinology* **36,** 891–897.

Gabriel, M., Burhans, L. & Kashef, A. (2003): Consideration of a unified model of amygdalar associative functions. *Ann. N.Y. Acad. Sci.* **985,** 206–217.

Gibboni, R.R., Zimmerman, P.E. & Gothard, K.M. (2009): Individual differences in scanpaths correspond with serotonin transporter genotype and behavioral phenotypes in rhesus monkeys *(Macaca mulatta). Front. Behav. Neurosci.* **3,** 50.

Giedd, J.N., Vaituzis, A.C., Hamburger, S.D., Lange, N., Rajapakse, J.C., Kaysen, D., *et al.* (1996): Quantitative MRI of the temporal lobe, amygdala, and hippocampus in normal human development: ages 4-18 years. *J. Compar. Neurol.* **366,** 223–230.

Giedd, J.N., Castellanos, F.X., Rajapakse, J.C., Vaituzis, A.C. & Rapoport, J.L. (1997): Sexual dimorphism of the developing human brain. *Prog. Neuropsychopharmacol. Biol. Psychiatry* **21,** 1185–1201.

Gloor, P. (1990): Experiential phenomena of temporal lobe epilepsy: facts and hypotheses. *Brain* **113,** 1673–1694.

Grelotti, D.J., Gauthier, I. & Schultz, R.T. (2002): Social interest and the development of cortical face specialization: what autism teaches us about face processing. *Dev. Psychobiol.* **40,** 213–225.

Hashimoto, T., Tavama, M., Murakawa, K., Yoshimoto, T., Mivazaki, M., Harada, M. & Kuroda, Y. (1995): Development of the brainstem and cerebellum in autistic patients. *J. Autism Dev. Disord.* **25,** 1–18.

Haznedar, M.M., Buchsbaum, M.S., Wei, T.C., Hof, P.R., Cartwright, C., Bienstock, C.A. & Hollander, E. (2000): Limbic circuitry in patients with autism spectrum disorders studied with positron emission tomography and magnetic resonance imaging. *Am. J. Psychiatry* **157,** 1994–2001.

Heimer, L., Van Hoesen, G.W., Trimble, M.R. & Zahm, D.S. (2008): *Anatomy of Neuropsychiatry. The New Anatomy of the Basal Forebrain and Its Implications for Neuropsychiatric Illness*, pp. 36. Netherlands: Elsevier.

Heinz, A., Braus, D.F., Smolka, M.N., Wrase, J., Puls, I., Hermann, D., *et al.* (2005): Amygdala-prefrontal coupling depends on a genetic variation of the serotonin transporter. *Nat. Neurosci.* **8,** 20–21.

Herbert, M.R., Ziegler, D.A., Deutsch, C.K., O'Brien, L.M., Lange, N., Bakardjiev, A., *et al.* (2003): Dissociations of cerebral cortex, subcortical and cerebral white matter volumes in autistic boys. *Brain* **126,** 1182–1192.

Hirata, T., Li, P., Lanuza, G.M., Cocas, L.A., Huntsman, M.H. & Corbin, J.G. (2009): Identification of distinct telencephalic progenitor pools for neuronal diversity in the amygdala. *Nat. Neurosci.* **2,** 141–149.

Hurlemann, R., Patin, A., Onur, O.A., Cohen, M.X., Baumgartner, T., Metzler, S., *et al.* (2010): Oxytocin enhances amygdala-dependent, socially reinforced learning and emotional empathy in humans. *J. Neurosci.* **30,** 4999–5007.

Jou, R.J., Jackowski, A.P., Papademetris, X., Rajeevan, N., Staib, L.H., Volkmar & F.R. (2011): Diffusion tensor imaging in autism spectrum disorders: preliminary evidence of abnormal neural connectivity. *Aust. N. Z. J. Psychiatry* **45,** 153–162.

Juranek, J., Filipek P.A., Berenji, G.R., Modahl, C., Osann, K. & Spence, M.A. (2006): Association between amygdala volume and anxiety level: magnetic resonance imaging (MRI) study in autistic children. *J. Child Neurol.* **21,** 1051–1058.

Kalin, N.H. (2001): The primate amygdala mediates acute fear but not the behavioral and physiological component of anxious temperament. *J. Neurosci.* **21,** 2067–2074.

Kanwisher, N., McDermott, J. & Chun, M.M. (1997): The fusiform face area: a module in human extrastriate cortex specialized for face perception. *J. Neurosci.* **17,** 4302–4311.

Kemper, T.L. & Bauman, M.L. (1993): The contribution of neuropathologic studies to the understanding of autism. *Neurol. Clin.* **11,** 175–187.

Kennedy, D., Glascher, J., Tyszka, M.J. & Adolphs, R. (2009): Personal space regulation by the human amygdala. *Nat. Neurosci.* **12,** 1226–1227.

Killgore, W.D., Oki, M. & Yurgelun-Todd, D.A. (2001): Sex-specific developmental changes in amygdala responses to affective faces. *Neuroreport* **12,** 427–433.

Kim, J.E., Lyoo, I.K., Estes, A.M., Renshaw, P.F., Shaw, D.W., Friedman, S.D., *et al.* (2010): Laterobasal amygdalar enlargement in 6- to 7-year-old children with autism spectrum disorder. *Arch. Gen. Psychiatry* **67,** 1187–1197.

Kim, M.J. & Whalen, P.J. (2009): The structural integrity of an amygdala-prefrontal pathway predicts trait anxiety. *J. Neurosci.* **29,** 11614–11618.

Kleinhans, N.M., Johnson, I.C., Richards, T., Mahurin, R., Greenson, J., Dawson, G. & Aylward, E. (2009): Reduced neural habituation in the amygdala and social impairments in autism spectrum disorders. *Am. J Psychiatry* **166,** 467–475.

Kling, A.S. & Brothers, L.A. (1992): The amygdala and social behavior. In: *The Amygdala: Neurobiological Aspects of Emotion, Memory, and Mental Dysfunction*, ed. J.P. Aggleton. New York: Wiley–Liss.

LaBar, K.S., Gatenby, J.C., Gore, J.C., LeDoux, J.E. & Phelps, E.A. (1998): Human amygdala activation during conditioned fear acquisition and extinction: a mixed-trial fMRI study. *Neuron* **20,** 937–945.

Laming, D. (2004): *Understanding Human Motivation: What Makes People Tick?*, p. 6. Wiley–Blackwell.

LeDoux, J. (2007): The amygdala. *Curr. Biol.* **17,** 868–874.

Leinhart, J.E., Piven, J., Wzorek, M., Landa, R., Santangelo, S.L., Coon, H. & Folstein, S.E.(1997): Macrocephaly in children and adults with autism. *J. Am. Acad. Child Adolesc. Psychiatry* **36,** 282–290.

Machado, C.J. & Bachevalier, J. (2006): The impact of selective amygdala, orbital frontal cortex, or hippocampal formation lesions on established social relationships in rhesus monkeys. *Behav. Neurosci.* **120,** 761–786.

Machado, C.J., Snyder, A.Z., Cherry, S.R., Lavenex, P. & Amaral, D.G. (2008a): Effects of neonatal amygdala or hippocampus lesions on resting brain metabolism in the macaque monkey: a microPET imaging study. *Neuroimage* **39,** 832–846.

Machado, C.J., Emery, N.J., Capitanio, J.P., Mason, W.A., Mendoza, S.P. & Amaral, D.G. (2008b): Bilateral neurotoxic amygdala lesions in rhesus monkeys *(Macaca mulatta)*: consistent pattern of behavior across different social contexts. *Behav. Neurosci.* **122,** 251–266.

Machado, C.J., Kazama, A.M. & Bachevalier, J. (2009): Impact of amygdala, orbital frontal, or hippocampal lesions on threat avoidance and emotional reactivity in nonhuman primates. *Emotion* **9,** 147–163.

Machado, C.J., Emery, N.J., Mason, W.A. & Amaral, D.G. (2010): Selective changes in foraging behavior following bilateral neurotoxic amygdala lesions in rhesus monkeys. *Behav. Neurosci.* **124,** 761–772.

Martin-Soelch, C., Linthicum, J. & Ernst, M. (2007): Appetitive conditioning: neural bases and implications for psychopathology. *Neurosci. Biobehav. Rev.* **31,** 426–440.

Mason, W.A., Capitanio, J.P., Machado, C.J., Mendoza, S.P. & Amaral, D.G. (2006): Amygdalactomy and responsiveness to novelty in rhesus monkeys *(Macaca mulatta)*: generality and individual consistency of effects. *Emotion* **6,** 73–81.

Mayberg, H.S., Liotti, M., Brannan, S.K., McGinnis, S., Mahurin, R.K., Jerabek, P.A., *et al.* (1999): Reciprocal limbic-cortical function and negative mood: converging PET findings in depression and normal sadness. *Am. J. Psychiatry* **156,** 675–682.

Medina, L., Legaz, I., González, G., De Castro, F., Rubenstein, J.L. & Puelles, L. (2004): Expression of Dbx1, Neurogenin 2, Semaphorin 5A, Cadherin 8 and Emx1 distinguish ventral and lateral pallial histogenetic divisions in the developing mouse claustroamygdaloid complex. *J. Comp. Neurol.* **474,** 504–523.

Monk, C.S., McClure, E.B., Nelson, E.E., Zarahn, E., Bilder, R.M., Leibenluft, E., *et al.* (2003): Adolescent immaturity in attention-related brain engagement to emotional facial expressions. *Neuroimage* **20,** 420–428.

Monk, C.S., Telzer, E.H., Mogg, K., Bradley, B.P., Mai, X., Louro, H.M., *et al.* (2008): Amygdala and ventrolateral prefrontal cortex activation to masked angry faces in children and adolescents with generalized anxiety disorder. *Arch. Gen. Psychiatry* **65,** 568–576.

Morgane, P.J., Galler, J.R. & Mokler, D.J. (2005): A review of systems and networks of the limbic forebrain/limbic midbrain. *Prog. Neurobiol.* **75,** 143–160.

Mosconi, M.W., Cody-Hazlett, H., Poe, M., Gerig, G., Gimpel-Smith, R. & Piven, J. (2009): Longitudinal study of amygdala volume and joint attention in 2- to 4-year-old children with autism. *Arch. Gen. Psychiatry* **66,** 509–516.

Mumby, D.G. & Pinel, J.P.J. (1994): Rhinal cortex lesions and object recognition in rats. *Behav. Neurosci.* **108,** 11–18.

Munk, M.H.J., Roelfsema, P.R., Konig, P., Engel, A.K. & Singer, W. (1996): Role of reticular activation in the modulation of intracortical synchronization. *Science* **272,** 271–273.

Munson, J., Dawson, G., Abbott, R., Faja, S., Webb, S.J., Friedman, S.D., *et al.* (2006): Amygdalar volume and behavioral development in autism. *Arch. Gen. Psychiatry* **63,** 686–693.

Muris, P., Steerneman, P., Merckelbach, H., Holdrinet, I. & Meesters, C. (1998): Comorbid anxiety symptoms in children with pervasive developmental disorders. *J. Anxiety Disord.* **12,** 387–393.

Nacewicz, B.M., Dalton, K.M., Johnstone, T., Long, M.T., McAuliff, E.M., Oakes, T.R., *et al.* (2006): Amygdala volume and nonverbal social impairment in adolescent and adult males with autism. *Arch. Gen. Psychiatry* **63,** 1417–1428.

Nordahl, C.W., Simon, T.J., Camilleri, K., Rogers, S.J., Ozonoff, S. & Amaral, D.G. (2009): Cerebral organization in young children with autism. Paper presented at the International Meeting for Autism Research (IMFAR), Chicago, May, 2009.

Ostby, Y., Tamnes, C.K., Fjell, A.M., Westlye, L.T., Due-Tonnessen, P., Walhovd & K.B. (2009): Heterogeneity in subcortical brain development: a structural magnetic resonance imaging study of brain maturation from 8 to 30 years. *J. Neurosci.* **29,** 11772–11782.

Pacheco, J., Beevers, C.G., Benavides, C., McGeary, J., Stice, E. & Schnyer, D.M. (2009): Frontal-limbic white matter pathway associations with the serotonin transporter gene promoter region (5-HTTLPR) polymorphism. *J. Neurosci.* **29,** 6229–6233.

Paul, L.K., Corsello, C., Tranel, D. & Adolphs, R. (2010): Does bilateral damage to the human amygdala produce autistic symptoms? *J. Neurodev. Disord.* **2,** 165–173.

Pelphrey, K.A., Morris, J.P., McCarthy, G. & LaBar, K.S. (2007): Perception of dynamic changes in facial affect and identity in autism. *SCAN* **2,** 140–150.

Pelphrey, K.A., Sasson, N.J., Reznick, J.S., Paul, G., Goldman, B.D. & Piven, J. (2002): Visual scanning of faces in autism. *J. Autism Dev. Disord.* **32,** 249–261.

Pessoa, L. (2010): Emotion and cognition and the amygdala: from 'what is it?' to 'what's to be done?' *Neuropsychologia* **48,** 3416–3429.

Pessoa, L. & Adolphs, R. (2010): Emotion processing and the amygdala: from a 'low road' to 'many roads' of evaluating biological significance. *Nat. Rev Neurosci.* **11,** 773–783.

Pezawas, L., Meyer-Lindenberg, A., Drabant, E.M., Verchinski, B.A., Munoz, K.E, Kolachana B.S., *et al.* (2005): 5-HTTLPR polymorphism impacts human cingulate-amygdala interactions: a genetic susceptibility mechanism for depression. *Nat. Neurosci.* **8,** 828–834.

Pierce, K., Muller, R.A., Ambrose, J., Allen, G. & Courchesne, E. (2001): Face processing occurs outside the fusiform 'face area' in autism: evidence from functional MRI. *Brain* **124,** 2059–2073.

Pierce, K., Haist, F., Sedaghat, F. & Courchesne, E. (2004): The brain response to personally familiar faces in autism: findings of fusiform activity and beyond. *Brain* **127,** 2703–2716.

Pitkänen, A., Savander, M., Nurminen, N. & Ylinen, A. (2003): Intrinsic synaptic circuitry of the amygdala. *Ann. N.Y. Acad. Sci.* **985,** 34–49.

Prather, M.D., Lavenex, P., Mauldin-Jourdain, M.L., Mason, W.A., Capitanio, J.P., Mendoza, S.P. & Amaral, D.G. (2001): Increased social fear and decreased fear of objects in monkeys with neonatal amygdala lesions. *Neuroscience* **106,** 653–658.

Richell, R.A., Mitchell, D.G.V., Newman, C., Leonard, A., Baron-Cohen, S. & Blair, R.J. (2003): Theory of mind and psychopathy: can psychopathic individuals read the 'language of the eyes'? *Neuropsychologia* **41,** 523–526.

Roiser, J.P., DeMartino, B., Tan, G.C.Y., Kumaran, D., Seymour, B., Wood, N.W. & Dolan, R.J. (2009): A genetically mediated bias in decision making driven by failure of amygdala control. *J. Neurosci.* **29,** 5985–5991.

Roozendaal, B. (2009): Emotional learning/memory. In: *Encyclopedia of Neuroscience*, eds. U. Windhorst, M. Binder & N. Hirokawa. Springer Verlag [online].

Rosvold, H.E., Mirsky, A.F. & Pribram, K. (1954): Influence of amygdalactomy on social behavior in monkeys. *J. Comp. Physiol. Psychol.* **47,** 173–178.

Sah, P., Faber, E.S.L., De Armentia, L.M. & Power, J. (2003): The amygdaloid complex: anatomy and physiology. *Physiol. Rev.* **83,** 803–834.

Saitoh, O., Karns, C.M. & Courchesne, E. (2001): Development of the hippocampal formation from 2 to 42 years: MRI evidence of smaller area dentata in autism. *Brain* **24,** 1317–1324.

Schultz, R.T. (2005): Developmental deficits in social perception in autism: the role of the amygdala and fusiform face area. *Int. J. Dev. Neurosci.* **23,** 125–141.

Schultz, R.T., Gauthier, I., Klin, A., Fulbright, R.K., Anderson, A.W., Volkmar, F., *et al.* (2000): Abnormal ventral temporal cortical activity during face discrimination among individuals with autism and Asperger syndrome. *Arch. Gen. Psychiatry* **57,** 331–340.

Schumann, C.M. & Amaral, D.G. (2006): Stereological analysis of amygdala neuron number in autism. *J. Neurosci.* **26,** 7674–7679.

Schumann, C.M., Hamstra, J., Goodlin-Jones, B.L., Lotspeich, L.J., Kwon, H., Buonocore, M.H., *et al.* (2004): The amygdala is enlarged in children but not adolescents with autism: the hippocampus is enlarged at all ages. *J. Neurosci.* **24,** 6392–6401.

Schumann, C.M., Barnes, C.C., Lord, C. & Courchesne, E. (2009): Amygdala enlargement in toddlers with autism related to severity of social and communication impairments. *Biol. Psychiatry* **66,** 942–949.

Schumann, C.M., Bauman, M.D. & Amaral, D.G. (2011): Abnormal structure or function of the amygdala is a common component of neurodevelopmental disorders. *Neuropsychologia* **49,**745-59.

Shumyatsky, G.P., Malleret, G., Shin, R.M., Takizawa, S., Tully, K., Tsvetkov, E., *et al.* (2005): Stathmin, a gene enriched in the amygdala, controls both learned and innate fear. *Cell* **123,** 697–709.

Sparks, B.F., Friedman, S.D., Shaw, D.W., Aylward, E.H., Echelard, D., Artru, A.A., *et al.* (2002): Brain structural abnormalities in young children with autism spectrum disorder. *Neurology* **59,** 184–192.

Spezio, M.L., Adolphs, R., Hurley, R.S. & Piven, J. (2007a): Abnormal use of facial information in high-functioning autism. *J. Autism Dev. Disord.* **37,** 929–939.

Spezio, M.L., Adolphs, R., Hurley, R.S. & Piven, J. (2007b): Analysis of face gaze in autism using 'bubbles'. *Neuropsychologia* **45,** 144–151.

Steklis, H.D. & Kling, A. (1985): Neurobiology of affiliative behavior in nonhuman primates. In: *The Psychobiology of Attachment and Separation*, ed. R. Martin &T. Field, pp. 93–131. Orlando, FL: Academic Press.

Stephan, H., Frahm, H.D. & Baron, G. (1987): Comparison of brain structure volumes in Insectivora and primates. VII. Amygdaloid components. *J. Hirnforsch.* **28,** 571–584.

Stone, V.E., Baron-Cohen, S., Calder, A., Keane, J. & Young, A. (2003): Acquired theory of mind impairments in individuals with bilateral amygdala lesions. *Neuropsychologia* **41,** 209–220.

Suslow, T., Ohrmann, P., Bauer, J., Rauch, A.V., Schwindt, W., Arolt, V., *et al.* (2006): Amygdala activation during masked presentation of emotional faces predicts conscious detection of threat-related faces. *Brain Cognit.* **61,** 243–248.

Suzuki, W.A. & Amaral, D.G. (1994): Topographic organization of the reciprocal connections between the monkey entorhinal cortex and the perirhinal and parahippocampal cortices. *J. Neurosci.* **14,** 1856–1877.

Swanson, L.W. & Petrovich, G.D. (1998): What is the amygdala? *Trends Neurosci.* **21,** 323–331.

Thomas, K.M., Drevets, W.C., Whalen, P.J., Eccard, C.H., Dahl, R.E., Ryan, N.D. & Casey, B.J. (2001): Amygdala response to facial expressions in children and adults. *Biol. Psychiatry* **49,** 309–316.

Thompson, C.I. (1981): Learning in rhesus monkeys after amygdalactomy in infancy or adulthood. *Behav. Brain Res.* **2,** 81–101.

Thompson, C.I., Schwartzbaum, J.S. & Harlow, H.F. (1969): Development of social fear after amygdalactomy in infant rhesus monkeys. *Physiol. Behav.* **4,** 249–254.

Toscano, J.E., Bauman, M.D., Mason, W.A. & Amaral, D.G. (2009): Interest in infants by female rhesus monkeys with neonatal lesions of the amygdala or hippocampus. *Neuroscience* **162,** 881–891.

Ulfig, N., Setzer, M. & Bohl, J. (1999): Distribution of GAP-43-immunoreactive structures in the human fetal amygdala. *Eur. J Histochem.* **43,** 19–28.

Ulfig, N., Setzer, M. & Bohl, J. (2003): Ontogeny of the human amygdala. *Ann. N.Y. Acad. Sci.* **985,** 22–33.

van Kooten, I.A., Palmen, S.J., von Cappeln, P., Steinbusch, H.W., Korr, H., Heinsen, H., *et al.* (2008): Neurons in the fusiform gyrus are fewer and smaller in autism. *Brain* **131,** 987–999.

Vygotsky, L. S. (1934): Thought in schizophrenia. *Arch. Neurol. Psychiatry* **1,** 1063–1077.

Wang, A.T., Dapretto, M., Hariri, A.R., Sigman, M. & Bookheimer, S.Y. (2004): Neural correlates of facial affect processing in children and adolescents with autism spectrum disorder. *J. Am. Acad. Child Adolesc. Psychiatry* **43,** 481–490.

White, S., Hill, E., Winston, J. & Frith, U. (2006): An islet of social ability in Asperger syndrome: judging social attributes from faces. *Brain Cognit.* **61,** 69–77.

Wing, L. & Gould, J. (1979): Severe impairments of social interaction and associated abnormalities in children: epidemiology and classification. *J. Autism Child. Schizophrenia* **9,** 11–29.

Winston, J.S., Strange, B.A. & O'Doherty, J. (2002): Automatic and intentional brain responses during evaluation of trustworthiness of faces. *Nat. Neurosci.* **5,** 277–283.

Zirlinger, M., Kreiman, G. & Anderson, D.J. (2001): Amygdala-enriched genes identified by microarray technology are restricted to specific amygdaloid subnuclei. *Proc. Natl. Acad. Sci. USA* **98,** 5270–5275.

Brain Lesion Localization and Developmental Functions, D. Riva, C. Njiokiktjien and S. Bulgheroni (eds.)

Chapter 16

Long-term neurobiologic impact of extreme early institutional deprivation in the English and Romanian Adoptees study: initial findings and future plans

Edmund J.S. Sonuga-Barke[*,o], Robert Kumsta[#] and Mitul A. Mehta[§]

**Developmental Brain-Behaviour Laboratory, School of Psychology, University of Southampton, Southampton S017 1BJ, United Kingdom;*
[o]Department of Experimental Clinical & Health Psychology, Ghent University, Ghent, Belgium;
[#]Department of Psychology, Laboratory for Biological and Personality Psychology, University of Freiburg, Freiburg, Germany;
[§]Department of Neuroimaging, Institute of Psychiatry, Kings College London, London, United Kingdom
ejb3@soton.ac.uk

Summary

Studies of the effects of early and extreme maltreatment on human brain development rely on the occurrence of natural experiments, whereby the effects of early risk can be separated from those associated with continuing exposure. The large-scale adoption of young children from the orphanages of the communist regime in Romania at the end of the 1980s represents one such natural experiment in which the passage from extremely depriving to above-average family homes in other countries could be precisely timed. The English and Romanian Adoptees study (ERA) was established to follow the development of a cohort of such children adopted by UK families before the age of 43 months. There was an initial devastating impact of deprivation seen at the time of adoption for most children, which, despite remarkable catch-up and recovery, left severe residual problems in a substantial minority of individuals in cognitive, social and mental health domains – effects that persisted into mid-adolescence. This chapter specifically reviews evidence of institutional deprivation on brain development. A number of important findings have been reported. First, deprivation had a substantial and lasting effect on head circumference (an indirect measure of brain size), which was strongly related to the duration of deprivation experienced. Despite substantial catch-up from the time of adoption, the head circumference at age 15 of children who suffered more than 6 months of deprivation in institutions was more than 1 standard deviation (SD) below the UK head circumference norms at the same age. Second, these effects of deprivation on head circumference partially mediated negative cognitive and mental health outcomes in adolescence. Third, the effects of deprivation were not fully accounted for by prior inadequate nutrition (as estimated on the basis of weight at the time of entry to the UK). Fourth, pilot imaging data provided initial evidence of structural alterations in a brain region involved in the processing of negative stimuli (*i.e.*, the amygdala). Fifth, functional alterations were seen in regions processing positive stimuli during reward tasks (*i.e.*, the nucleus accumbens) and possibly those involved in inhibitory control. Building on these findings in the future, we plan a large-scale imaging study using a range of structural and functional techniques and tasks to address key questions about the long-term impact of institutional deprivation on brain development.

Background

The majority of children are loved and nurtured by their families, but others are not so fortunate. For those who are maltreated within their families or grow up in institutions, deprived of the love and care normally provided by families, the future may be bleak. Because neglect and abuse exact an enormous human and economic toll (Bonomi *et al.*, 2008; Wang & Holton, 2007), improving children's care and protection is a major social and health policy priority, both nationally (Parton, 2006) and internationally (Kamerman *et al.*, 2009). A better scientific understanding of the effects of severe childhood adversity can both inform remedial interventions and answer fundamental questions about early influences. The study of the long-term effects of such maltreatment on brain development may be especially important (Nelson *et al.*, in press) in that it informs our general understanding of the way that the environment shapes brain structure and function and how these effects mediate behaviour, cognition, and well-being (Grossman *et al.*, 2003). It can help answer questions about the neurodevelopmental timing of environmental influences and the presumed primacy of the effects of early as opposed to late experience (Fox *et al.*, 2010). More practically, this information highlights the enormous human toll of maltreatment (Bonomi *et al.*, 2008; Wang & Holton, 2007) and motivates attempts to improve child care and protection – a major social and health policy priority (Kamerman *et al.*, 2009; Parton, 2006). By illuminating the putative biological mediators of maltreatment such study also promotes potential therapeutic innovation by identifying new targets for treatment (McCrory *et al.*, 2010).

For obvious practical and ethical reasons, experimental studies of the impact of child maltreatment on brain development have relied on animal models that involve the systematic manipulation of early adversity factors and precise measurement of their effects using invasive techniques. Such methods and models have provided basic insights into the neurobiology of maltreatment (Teicher *et al.*, 2006). However, translating these insights to benefit maltreated children also requires studies in humans. The small number of human studies that have been carried out are perforce retrospective, yet have provided important insights, although these findings are difficult to interpret because of a number of common methodologic limitations, including small and heterogeneous samples, the fact that retrospective assessment of maltreatment lacks precision and reliability in the measurement of its timing and severity, and the difficulty of disentangling early adversity from subsequent chronic continuing risk as well as the impact of risk and disorder that so often co-occur (Tarullo & Gunnar, 2006). In order to study this ethically, we need to identify 'natural experiments' in which the effects of exposure to *early* adversity can be isolated from those of *continuing* adversity.

One of the most compelling examples of such a situation was the large-scale adoption of children who spent their early years in the extremely depriving Romanian orphanages following the fall of the Ceauşescu regime in 1989 (Johnson *et al.*, 1992). Most Romanian 'orphans' experienced global institutional deprivation, often secured to cots during the day and deprived of sufficient food, with minimal human contact and cognitive stimulation during their early years (Sonuga-Barke *et al.*, 2008). Adoption from abroad gave many 'orphans' a chance in life; at a moment easily pinpointed in terms of their chronological age, they experienced a sudden, radical change from a profoundly deprived institutional environment to an above-average home with adoptive families.

The English and Romanian Adoptees (ERA) study: design and overview of findings

The circumstances just outlined supported the establishment of the English and Romanian Adoptees study (ERA). This is the largest and most comprehensive developmental study (Rutter, 1998) of this cohort of children including, as it does, 165 Romanian adoptees who experienced between 2 weeks and 43 months of deprivation. These children, and a comparison group of 52 UK children adopted before the age of 6 months, have been followed up at ages 4, 6, 11, and 15 years. Together with other studies (McCall, 2011), the ERA study provides seminal insights into the effect of early global deprivation (Rutter & Sonuga-Barke, 2010). These include findings of:

(i) a devastating initial impact of deprivation on cognitive and social development for the majority of children (Rutter, 1998);

(ii) marked heterogeneity of later outcome in terms of both severity and type of problems;

(iii) a remarkable degree of catch-up for most individuals (Rutter *et al.*, 2001); but

(iv) a residual pattern of developmentally persistent severe deprivation-specific problems in a substantial minority (33 per cent at age 15), leading to a great need for clinical and special education (Beckett *et al.*, 2010). The problems evinced by these children had at their core an inappropriate social approach to strangers, that is, disinhibited attachment [DA] (Rutter *et al.*, 2007a) and quasi-autistic [Q-A] (Rutter *et al.*, 1999; Rutter *et al.*, 2007b) features often combined with inattention/overactivity [I/O] and cognitive impairment [CI] (Kreppner *et al.*, 2010; Kumsta *et al.*, 2010a), termed deprivation-specific patterns [DSPs];

(v) a link between DSP and deprivation duration – 50 per cent of children with more than 6 months' deprivation displayed DSP compared to 7 per cent of others (Kreppner *et al.*, 2007);

(vi) adolescent-onset emotional and peer problems in children with prior DSP (Sonuga-Barke *et al.*, 2010a);

(vii) little evidence of long-term difficulties in attachment to adoptive parents (Kreppner *et al.*, 2010) despite persistent DA (Kreppner *et al.*, 2010); and

(viii) moderation of outcomes primarily by genetic factors (Kumsta *et al.*, 2010b; Stevens *et al.*, 2009), and only minimally by postadoption family factors (Castle *et al.*, 2010).

Deprivation-related stunting of brain growth seen in the ERA study

Conclusive evidence now exists of the persistent negative impact of early severe deprivation (Rutter *et al.*, 2010a); there is also considerable continuity of problems in individual cases (Kreppner *et al.*, 2007). Together this has led to a strong hypothesis that the effects of institutional deprivation are due to fundamental neurobiologic alterations (Mehta *et al.*, 2009). To date, the strongest evidence for the neurobiologic hypothesis in ERA comes from the persistent effect of deprivation on brain growth as indexed by head circumference. Despite marked catch-up after adoption, deprivation still had a profound effect on all aspects of physical growth measures (height, weight, and head circumference) (Sonuga-Barke *et al.*, 2008) at age 6 years. Romanian adoptees had smaller heads (and therefore we can infer smaller brains) than UK adoptees in general. Furthermore, those suffering the most deprivation had the smallest heads of all – those with deprivation for more than 24 months were on average 2 standard deviations below the UK norms. Between 6 and 15 years there was further substantial catch-up in head circumference, so that those adoptees experiencing fewer than 6 months' deprivation have normal head circumference by age 15 years. For those exposed to more than 6 months' deprivation, major stunting is still apparent. Interestingly, these head circumference effects were rather different from other trajectories of growth (*i.e.*, height and weight). For children with fewer than 6 months' deprivation, height and weight were largely normalized by age 6 years. For those experiencing more than 6 months' deprivation, catch-up seemed complete by age 11 years – however, for this group there was a surprising deceleration in growth trajectory between 11 and 15 years, with most of the gains made between 6 and 11 lost again. Interestingly the most profound effects of deprivation on head growth were found with those children who had prior patterns of DSP (Sonuga-Barke *et al.*, 2010b).

The association between head growth stunting and DSP raises an obvious question: *Are the effects of deprivation on behavior and functioning, as manifest in DSP, mediated by its effects on developmental growth of the brain (as measured by head circumference)?* Overall stunting of the brain in general would be one way in which deprivation could fundamentally alter the brain to *cause* persistent deprivation-specific problems (DSPs). Our results have been mixed in this regard. In our first set of analyses using data obtained at age 11, there was no evidence that the effects of deprivation on head circumference mediated the emergence of DSPs (Sonuga-Barke *et al.*, 2008). However, in a more recent analysis using more powerful path-analytic techniques and age-15 head circumference data, we found somewhat different results. As predicted, there was a strong direct effect of duration of deprivation on the presence of DSPs. This effect remained significant when head circumference at age 6 years was introduced into the models as a second pathway. However, this second 'head circumference' pathway also accounted for a highly significant proportion of variance in DSPs in its own right. This effect was especially marked with regard to DA (rather than Q-A) patterns with approximately 20 per cent of the effect of duration of deprivation on this variable accounted for by head circumference.

The effects of deprivation on brain growth are *not* simply due to malnutrition

The Romanian adoptees were exposed to multiple putative risks of diverse kinds in the institutions (Rutter *et al.*, 2010b). Therefore, from the findings we have presented so far it is unclear which aspect of deprivation-related risk is responsible for poor outcomes in general and DSP in particular. There was, of course, psychosocial deprivation associated with extremely low levels of social contact and emotional support. There was also very limited intellectual stimulation (Castle *et al.* 1999). Although, perhaps less pervasive across institutions, severe levels of subnutrition were seen in many children on account of the very poor diets in many orphanages. These effects can be seen from the severely stunted growth of adoptees at the time of their placement in families (Sonuga-Barke *et al.*, 2008). Both nutritional and the psychosocial/cognitive deprivations have been implicated in negative long-term psychological outcomes in previous samples of deprived children. Brain development is inhibited by early-life subnutrition, which can cause long-term cognitive deficits and lessened well-being (Liu & Raine, 2006; Liu *et al.*, 2004). Studies of both patient populations (Pears & Fisher, 2005; Teicher *et al.*, 2003) and animal models (de Kloet *et al.*, 2005; Rosenzweig & Bennett, 1996) support this finding that early-life experience in impoverished environments is associated with smaller brains and altered brain structure and function, even when nutritional effects are controlled.

In the ERA study we have used a model of nutritional effects based on reduced weight at the time of entry into the UK, standardized in relation to UK norms and using a relatively liberal cut-off (1.5 standard deviations below the UK norm). Psychosocial and nutritional deprivation are clearly related, but we argue that if deficits are found in children of normal weight, then psychosocial deprivation must be operating through some mechanism other than low caloric intake. We use the term *subnutrition* rather than malnutrition because basing our analyses on weight at entry can tell us little about the role of specific nutritional imbalance and deficits: a diet may be fine in terms of the quantity of food, but low in nutritional value. With this definition in hand we went on to reassess the effects of duration of deprivation on head circumference at age 11 years, partitioning effects by nutritional status (Sonuga-Barke *et al.*, 2008). There were a number of striking results: (*1*) Head circumference was not substantially reduced in the non-subnourished group with less than 6 months' deprivation. (*2*) Subnourished children, irrespective of duration of deprivation, displayed head-growth stunting. (*3*) Crucially, children who were not subnourished, but who had experienced extended deprivation, also showed stunting. Psychosocial risk of sufficient duration (*i.e.*, more than 6 months) apparently had an effect on brain development that was independent of nutritional risk, at least as indexed by weight at entry into the UK. In a more recent analysis using data obtained at age 15, we explored the role of the presence of DSPs on the effects of duration of deprivation and subnutrition on head circumference. This analysis confirmed the effects of duration of deprivation independent of subnutrition. Strikingly subnutrition did not increase the risk of the development of DSPs or their subcomponents (Q-A, DA, CI, or IO) in the group of Romanian adoptees who had experienced greater than 6 months' deprivation.

In summary, the effects of early deprivation on overall brain growth appear to be profound and persistent, despite substantial catch-up in those exposed to the least degree of deprivation. If anything, the effects are more substantial than those for height and weight. The effects were observed even in the absence of subnutrition, which reinforces the view that *psychosocial*, as well as nutritional, risks can produce fundamental alterations in brain size, consistent with the notion that psychosocial deprivation appears to have a pervasive effect across biologic and psychological systems, independent of the nutritional risk often associated with institutional living. This view is supported by our mediational analyses, where the indirect path *via* head circumference, although less important than the direct pathway, still accounted for around 20 per cent of the effects.

Putative deprivation-sensitive brain networks

Prior research suggests that the sorts of institutional deprivation to which the Romanian adoptees were exposed in the early years of their lives is likely to result in more subtle structural and functional alterations in the brain as well as the gross effects on overall size reported above. The human brain is organized into interrelated, but functionally segregated brain networks underpinning distinctive neuropsychological processes that operate in concert to regulate behaviour and cognition (Bressler & Menon, 2010). Given the global nature of the deprivation to which many of the Romanian adoptees were exposed and the broad patterns of impairment suffered, we predict deprivation-specific alterations across a number of brain networks. Here we focus on three of the most plausible putative deprivation-sensitive brain networks. Each (i) is sensitive to early adversity similar to that suffered by the Romanian adoptees, (ii) underpins important socio-emotional regulatory functions, and (iii) is disrupted in clinical groups with problems overlapping with those presented by the adoptees.

Processing of negative stimuli (PoNS)

The hippocampus, amygdala, and, to a lesser extent, the corpus callosum (CC) form a network of putative deprivation-sensitive limbic regions (Sanchez *et al.*, 1998; Suomi, 1997; Teicher *et al.*, 2003). The CC is the major commissure connecting the cerebral hemispheres crucial for effective interhemispheric connectivity (Gazzaniga, 2000; Tomasch, 1954). The hippocampus and amygdala are medial temporal lobe structures implicated in the processing of negative experiences, such as those associated with aversive social and emotional stimuli and guiding behaviour to social threat (Adolphs & Spezio, 2006; Strange & Dolan, 2006), punishment (Vrticka *et al.*, 2008) and stress (Herman *et al.*, 2003). Neurochemically, serotonin functions as a key modulator of the processing of negative experiences by this network (Holmes, 2008; McEwen, 2003). Human and animal studies demonstrate the sensitivity of temporal lobe (Bremner, 1999, 2001, 2007; Bremner *et al.*, 1995, 1997, 1999; Vythilingam *et al.*, 2002) and CC structures (De Bellis *et al.*, 1999; Teicher *et al.*, 1997, 2004) to early adversity such as neglect and abuse. One possible mechanism by which early institutional deprivation could lead to lasting alterations in brain structure and function might involve psychosocial stress associated with institutional rearing and associated prolonged activation and inadequate regulation of the hypothalamus-pituitary-adrenal (HPA) axis. Animal models support the existence of long lasting effects of early stress on brain development and on later psychological and behavioural functioning, including altered structure and function of HPA axis associated brain structures, *e.g.*, the hippocampus (Sapolsky, 1985; Sapolsky *et al.*, 1990; Uno *et al.*, 1989), as well as effects on catecholaminergic neurotransmitter branches and neurocircuitry in dorsal striatum and prefrontal cortex (McEwen, 1999; Sanchez *et al.*, 2001; Teicher *et al.*, 2003). Indeed, there is some evidence suggesting inadequate HPA axis regulation as a consequence of institutional rearing (Carlson & Earls, 1997; Fries *et al.*, 2008). However, a recent study in a sample of post-institutionalized children showed no differences in cortisol levels following a laboratory stress protocol (Gunnar *et al.*, 2009). This does not preclude altered stress responsivity in these cohorts, although longitudinal studies charting stress responses in post-institutionalized children would be required to fully appreciate the effects on the HPA axis.

Functional alterations have also been demonstrated. Maheu *et al.* (2010) found a link between early emotional neglect and increased left amygdala and left anterior hippocampus activation to social threat. In groups of Romanian adoptees there is preliminary evidence of limbic emotional network involvement. We have found deficits in emotion processing in the ERA sample (Colvert *et al.*, 2008a). Altered amygdala volumes (Tottenham *et al.*, 2010), reduced glucose metabolism in the left medial temporal lobe area (including the hippocampus and amygdala [Chugani *et al.*, 2001]) and reduced integrity of the uncinate fasciculus, which connects inferior frontal lobe and anterior temporal lobe areas including the amygdala (Eluvathingal *et al.*, 2006) have also been found. Structural and functional alterations are found in patients with unipolar (Drevets, 2001; Mitterschiffthaler *et al.*, 2006) and bipolar depression (Pan *et al.*, 2009; Savitz & Drevets, 2009) and personality disorders (Buchheim *et al.*, 2008). Furthermore, the response of the amygdala to social punishment is influenced by attachment security (Lemche *et al.*, 2006). Our report that polymorphisms in the 5-HTT gene moderate the effects of deprivation with regard to emotional problems further strengthens the notion of PoNS-related structures as putative deprivation-sensitive brain regions (Kumsta *et al.*, 2010b).

Processing of positive stimuli (PoPS)

Working in concert with PoNS, with which it is functionally and structurally linked, a second brain network is implicated in the regulation of positive social encounters and social reward (O'Doherty, 2004; Schultz, 2006). This network includes the ventral tegmental area, ventral components of both basal ganglia (*e.g.*, nucleus accumbens), and anterior cingulate and orbitofrontal cortex – all heavily modulated by mesolimbic dopaminergic inputs (Wise, 2004; Wise & Bozarth, 1982). Animal models demonstrate the sensitivity of these regions to early social adversity (Hall *et al.*, 1998; Jones *et al.*, 1990, 1992; Powell *et al.*, 2003; Sahakian *et al.*, 1975) with abnormal mesolimbic dopamine function, including that in the nucleus accumbens and the prefrontal cortex (Fulford & Marsden, 1998; Jones *et al.*, 1992), altered responses to amphetamine and dopamine agonists (Ahmed *et al.*, 1995; Jones *et al.*, 1990; Phillips *et al.*, 1994; Sahakian *et al.*, 1975; Weiss *et al.*, 2001). Hanson *et al.* (2010) found alterations in orbitofrontal cortex activity related to long-term social functioning in previously abused adolescents. Shin and Liberzon (2010) reported effects of early trauma manifest in the rostral portion of the cingulate cortex. Abused and neglected children have been shown to have deficits in reward processing (Guyer *et al.*, 2006), which Dillon and colleagues linked to reduced activity in the pallidum (Dillon *et al.*, 2009). Furthermore, Chugani *et al.* (2001) found reduced glucose metabolism in the left orbitofrontal cortex in Romanian adoptees with a history of deprivation. Altered PoPS structure and activity have been implicated in disorders overlapping with DSPs, especially ADHD. Finally PoPS activation to social reward appears to underpin mechanisms regulating reward-positive social encounters (Vrticka *et al.*, 2008) and the development of trust (Krueger *et al.*, 2007). Our report that polymorphisms in the DAT1 gene, which regulates ventral striatal dopamine function, also moderate DSPs shows this to be a potential candidate network of interest (Stevens *et al.*, 2009).

Executive control of inappropriate responses (ECIR)

The social and emotional dysregulation associated with DSPs may result from deficient 'top down' executive control, leading to failure to inhibit inappropriate responses. A brain network incorporating projections from dorsolateral prefrontal cortex, to rostral and dorsal components of the anterior cingulate cortex and the striatum (*i.e.*, the caudate) is implicated in inhibitory-based executive control of inappropriate responses. Carrion *et al.* (2001) found structural frontal lobe abnormalities (especially altered patterns of asymmetry) in children exposed to severe abuse and neglect. Mueller *et al.* (2010) found reduced cognitive control in a maltreated group who showed reduced activation in frontostriatal networks. In resting EEGs, Miskovic *et al.* (2010) found reduced alpha coherence in adolescents with a history of abuse. Tomoda *et al.* (2009) found reduced grey matter in frontal regions of the cortex in children exposed to extremely harsh discipline. Carrion *et al.* (2007) found that adolescents with a history of maltreatment displayed reduced middle frontal cortex activation. Our own data suggest specific deficits in inhibitory control and executive functions more generally (Colvert *et al.*, 2008b; Sonuga-Barke & Rubia, 2008). ECIR has been implicated in disinhibitory disorders such as ADHD, conduct disorder, and severe emotional dysregulation (Rubia, 2010; Berna *et al.*, 2010; Brooks *et al.*, 2010).

The ERA Imaging Pilot

We have conducted a pilot study to help guide the ERA brain imaging strategy (*i.e.*, the choice of imaging tasks and techniques for a large-scale study). Fourteen Romanian adoptees from the ERA cohort who had experienced extended deprivation (> 6 months) and who had a range of different types and severity of DSPs were compared with 11 age-equivalent normal controls with no history of deprivation or adoption. Both structural and functional protocols were run.

Three tasks were included for the functional analysis: a reward cue processing task (Monetary Incentive Delay or MID [Knutson *et al.*, 2001]); an inhibitory control task (Stop Signal Task or SST [Rubia *et al.*, 2003]); and a social inference task (Schultz *et al.*, 2003).

Initial structural findings

Consistent with the ERA head circumference finding, the total brain volume was lower in the adoptees than in controls (Mehta *et al.*, 2009). In a region of interest (ROI) analysis targeting the PoNS regions, we found the Romanian adoptees group had a larger relative amygdala volume, these effects being greater for the right amygdala (Mehta *et al.*, 2009). We also found a significant negative relationship between the volume of the left amygdala and time spent in institutions. There was no evidence for altered CC mid-sagittal area or hippocampal volume – these effects may emerge later or may not be detected in the pilot study, given its limited power. Indeed, when the cohort from our pilot study is segregated by the degree of current problems, CC abnormalities were detectable, indicating that the more sophisticated analyses afforded by larger sample sizes will be important. A whole-brain voxel-wise analysis of grey matter volume using voxel-based morphometry (Mehta *et al.*, in preparation) confirmed the amygdala finding, although significance did not survive correction for multiple testing. Additionally, in the same analysis (Mehta *et al.*, in preparation), we found a range of effects in structures implicated in our putative deprivation-specific networks. These included especially strong effects in the thalamus, and the dorsal striatum. This analysis reveals previously unseen alterations in brain structure in the Romanian adoptees, implicating the basal ganglia and frontal lobes, regions critical for the regulation of social behaviour and emotional processing.

Initial functional findings

Two of the three tasks were implemented successfully within the imaging protocol producing expected activation patterns in controls. For the MID, controls activated the PoPS network as expected to signals predicting future rewards. Furthermore activation increased monotonically with increasing rewards. In contrast Romanian adoptees exhibited a very striking pattern of PoPS hyporesponsiveness, especially in the ventral striatum, and reward size had no effect on activation (Mehta *et al.*, 2010), despite normal reaction times and accuracy. On the SST, controls once again activated the expected regions on the ECIR networks with activations in the inferior prefrontal cortex and the dorsal striatum (Mehta *et al.*, unpublished data). For the Romanian adoptees who were able to perform the task to the required accuracy criteria, activation of the inferior frontal gyrus was impaired during inhibition. In the group of Romanian adoptees, the size of activation deficits was not significantly correlated with either duration of deprivation (although all included were over the 6-month threshold) or the presence of DSPs (or correlated with continuous measures of problems). The final task included was a measure of social intention, which was included to tap into the theory of mind concept. It failed to either activate the expected network or show differences between adoptees and controls.

ERA brain imaging: the future

This pilot study, despite its limited size and scope, (i) underscored the value of MRI approaches to tackling the question of the long-term effects of deprivation on the brain; (ii) demonstrated the feasibility of imaging this sample of vulnerable individuals; (iii) highlighted the value of structural analytical approaches sensitive enough to capture the long-term effects of deprivation;

(iv) allowed us to identify two tasks (tapping putative deprivation-sensitive brain networks) showing differences between deprived and nondeprived individuals. It therefore provided a promising platform for a larger-scale study. However, much larger numbers of subjects will be required (1) to fully characterize the functional and structural alterations in the Romanian adoptees with a greater degree of confidence; (2) to explore interactions within and between different brain networks; (3) to test for dose-response relations between time spent in institutions and brain structure and function; and (4) to examine whether particular brain alterations specifically mediate the effects of deprivation on specific DSPs. Furthermore, the pilot design did not allow us to (*a*) explore the effects of deprivation independent of adoption (given that it only included a nonadopted control group) and so differences reported could be the result of early deprivation or subsequent adoption; (*b*) effectively cover all brain networks of interest; and (*c*) examine patterns of functional connectivity in the resting brain within key brain networks. In the light of the human and animal literature and our own pilot data, we are aiming to conduct a large-scale imaging study employing a range of structural and functional imaging techniques to explore the long-term impact of severe early institutional deprivation across the whole brain, specifically in relation to the putative deprivation-sensitive brain networks: those involved in the processing of negative stimuli, the processing of positive stimuli, and the executive control of inappropriate responses.

References

Adolphs, R. & Spezio, M. (2006): Role of the amygdala in processing visual social stimuli. *Prog. Brain Res.* **156,** 363–378.

Ahmed, S.H., Stinus, L., Le Moal, M. & Cador, M. (1995): Social deprivation enhances the vulnerability of male Wistar rats to stressor- and amphetamine-induced behavioral sensitization. *Psychopharmacology (Berl.)* **117,** 116–124.

Beckett, C., Castle, J., Rutter, M. & Sonuga-Barke, E. J. (2010): VI. Institutional deprivation, specific cognitive functions, and scholastic achievement: English and Romanian Adoptee (ERA) study findings. *Monogr. Soc. Res. Child Dev.* **75,** 125–142.

Berna, C., Leknes, S., Holmes, E.A., Edwards, R.R., Goodwin, G. M. & Tracey, I. (2010): Induction of depressed mood disrupts emotion regulation neurocircuitry and enhances pain unpleasantness. *Biol Psychiatry* **67,** 1083–1090.

Bonomi, A.E., Anderson, M.L., Rivara, F.P., Cannon, E.A., Fishman, P.A., Carrell, D., *et al.* (2008): Health care utilization and costs associated with childhood abuse. *J. Gen. Intern. Med.* **23,** 294–299.

Bremner, J.D. (1999): Alterations in brain structure and function associated with post-traumatic stress disorder. *Semin. Clin Neuropsychiatry.* **4,** 249–255.

Bremner, J.D. (2001): Hypotheses and controversies related to effects of stress on the hippocampus: an argument for stress-induced damage to the hippocampus in patients with posttraumatic stress disorder. *Hippocampus* **11,** 75–81; discussion 82–84.

Bremner, J.D. (2007): Neuroimaging in posttraumatic stress disorder and other stress-related disorders. *Neuroimaging Clin. N. Am.* **17,** 523–538, ix.

Bremner, J.D., Randall, P., Scott, T.M., Bronen, R.A., Seibyl, J.P., Southwick, S.M., *et al.* (1995): MRI-based measurement of hippocampal volume in patients with combat-related posttraumatic stress disorder. *Am. J. Psychiatry* **152,** 973–981.

Bremner, J.D., Randall, P., Vermetten, E., Staib, L., Bronen, R.A., Mazure, C., *et al.* (1997): Magnetic resonance imaging-based measurement of hippocampal volume in posttraumatic stress disorder related to childhood physical and sexual abuse – a preliminary report. *Biol. Psychiatry* **41,** 23–32.

Bremner, J.D., Narayan, M., Staib, L.H., Southwick, S.M., McGlashan, T. & Charney, D.S. (1999): Neural correlates of memories of childhood sexual abuse in women with and without posttraumatic stress disorder. *Am. J. Psychiatry* **156,** 1787–1795.

Bremner, J.D., Elzinga, B., Schmahl, C. & Vermetten, E. (2008): Structural and functional plasticity of the human brain in posttraumatic stress disorder. *Prog. Brain Res.* **167,** 171–186.

Bressler, S.L. & Menon, V. (2010): Large-scale brain networks in cognition: emerging methods and principles. *Trends Cognit. Sci.* **14,** 277–290.

Brooks, J.O., 3rd, Bearden, C.E., Hoblyn, J.C., Woodard, S.A. & Ketter, T.A. (2010): Prefrontal and paralimbic metabolic dysregulation related to sustained attention in euthymic older adults with bipolar disorder. *Bipolar Disord.* **12,** 866–874.

Buchheim, A., Erk, S., George, C., Kachele, H., Kircher, T., Martius, P., *et al.* (2008): Neural correlates of attachment trauma in borderline personality disorder: a functional magnetic resonance imaging study. *Psychiatry Res.* **163,** 223–235.

Carlson, M. & Earls, F. (1997): Psychological and neuroendocrinological sequelae of early social deprivation in institutionalized children in Romania. *Ann. N. Y. Acad. Sci.* **807,** 419–428.

Carrion, V.G., Weems, C.F., Eliez, S., Patwardhan, A., Brown, W., Ray, R.D. & Reiss, A.L. (2001): Attenuation of frontal asymmetry in pediatric posttraumatic stress disorder. *Biol. Psychiatry* **50,** 943–951.

Carrion, V.G., Weems, C.F. & Reiss, A.L. (2007): Stress predicts brain changes in children: a pilot longitudinal study on youth stress, posttraumatic stress disorder, and the hippocampus. *Pediatrics* **119,** 509–516.

Castle, J., Groothues, C., Bredenkamp, D., Beckett, C., O'Connor, T. & Rutter, M. (1999): Effects of qualities of early institutional care on cognitive attainment. E.R.A. Study Team. English and Romanian Adoptees. *Am. J. Orthopsychiatry* **69,** 424–437.

Castle, J., Beckett, C., Rutter, M. & Sonuga-Barke, E.J. (2010): VIII. Postadoption environmental features. *Monogr. Soc. Res. Child Dev.* **75,** 167–186.

Chugani, H.T., Behen, ME., Muzik, O., Juhasz, C., Nagy, F. & Chugani, D.C. (2001): Local brain functional activity following early deprivation: a study of postinstitutionalized Romanian orphans. *NeuroImage* **14,** 1290–1301.

Colvert, E., Rutter, M., Beckett, C., Castle, J., Groothues, C., Hawkins, A., *et al.* (2008a): Emotional difficulties in early adolescence following severe early deprivation: findings from the English and Romanian adoptees study. *Dev. Psychopathol.* **20,** 547–567.

Colvert, E., Rutter, M., Kreppner, J., Beckett, C., Castle, J., Groothues, C., *et al.* (2008b): Do theory of mind and executive function deficits underlie the adverse outcomes associated with profound early deprivation?: findings from the English and Romanian adoptees study. *J. Abnorm. Child Psychol.* **36,** 1057–1068.

De Bellis, M.D., Keshavan, M.S., Clark, D.B., Casey, B.J., Giedd, J.N., Boring, A.M., *et al.* (1999): A.E. Bennett Research Award. Developmental traumatology. Part II: Brain development. *Biol. Psychiatry* **45,** 1271–1284.

de Kloet, E.R., Sibug, R.M., Helmerhorst, F.M. & Schmidt, M.V. (2005): Stress, genes and the mechanism of programming the brain for later life. *Neurosci. Biobehav. Rev.* **29,** 271–281.

Dillon, D.G., Holmes, A.J., Birk, J.L., Brooks, N., Lyons-Ruth, K. & Pizzagalli, D.A. (2009): Childhood adversity is associated with left basal ganglia dysfunction during reward anticipation in adulthood. *Biol. Psychiatry.* **66,** 206–213.

Drevets, W.C. (2001): Neuroimaging and neuropathological studies of depression: implications for the cognitive-emotional features of mood disorders. *Curr. Opin. Neurobiol.* **11,** 240–249.

Eluvathingal, T.J., Chugani, H.T., Behen, M.E., Juhasz, C., Muzik, O., Maqbool, M., *et al.* (2006): Abnormal brain connectivity in children after early severe socioemotional deprivation: a diffusion tensor imaging study. *Pediatrics* **117,** 2093–2100.

Fox, S.E., Levitt, P. & Nelson, C.A., 3rd (2010): How the timing and quality of early experiences influence the development of brain architecture. *Child Dev.* **81,** 28–40.

Fries, A.B., Shirtcliff, E.A. & Pollak, S.D. (2008): Neuroendocrine dysregulation following early social deprivation in children. *Dev. Psychobiol.* **50,** (6), 588–599.

Fulford, A.J. & Marsden, C.A. (1998): Effect of isolation-rearing on conditioned dopamine release in vivo in the nucleus accumbens of the rat. *J. Neurochem.* **70,** 384–390.

Gazzaniga, M.S. (2000): Cerebral specialization and interhemispheric communication: does the corpus callosum enable the human condition? *Brain* **123** (Pt 7), 1293–1326.

Grossman, A.W., Churchill, J.D., McKinney, B.C., Kodish, I.M., Otte, S.L. & Greenough, W.T. (2003): Experience effects on brain development: possible contributions to psychopathology. *J. Child Psychol. Psychiatry* **44,** 33–63.

Gunnar M.R., *et al.* (2009): Moderate versus severe early life stress: Associations with stress reactivity and regulation in 10-12-year-old children. *Psychoneuroendocrinology* **34,** 62–75.

Guyer, A.E., Kaufman, J., Hodgdon, H.B., Masten, C.L., Jazbec, S., Pine, D.S. & Ernst, M. (2006): Behavioral alterations in reward system function: the role of childhood maltreatment and psychopathology. *J. Am. Acad. Child Adolesc. Psychiatry* **45,** 1059–1067.

Hall, F.S., Wilkinson, L.S., Humby, T., Inglis, W., Kendall, D.A., Marsden, C.A. & Robbins, T.W. (1998): Isolation rearing in rats: pre- and postsynaptic changes in striatal dopaminergic systems. *Pharmacol. Biochem. Behav.* **59,** 859–872.

Hanson, J.L., Chung, M.K., Avants, B.B., Shirtcliff, E.A., Gee, J.C., Davidson, R.J. & Pollak, S.D. (2010): Early stress is associated with alterations in the orbitofrontal cortex: a tensor-based morphometry investigation of brain structure and behavioral risk. *J. Neurosci.* **30,** 7466–7472.

Herman, J.P., Figueiredo, H., Mueller, N.K., Ulrich-Lai, Y., Ostrander, M.M., Choi, D.C. & Cullinan, W.E. (2003): Central mechanisms of stress integration: hierarchical circuitry controlling hypothalamo-pituitary-adrenocortical responsiveness. *Frontiers Neuroendocrinol.* **24,** 151–180.

Holmes, A. (2008): Genetic variation in cortico-amygdala serotonin function and risk for stress-related disease. *Neurosci. Biobehav. Rev.* **32,** 1293–1314.

Johnson, D.E., Miller, L.C., Iverson, S., Thomas, W., Franchino, B., Dole, K., *et al.* (1992): The health of children adopted from Romania. *JAMA* **268,** 3446–3451.

Jones, G.H., Marsden, C.A. & Robbins, T.W. (1990): Increased sensitivity to amphetamine and reward-related stimuli following social isolation in rats: possible disruption of dopamine- dependent mechanisms of the nucleus accumbens. *Psychopharmacology* **102,** 364–372.

Jones, G.H., Hernandez, T.D., Kendall, D.A., Marsden, C.A. & Robbins, T.W. (1992): Dopaminergic and serotonergic function following isolation rearing in rats: study of behavioural responses and postmortem and in vivo neurochemistry. *Pharmacol. Biochem. Behav.* **43,** 17–35.

Kamerman, S., Phipps, S. & Ben-Arieh, A., eds. (2009a): *From Child Welfare to Child Well-Being: An International Perspective on Knowledge in the Service of Policy Making.* New York: Springer.

Knutson, B., Adams, C.A., Fong, G.W. & Hommer, D. (2001): Anticipation of increasing monetary reward selectively recruits nucleus accumbens. *J. Neurosci.* **21,** RC159 (1–5).

Kreppner, J.M., Rutter, M., Beckett, C., Castle, J., Colvert, E., Groothues, C., *et al.* (2007): Normality and impairment following profound early institutional deprivation: a longitudinal follow-up into early adolescence. *Dev. Psychol.* **43,** 931–946.

Kreppner, J., Kumsta, R., Rutter, M., Beckett, C., Castle, J., Stevens, S. & Sonuga-Barke, E.J. (2010): IV. Developmental course of deprivation-specific psychological patterns: early manifestations, persistence to age 15, and clinical features. *Monogr. Soc. Res. Child Dev.* **75,** 79–101.

Krueger, F., McCabe, K., Moll, J., Kriegeskorte, N., Zahn, R., Strenziok, M., *et al.* (2007): Neural correlates of trust. *Proc. Natl. Acad. Sci. USA* **104,** 20084–20089.

Kumsta, R., Kreppner, J., Rutter, M., Beckett, C., Castle, J., Stevens, S. & Sonuga-Barke, E.J. (2010a): III. Deprivation-specific psychological patterns. *Monogr. Soc. Res. Child Dev.* **75,** 48–78.

Kumsta, R., Stevens, S., Brookes, K., Schlotz, W., Castle, J., Beckett, C., *et al.* (2010b): 5HTT genotype moderates the influence of early institutional deprivation on emotional problems in adolescence: evidence from the English and Romanian Adoptee (ERA) study. *J. Child Psychol. Psychiatry* **51,** 755–762.

Lemche, E., Giampietro, V.P., Surguladze, S.A., Amaro, E.J., Andrew, C.M., Williams, S.C., *et al.* (2006): Human attachment security is mediated by the amygdala: evidence from combined fMRI and psychophysiological measures. *Hum. Brain Mapp.* **27,** 623–635.

Liu, J. & Raine, A. (2006): The effect of childhood malnutrition on externalizing behavior. *Curr. Opin. Pediatr.* **18,** 565–570.

Liu, J., Raine, A., Venables, P.H. & Mednick, S.A. (2004): Malnutrition at age 3 years and externalizing behavior problems at ages 8, 11, and 17 years. *Am. J. Psychiatry* **161,** 2005–2013.

Maheu, F.S., Dozier, M., Guyer, A.E., Mandell, D., Peloso, E., Poeth, K., *et al.* (2010): A preliminary study of medial temporal lobe function in youths with a history of caregiver deprivation and emotional neglect. *Cogn. Affect. Behav. Neurosci.* **10,** 34–49.

McCall, R. (2011): Children without permanent parental care: research, practice, and policy. *Monogr. Soc. Res. Child Dev.* In press.

McCrory, E., De Brito, S.A. & Viding, E. (2010): Research review: the neurobiology and genetics of maltreatment and adversity. *J. Child Psychol. Psychiatry* **51,** 1079–1095.

McEwen, B. (1999): Development of the cerebral cortex: XIII. Stress and brain development: II. *J. Am. Acad. Child Adolesc. Psychiatry* **38,** 101–103.

McEwen, B.S. (2003): Early life influences on life-long patterns of behavior and health. *Ment. Retard. Dev. Disabil. Res. Rev.* **9,** 149–154.

Mehta, M.A., Golembo, N.I., Nosarti, C., Colvert, E., Mota, A., Williams, S.C., *et al.* (2009): Amygdala, hippocampal and corpus callosum size following severe early institutional deprivation: the English and Romanian Adoptees study pilot. *J. Child Psychol. Psychiatry* **50,** 943–951.

Mehta, M.A., Gore-Langton, E., Golembo, N., Colvert, E., Williams, S.C. & Sonuga-Barke, E. (2010): Hyporesponsive reward anticipation in the basal ganglia following severe institutional deprivation early in life. *J. Cognit. Neurosci.* **22,** 2316–2325.

Miskovic, V., Schmidt, L.A., Georgiades, K., Boyle, M. & Macmillan, H.L. (2010): Adolescent females exposed to child maltreatment exhibit atypical EEG coherence and psychiatric impairment: linking early adversity, the brain, and psychopathology. *Dev. Psychopathol.* **22,** 419–432.

Mitterschiffthaler, M.T., Ettinger, U., Mehta, M.A., Mataix-Cols, D. & Williams, S.C. (2006): Applications of functional magnetic resonance imaging in psychiatry. *J. Magn. Reson. Imaging* **23,** 851–861.

Mueller, S.C., Maheu, F.S., Dozier, M., Peloso, E., Mandell, D., Leibenluft, E., *et al.* (2010): Early-life stress is associated with impairment in cognitive control in adolescence: an fMRI study. *Neuropsychologia* **48,** 3037–3044.

Nelson, C.A., III, Bos, K., Gunnar, M.R. & Sonuga-Barke, E. (In press): The neurobiological toll of early human deprivation. *Monogr. Soc. Res. Child Dev.*

O'Doherty, J.P. (2004): Reward representations and reward-related learning in the human brain: insights from neuroimaging. *Curr. Opin. Neurobiol.* **14,** 769–776.

Pan, L., Keener, M.T., Hassel, S. & Phillips, M.L. (2009): Functional neuroimaging studies of bipolar disorder: examining the wide clinical spectrum in the search for disease endophenotypes. *Int. Rev. Psychiatry* **21,** 368–379.

Parton, N. (2006): Every child matters: the shift to prevention whilst strengthening protection in children's services in England. *Child. Youth Serv. Rev.* **28,** 976–992.

Pears, K. & Fisher, P.A. (2005): Developmental, cognitive, and neuropsychological functioning in preschool-aged foster children: associations with prior maltreatment and placement history. *J. Dev. Behav. Pediatr.* **26,** 112–122.

Phillips, G.D., Howes, S.R., Whitelaw, R.B., Wilkinson, L.S., Robbins, T.W. & Everitt, B.J. (1994): Isolation rearing enhances the locomotor response to cocaine and a novel environment, but impairs the intravenous self-administration of cocaine. *Psychopharmacology (Berl.)* **115,** 407–418.

Powell, S.B., Geyer, M.A., Preece, M.A., Pitcher, L.K., Reynolds, G.P. & Swerdlow, N.R. (2003): Dopamine depletion of the nucleus accumbens reverses isolation-induced deficits in prepulse inhibition in rats. *Neuroscience* **119,** 233–240.

Rosenzweig, M.R. & Bennett, E.L. (1996): Psychobiology of plasticity: effects of training and experience on brain and behavior. *Behav. Brain Res.* **78,** 57–65.

Rubia, K. (2010): 'Cool' inferior Frontostriatal dysfunction in attention-deficit/hyperactivity disorder *versus* 'hot' ventromedial orbitofrontal-limbic dysfunction in conduct disorder: a review. *Biol. Psychiatry* **69,** E69–E87.

Rubia, K., Smith, A.B., Brammer, M.J. & Taylor, E. (2003): Right inferior prefrontal cortex mediates response inhibition while mesial prefrontal cortex is responsible for error detection. *NeuroImage* **20,** 351–358.

Rutter, M. (1998): Developmental catch-up, and deficit, following adoption after severe global early privation. English and Romanian Adoptees (ERA) Study Team. *J. Child Psychol. Psychiatry* **39,** 465–476.

Rutter, M., Andersen-Wood, L., Beckett, C., Bredenkamp, D., Castle, J., Groothues, C., *et al.* (1999): Quasi-autistic patterns following severe early global privation. English and Romanian Adoptees (ERA) Study Team. *J. Child Psychol. Psychiatry* **40,** 537–549.

Rutter, M.L., Kreppner, J.M. & O'Connor, T.G. (2001): Specificity and heterogeneity in children's responses to profound institutional privation. *Br. J. Psychiatry* **179,** 97–103.

Rutter, M., Colvert, E., Kreppner, J., Beckett, C., Castle, J., Groothues, C., *et al.* (2007a): Early adolescent outcomes for institutionally-deprived and non-deprived adoptees. I: Disinhibited attachment. *J. Child Psychol. Psychiatry* **48,** 17–30.

Rutter, M., Kreppner, J., Croft, C., Murin, M., Colvert, E., Beckett, C., *et al.* (2007b): Early adolescent outcomes of institutionally deprived and non-deprived adoptees. III. Quasi-autism. *J. Child Psychol. Psychiatry* **48,** 1200–1207.

Rutter, M. & Sonuga-Barke, E.J. (2010): X. Conclusions: overview of findings from the era study, inferences, and research implications. *Monogr. Soc. Res. Child Dev.* **75,** 212–229.

Rutter, M., Sonuga-Barke, E.J., Castle, J., Kreppner, J., Kumsta, R., Schlotz, W., Stevens, S. & Bell, C.A. (2010a): Deprivation-specific psychological patterns: effects of institutional deprivation. *Monogr. Soc. Res. Child Dev.* **75,** 1–252.

Rutter, M., Sonuga-Barke, E.J. & Castle, J. (2010b): I. Investigating the impact of early institutional deprivation on development: background and research strategy of the English and Romanian Adoptees (ERA) study. *Monogr. Soc. Res. Child Dev.* **75,** 1–20.

Sahakian, B.J., Robbins, T.W., Morgan, M.J. & Iversen, S.D. (1975): The effects of psychomotor stimulants on stereotypy and locomotor activity in socially-deprived and control rats. *Brain Res.* **84,** 195–205.

Sanchez, M.M., Hearn, E.F., Do, D., Rilling, J.K. & Herndon, J.G. (1998): Differential rearing affects corpus callosum size and cognitive function of rhesus monkeys. *Brain Res.* **812,** 38–49.

Sanchez, M.M., Ladd, C.O. & Plotsky, P.M. (2001). Early adverse experience as a developmental risk factor for later psychopathology: evidence from rodent and primate models. *Dev. Psychopathol.* **13**(3), 419–449.

Sapolsky, R.M. (1985): Glucocorticoid toxicity in the hippocampus: temporal aspects of neuronal vulnerability. *Brain Res.* **359,** 300–305.

Sapolsky, R.M., Uno, H., Rebert, C.S. & Finch, C.E. (1990): Hippocampal damage associated with prolonged glucocorticoid exposure in primates. *J. Neurosci.* **10,** 2897–2902.

Savitz, J. & Drevets, W.C. (2009): Bipolar and major depressive disorder: neuroimaging the developmental-degenerative divide. *Neurosci. Biobehav. Rev.* **33,** 699–771.

Schultz, R.T., Grelotti, D.J., Klin, A., Kleinman, J., Van der Gaag, C., Marois, R. & Skudlarski, P. (2003): The role of the fusiform face area in social cognition: implications for the pathobiology of autism. *Philos. Trans. R. Soc. Lond. B. Biol. Sci.* **358,** 415–427.

Schultz, W. (2006): Behavioral theories and the neurophysiology of reward. *Annu. Rev. Psychol.* **57,** 87–115.

Shin, L.M. & Liberzon, I. (2010): The neurocircuitry of fear, stress, and anxiety disorders. *Neuropsychopharmacology* **35,** 169–191.

Sonuga-Barke, E.J. & Rubia, K. (2008): Inattentive/overactive children with histories of profound institutional deprivation compared with standard ADHD cases: a brief report. *Child Care Health Dev.* **34,** 596–602.

Sonuga-Barke, E.J., Beckett, C., Kreppner, J., Castle, J., Colvert, E., Stevens, S., *et al.* (2008): Is sub-nutrition necessary for a poor outcome following early institutional deprivation? *Dev. Med. Child. Neurol.* **50,** 664–671.

Sonuga-Barke, E.J., Schlotz, W. & Kreppner, J. (2010a): V. Differentiating developmental trajectories for conduct, emotion, and peer problems following early deprivation. *Monogr. Soc. Res. Child Dev.* **75,** 102–124.

Sonuga-Barke, E.J., Schlotz, W. & Rutter, M. (2010b): VII. Physical growth and maturation following early severe institutional deprivation: do they mediate specific psychopathological effects? *Monogr. Soc. Res. Child Dev.* **75,** 143–166.

Stevens, S.E., Kumsta, R., Kreppner, J.M., Brookes, K.J., Rutter, M. & Sonuga-Barke, E.J. (2009): Dopamine transporter gene polymorphism moderates the effects of severe deprivation on ADHD symptoms: developmental continuities in gene-environment interplay. *Am. J. Med. Genet. B Neuropsychiatr. Genet.* **150B,** 753–761.

Strange, B.A. & Dolan, R.J. (2006): Anterior medial temporal lobe in human cognition: memory for fear and the unexpected. *Cognit. Neuropsychiatry* **11,** 198–218.

Suomi, S.J. (1997) Long-term effects of different early rearing experiences on social, emotional, and physiological development in non-human primates. In: *Neurodevelopment and Adult Psychopathology*, eds. M.S. Keshevan & R.M. Murray, pp. 104–116. Cambridge, UK: Cambridge University Press.

Tarullo, A.R. & Gunnar, M.R. (2006): Child maltreatment and the developing HPA axis. *Horm. Behav.* **50,** 632–639.

Teicher, M.H., Ito, Y., Glod, C.A., Andersen, S.L., Dumont, N. & Ackerman, E. (1997): Preliminary evidence for abnormal cortical development in physically and sexually abused children using EEG coherence and MRI. *Ann. N.Y. Acad. Sci.* **821,** 160–175.

Teicher, M.H., Andersen, S.L., Polcari, A., Anderson, C.M., Navalta, C.P. & Kim, D.M. (2003): The neurobiological consequences of early stress and childhood maltreatment. *Neurosci. Biobehav. Rev.* **27,** 33–44.

Teicher, M.H., Dumont, N.L., Ito, Y., Vaituzis, C., Giedd, J.N. & Andersen, S.L. (2004): Childhood neglect is associated with reduced corpus callosum area. *Biol. Psychiatry* **56,** 80–85.

Teicher, M.H., Tomoda, A. & Andersen, S.L. (2006): Neurobiological consequences of early stress and childhood maltreatment: are results from human and animal studies comparable? *Ann. N.Y. Acad. Sci.* **1071,** 313–323.

Tomasch, J. (1954): Size, distribution, and number of fibres in the human corpus callosum. *Anat. Rec.* **119,** 119–135.

Tomoda, A., Suzuki, H., Rabi, K., Sheu, Y.S., Polcari, A. &.Teicher, M.H. (2009): Reduced prefrontal cortical gray matter volume in young adults exposed to harsh corporal punishment. *NeuroImage* **47** (Suppl. 2), T66–71.

Tottenham, N., Hare, T.A., Quinn, B.T., McCarry, T.W., Nurse, M., Gilhooly, T., *et al.* (2010): Prolonged institutional rearing is associated with atypically large amygdala volume and difficulties in emotion regulation. *Dev. Sci.* **13,** 46–61.

Uno, H., Tarara, R., Else, J.G., Suleman, M.A. & Sapolsky, R.M. (1989): Hippocampal damage associated with prolonged and fatal stress in primates. *J. Neurosci.* **9,** 1705–1711.

Vrticka, P., Andersson, F., Grandjean, D., Sander, D. & Vuilleumier, P. (2008): Individual attachment style modulates human amygdala and striatum activation during social appraisal. *PLoS One* **3,** e2868.

Vythilingam, M., Heim, C., Newport, J., Miller, A.H., Anderson, E., Bronen, R., *et al.* (2002): Childhood trauma associated with smaller hippocampal volume in women with major depression. *Am. J. Psychiatry* **159,** 2072–2080.

Wang, C. & Holton, J. (2007): *Total Estimated Cost of Child Abuse and Neglect in the United States: Economic Impact Study.* Chicago, Illinois: Prevent Child Abuse America.

Weiss, I.C., Domeney, A.M., Heidbreder, C.A., Moreau, J.L. & Feldon, J. (2001): Early social isolation, but not maternal separation, affects behavioral sensitization to amphetamine in male and female adult rats. *Pharmacol. Biochem. Behav.* **70,** 397–409.

Wise, R.A. (2004): Dopamine, learning and motivation. *Nat. Rev. Neurosci.* **5,** 483–494.

Wise, R.A. & Bozarth, M.A. (1982): Action of drugs of abuse on brain reward systems: an update with specific attention to opiates. *Pharmacol. Biochem. Behav.* **17,** 239–243.

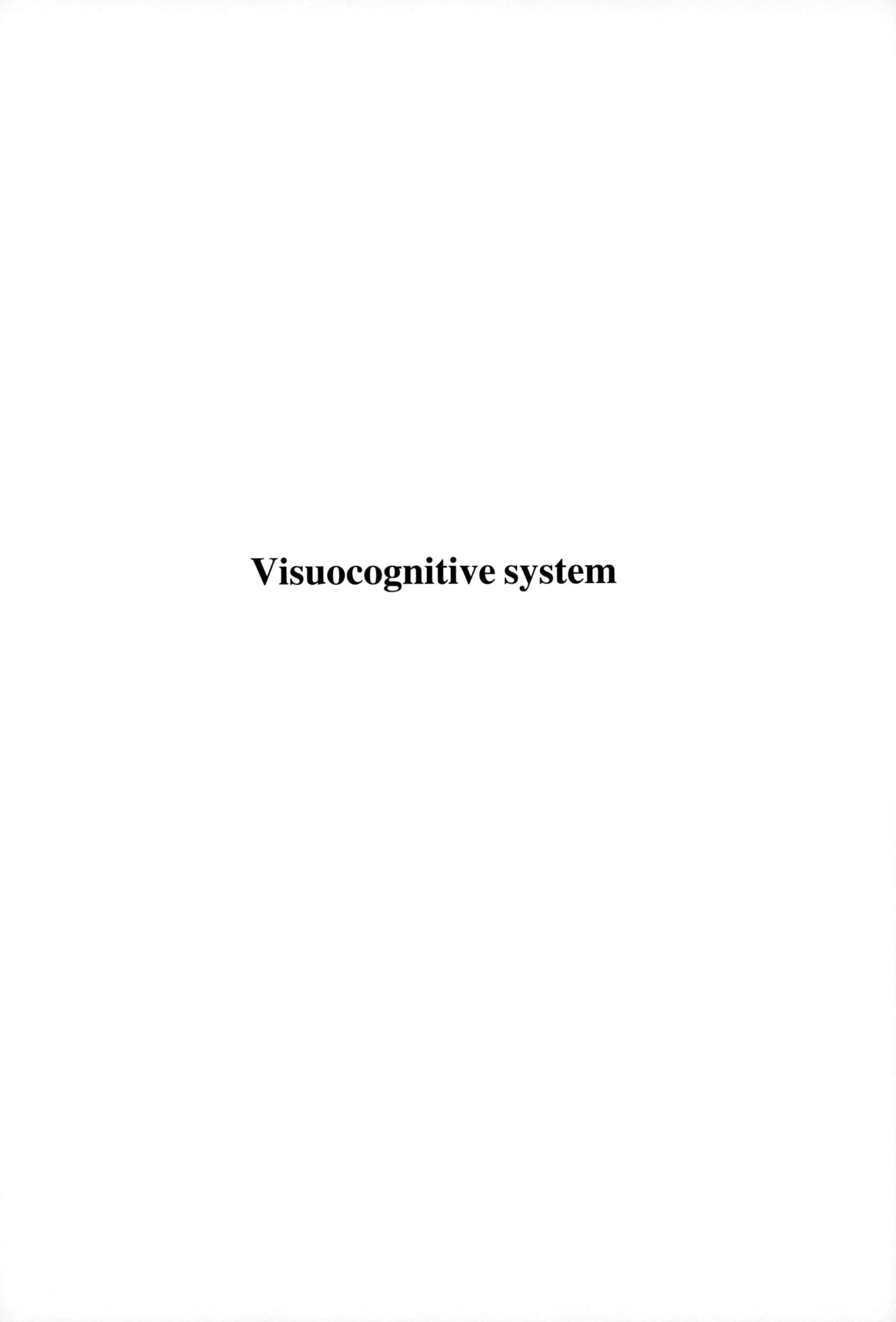

Visuocognitive system

Brain Lesion Localization and Developmental Functions, D. Riva, C. Njiokiktjien and S. Bulgheroni (eds.)

Chapter 17

Visual field defects and visual search abilities in children with focal brain lesions

Giovanni Cioni[*,o] and Francesca Tinelli[*,#]

**Department of Developmental Neuroscience, Fondazione IRCCS Stella Maris, via dei Giacinti 2, 56128 Calambrone, Pisa, Italy;*
[o]Division of Child Neurology and Psychiatry, University of Pisa, Pisa, Italy;
[#]Department of Psychology, University of Florence, Florence, Italy
gcioni@inpe.unipi.it

Summary

Different processes of visual brain plasticity can be observed after early damage, as opposed to damage that occurs during adulthood. Some of the neuroplastic mechanisms adopted by the brain after early damage to the visual system are unavailable at a later stage. The young brain also uses the same mechanisms available at later stages of development, but in a more efficient way. For example, patients with visual field defects of central origin show a greater anatomic expansion of the extrastriatal visual network after an early lesion than after a later one, which results in more efficient mechanisms of visual exploration of the blind field. We have studied visual search abilities in children with congenital or acquired cerebral lesions, with and without visual field defects. Children with acquired lesions and visual field defects had longer reaction times (RTs) in the contralesional visual field compared with the ipsilesional; conversely, those with congenital lesions and visual field defects did not have differences in RTs between the contralateral and ipsilateral visual fields and have a visual search pattern similar to that of children without a visual field defect. These findings support the hypothesis of more effective mechanisms of functional compensation and reorganization of the visual system in children with very early brain lesions, as opposed to those with later damage.

Introduction

The presence of more powerful mechanisms of neuronal plasticity during early development should imply that recovery from brain damage is more effective after early lesions than after lesions occurring later in life. Today, there is general agreement that the way the brain reacts to damage is influenced by the timing of the insult, both in the domain of language and for the motor and somatosensory system, but only at a lesser extent for the visual system. In this chapter the literature will be briefly reviewed about different mechanisms of visual system plasticity in children with congenital and acquired focal brain lesions.

Main findings in the literature

Several studies have reported abnormalities of visual function in adults who suffered ischaemic brain stroke and in children with stroke acquired after the neonatal period. In those patients lesions affecting the striate occipital cortex and the optic radiations were nearly invariably associated with contralateral hemianopia, that is, the loss, in part or completely, of vision in the visual field contralateral to the side of the lesion, whereas lesions affecting the parietal lobe generally resulted in abnormal visual attention and, in the most severe cases, in contralateral visual neglect. Studies in adults have shown that unilateral damage to the post-chiasmal visual pathway is also often associated with visual search disorders (Cornette *et al.*, 1998) and so these persons cannot process images in the same way as do normal controls and usually have difficulties with reading, detecting stimuli, or finding objects in the visual space corresponding to the affected field. Their fixations typically dwell in the intact hemifield and their search pattern is characterized by frequent exploratory saccades into the blind part of the visual field (Tant *et al.*, 2002; Zangemeister *et al.*, 1982; Zihl, 1995), with repeated saccades and fixations to the same object, resulting in overall longer visual search times (Chedru *et al.*, 1973; Pambakian *et al.*, 2000; Zihl, 1995). This phenomenon has been defined by Zihl (1995) as 'slowness of vision' in the contralateral hemifield to the side of the lesion.

Ischaemic stroke can also occur in newborns around term age, and during the preterm period, which are often related to transient or genetic prothrombotic abnormalities of coagulation (Kirton & deVeber, 2009). However, in infants with neonatal stroke the correlation between neurobehavioural visual tests and neonatal magnetic resonance imaging (MRI) is not always consistent (Mercuri *et al.*, 1996a): acuity and ocular movements are usually normal, while other aspects of visual function, such as visual fields and visual attention, can be impaired. In our experience (Mercuri *et al.*, 1996b), the risk of developing visual abnormalities is higher in children who develop hemiplegia (33 per cent) than it is in those with normal motor outcome. This reflects the importance of the extent of the lesion, as demonstrated by the fact that visual abnormalities are significantly more frequently associated with lesions involving the main branch of the medial cerebral artery (MCA), than to those localised in the territory of one of the cortical branches of MCA (75 *vs.* 32 per cent).

However, when the same infants were tested at school age, the proportion of children with visual abnormalities was found to be lower than at the early assessment (Mercuri *et al.*, 2003). The low incidence of abnormal visual functions in children after cortical infarction, compared with adults with similar lesions, may be related to the existence of effective mechanisms of plasticity of the visual structures.

This is also evidenced by the presence of normal vision in children with damaged optic radiations and visual cortex. Werth (2008) described a child who underwent hemispherectomy when he was 4 months old but developed a normal visual field comparable to that of age-matched controls. More recently Muckli and colleagues (2009) performed an fMRI study using visual stimuli in a 10-year-old girl born with only the left hemisphere because the right hemisphere failed to develop after the seventh week of gestation: the spared hemisphere not only developed maps of the contralateral (right) visual hemifield, but also, surprisingly, maps of the ipsilateral hemifield.

These cases are probably exceptional, and homonymous hemianopia can be found in children with congenital cortico-subcortical lesions involving the posterior visual system on account of perinatal cerebral artery stroke, probably acquired during the late gestation period (Jacobson *et al.*, 2010). However, these children do not seem to have the same difficulties in moving around in the world and avoiding obstacles as adults with the same lesions. This suggests a strong plasticity and important, but still unexplained, functional visual capabilities.

Visual search abilities

One of the functions that can be studied in children with focal brain lesion and visual field defects to explain visual plasticity mechanisms is that of visual search. It refers to the capacity of a subject to find a target among simultaneously presented distractors (Treisman, 1982), and it is based on visual abilities such as a fast visual processing and an accurate control of ballistic eye movements (saccades) that guide the fovea to the target location (Findlay, 1995, 1997; Smith *et al.*, 1998). Many brain areas are involved in this type of task, particularly the two major visual intracortical streams, the so-called ventral and dorsal pathways, that transmit information from posterior sites (the primary visual areas) to anterior cortical regions. During visual search the two systems work in parallel, the ventral stream being involved in pattern recognition of the searched stimulus and the dorsal stream being responsible for its spatial localization.

To our knowledge only few studies have explored the possible effects of brain damage on visual search abilities when the lesion is acquired during childhood. Netelenbos and Van Rooij (2004) studied a small group of seven school-aged children with acquired unilateral brain lesions, but without visual field defect and sensory or motor deficits. They reported abnormal values on visual search tasks only in children with right hemispheric lesions. Different results were reported by Schatz and colleagues (2004), who studied thirty-three children (older than six) with acquired stroke secondary to sickle cell disease and found abnormally slow responses in the contralesional visual field, especially when the lesion involved the left hemisphere.

Very little is known on the possible effects of lesions occurring prenatally or around birth, when the nervous system is still largely immature and plastic reorganization might be expected to be more effective. Animal studies are strongly suggestive of a dramatically different effect of early brain damage on visual orienting, as opposed to the effect after later damage. Monkeys with unilateral surgical ablation of the striate cortex sustained at 5–6 weeks of age show residual abilities to detect and localize visual stimuli (lights) within the contralateral hemifield, whereas monkeys with lesions sustained in adulthood show a large impairment in visual orienting (Moore, 1996). Analogous studies on cats have reported a considerable sparing of visual functions following unilateral lesions in infancy extending to the occipital, parietal, and temporal cortices, while in the adult cats, the same lesion results in a dense blindness and incapacity to orient to contralateral visual stimuli (Rushmore & Payne, 2004). It has been suggested that modifications in circuits within the superior colliculus (SC) or involving efferent pathways from the contralateral intact hemisphere to the ipsilesional SC underlie the observed visual sparing (Ciaramitaro *et al.*, 1997; Hairston *et al.*, 2003; Lomber *et al.*, 1996).

Recently, we have investigated visual search abilities in 29 children (aged 6 to 16 years) with congenital or acquired cerebral lesions, with and without visual field defects by means of a visual search test battery consisting of four different tests based on the research of a target (apple, frog, smile, EF) among distractors (Tinelli *et al.*, 2011). We investigated the percentage of correct responses and we found no difference among ipsi- and contralesional visual field in all groups, whereas studying Z-Scores of the mean reaction times (recorded in milliseconds) and the standard error of the mean [SEM] at the four visual search tests, we found that children with acquired damage and visual field reduction show significantly longer reaction times when the target is presented in the hemianopic field, compared to the normal field. On the contrary, children with congenital damage and visual field reduction do not show significantly different performances between the ipsilesional and contralesional visual field (see Fig. 1). This striking result, suggesting a greater sparing of visual search abilities after early lesions, is also corroborated by the finding that the performance of children with congenital lesions and visual field reduction is comparable to the performance of children without visual field restriction.

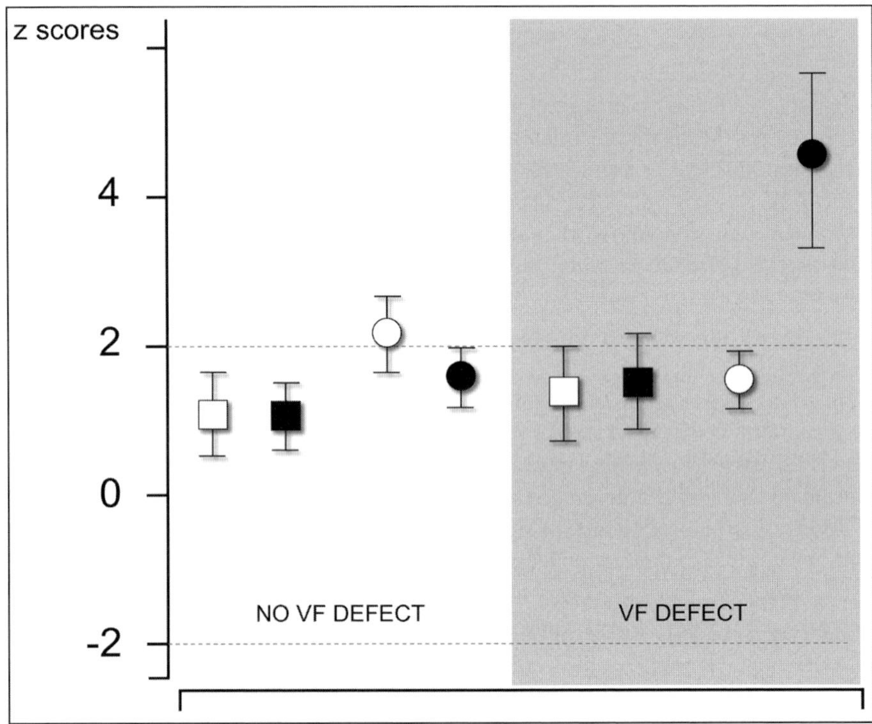

Fig. 1. Results obtained in 29 children with hemiplegia on a visual search battery consisting of four tests (Apple test: a yellow apple among red apples; Frog test: a green frog among green trees; Smile test: a sad face among happy ones; and an E–F test: a green 'F' among many green 'E') based on the research of a single target embedded among distractors. Z-Scores of the mean reaction times (± standard error of the mean [SEM]) at the four visual search tests are reported in children with visual field defects (grey background) and without visual field defect (white background). Z-Scores were obtained using data collected from 200 healthy control children of comparable age. Squares indicate children with congenital damage and circles indicate children with acquired damage. Open symbols indicate the exploration of the ipsilesional hemifield and filled symbols indicate the exploration of the contralesional hemifield. Only the children with acquired visual field defect have abnormal values in the field of visual presentation contralateral to the side of the lesion (modified from Tinelli et al., *2011).*

The different pattern of results observed in patients with visual field defect with acquired or congenital lesions cannot be ascribed to differences in the severity of the visual field defect or in the extent of the lesions. In fact, the two groups of patients were similar in terms of percentage of correct detections in the affected field. As for the extent of the brain lesion in patients with the acquired lesion, despite exhibiting a more compromised behavioural performance, overall they showed smaller lesions compared to those with the congenital lesions.

Conclusions

Our findings of a more effective visual search strategy in children with congenital brain damage, compared to patients with acquired ones, are in line with results in animal models, and they suggest the existence, in the case of early lesions, of a spontaneous functional reorganization, probably by means of subcortical structures, for the visual system also. On the contrary, in case of acquired lesions, spontaneous visual compensation is not so effective and visual search abilities are still impaired.

The question of why and to what extent the young visual brain reacts differently to damage is still open and will need extensive research to be answered. Only with this knowledge will we be able to modify the environment of infants with early brain damage to support and enhance the adaptive processes of visual reorganization at a time when brain plasticity potentials are highest (Guzzetta *et al.*, 2010).

Acknowledgments: The principal results reported in this paper have been obtained through research supported by the Mariani Foundation, Milan (Grant 2006) to G.C. and by Grant STANIB 229445 to F.T.

References

Chedru, F., Leblanc, M. & Lhermitte, F. (1973): Visual searching in normal and brain-damaged subjects: contribution to the study of unilateral inattention. *Cortex* **9,** 94–111.

Ciaramitaro, V.M., Todd, W.E. & Rosenquist, A.C. (1997): Disinhibition of the superior colliculus restores orienting to visual stimuli in the hemianopic field of the cat. *J. Comp. Neurol.* **387,** 568–587.

Cornette, L., Dupont, P., Rosier, A., Sunaert, S., Van Hecke, P., Michiels, J., *et al.* (1998): Human brain regions involved in direction discrimination. *J. Neurophysiol.* **79,** 2749–2765.

Findlay, J.M. (1995): Visual search: eye movements and peripheral vision. *Optom. Vis. Sci.* **72,** 461–466.

Findlay, J.M. (1997): Saccade target selection during visual search. *Vision Res.* **37,** 617–631.

Guzzetta, A., D'Acunto, G., Rose, S., Tinelli, F., Boyd, R. & Cioni, G. (2010): Plasticity of the visual system after early brain damage. *Dev. Med. Child Neurol.* **52,** 891–900.

Hairston, W.D., Laurienti, P.J., Mishra, G., Burdette, J.H. & Wallace, M.T. (2003): Multisensory enhancement of localization under conditions of induced myopia. *Exp. Brain Res.* **152,** 404–408.

Kirton, A. & deVeber, G. (2009): Advances in perinatal ischemic stroke [review]. *Pediatr. Neurol.* **40,** 205–214.

Jacobson, L., Rydberg, A., Eliasson, A.C., Kits, A. & Flodmark, O. (2010): Visual field function in school-aged children with spastic unilateral cerebral palsy related to different patterns of brain damage. *Dev. Med. Child Neurol.* **52,** e184–187.

Lomber, S.G., Payne, B.R. & Cornwell, P. (1996): Learning and recall of form discriminations during reversible cooling deactivation of ventral-posterior suprasylvian cortex in the cat. *Proc. Natl. Acad. Sci. USA* **93,** 1654–1658.

Mercuri, E., Atkinson, J., Braddick, O., Anker, S., Nokes, L., Cowan, F., *et al.* (1996a): Visual function and perinatal focal cerebral infarction. *Arch. Dis. Child: Fetal Neonatal Ed.* **75**: F76–81.

Mercuri, E., Spanò, M., Bruccini, G., Frisone, M.F., Trombetta, J.C., Blandino, A., *et al.* (1996b): Visual outcome in children with congenital hemiplegia: correlation with MRI findings. *Neuropediatrics* **27,** 184–188.

Mercuri, E., Anker, S., Guzzetta, A., Barnett, A., Haataja, L., Rutherford, M., *et al.* (2003): Neonatal cerebral infarction and visual function at school age. *Arch. Dis. Child: Fetal Neonatal. Ed.* **88,** F487–491.

Moore, T., Rodman, H.R., Repp, A.B., Gross, C.G. & Mezrich, R.S. (1996): Greater residual vision in monkeys after striate cortex damage in infancy. *J. Neurophysiol.* **76,** 3928–3933.

Muckli, L., Naumer, M.J. & Singer, W. (2009): Bilateral visual field maps in a patient with only one hemisphere. *Proc. Natl. Acad. Sci. USA* **106,** 13034–13039.

Netelenbos, J.B. & Van Rooij, L. (2004): Visual search in school-aged children with unilateral brain lesions. *Dev. Med. Child Neurol.* **46,** 334–339.

Pambakian, A.L., Wooding, D.S., Patel, N., Morland, A.B., Kennard, C. & Mannan, S.K. (2000): Scanning the visual world: a study of patients with homonymous hemianopia. *J. Neurol. Neurosurg. Psychiatry* **69,** 751–759.

Rushmore, R.J. & Payne, B.R. (2004): Neuroplasticity after unilateral visual cortex damage in the newborn cat. *Behav. Brain Res.* **153,** 557–565.

Schatz, J., Craft, S., Koby, M. & DeBaun, M.R. (2004): Asymmetries in visual-spatial processing following childhood stroke. *Neuropsychology* **18,** 340–352.

Smith, A.T., Greenlee, M.W., Singh, K.D., Kraemer, F.M. & Hennig, J. (1998): The processing of first- and second-order motion in human visual cortex assessed by functional magnetic resonance imaging (fMRI). *J. Neurosci.* **18,** 3816–3830.

Tant, M.L., Cornelissen, F.W., Kooijman, A.C. & Brouwer, W.H. (2002): Hemianopic visual field defects elicit hemianopic scanning. *Vision Res.* **42,** 1339–1348.

Tinelli, F., Guzzetta, A., Bertini, C., Ricci, D., Mercuri, E., Ladavas, E. & Cioni, G. (2011): Greater sparing of visual search abilities in children after congenital rather than focal brain damage. *Neurorehab. Neural Repair* Jun 6 [E-pub ahead of print].

Treisman, A. (1982): Perceptual grouping and attention in visual search for features and for objects. *J. Exp. Psychol. Hum. Percept. Perform.* **8,** 194–214.

Werth, R. (2008): Cerebral blindness and plasticity of the visual system in children: a review of visual capacities in patients with occipital lesions, hemispherectomy or hydranencephaly. *Restor. Neurol. Neurosci.* **26,** 377–389.

Zangemeister, W.H., Meienberg, O., Stark, L. & Hoyt, W.F. (1982): Eye-head coordination in homonymous hemianopia. *J. Neurol.* **226,** 243–254.

Zihl, J. (1995): Visual scanning behavior in patients with homonymous hemianopia. *Neuropsychologia* **33,** 287–303.

Brain Lesion Localization and Developmental Functions, D. Riva, C. Njiokiktjien and S. Bulgheroni (eds.)

Chapter 18

Neurophysiologic and behavioural aspects of visual assessment: correlation with neuroimaging

Oliver Braddick* and Janette Atkinson°

**Department of Experimental Psychology, University of Oxford, South Parks Road, Oxford OX1 3UD, United Kingdom;*
°Department of Developmental Science, University College, London, United Kingdom
oliver.braddick@psy.ox.ac.uk

Summary

Visual assessments can provide a unique window on the brain in early life and are sensitive indicators of broader neurocognitive development. We review the emergence during infancy of specific modes of processing in the visual cortex, assessed using visual event-related potentials (VERPs) and behavioural measures, and the subsequent development of the dorsal and ventral cortical streams. Using these measures we have shown 'dorsal stream vulnerability' in a range of genetic and acquired developmental disorders, where visual motion analysis in the dorsal stream is more vulnerable during development than is static form analysis in the ventral stream. Studies with infants born preterm (< 33 weeks' gestation) find that even healthy preterm infants show delay in the early development of cortical motion responses compared to orientation sensitivity. Over the first years of life, the development of cortical orientation responses, shifts of fixation (attention), functional vision and visuocognitive measures from the ABCDEFV battery, and early tests of attentional control (executive function) show impairment correlated with preterm infants' severity of brain damage (particularly in white matter). Follow-up study of a group of such children at 6–7 years shows specific impairment in attention, spatial cognition, spatial memory, motion coherence sensitivity and visuomotor skills – all functions associated with neural networks in the dorsal stream. New VERP methods have enabled us to isolate and map infants' responses to global motion and global form. These show (*a*) that both responses can be identified and are anatomically distinct in typically developing 5-month-olds; (*b*) that global motion processing precedes global form processing in development; and (*c*) that preterm-born infants show relatively immature global motion responses, possibly reflecting the delayed development of cortical feedback pathways. We conclude that visual measures in infancy and early childhood are providing increasingly rich and specific information about patterns of both visual and cognitive development following perinatal brain injury.

Introduction

Vision is an early-developing cerebral system in infancy and a key function for the child's developing interaction with his or her physical and social environment. Visual assessments can therefore provide a unique window on the brain in the first months of life and are a sensitive indicator of broader neurocognitive development throughout the pre-school and early school years. In this chapter we will discuss evidence on how visual measures can be linked with neuroimaging and other indicators of perinatal brain damage.

A range of evidence shows that the first months of life are marked by the emergence of specifically cortical modes of visual processing, and of the cortical modulation of subcortical processes (Atkinson, 1984, 2000). When we use visual measures to assess at-risk infants in this period, as indicators of cerebral integrity and as predictors of neurocognitive outcome, it is important to distinguish between those which are specific to cortical processing and those which can be mediated by earlier levels of the visual pathway (*i.e.*, by subcortical systems). We describe below the visual event-related potentials (VERPs) that are associated with lower and higher levels in the hierarchy of visual processing. We also distinguish between behavioural visual responses that are linked to cortical development (*e.g.*, fixation shifts [FS] under competition) and those that are less sensitive to cortical processing (*e.g.*, acuity measurement using the visual preferential looking technique).

Beyond primary visual cortex (known as V1), visual processing is divided between two cortical streams: the 'ventral stream', which underlies recognition of objects and faces, and the 'dorsal stream', which processes spatial relationships and motion and underlies visual control of action (Milner & Goodale, 1995; Mishkin *et al.*, 1983). These two streams have distinct developmental courses, and are differently vulnerable, in both acquired and genetic developmental disorders. We will present evidence that the development of various visual and visuocognitive functions associated with the dorsal stream is sensitive to perinatal brain insult and is seen in a wide range of other neurodevelopmental disorders.

Visual event-related potentials

Visual event-related potentials (VERPs), also known as visual evoked potentials (VEPs), represent electrical brain activity in response to visual stimulation recorded from electrodes placed on the surface of the scalp. They are a specialized form of EEG. Since the method is not dependent on cognitive or motor skills beyond looking at a large display screen, it can be used to assess visual functions over a wide range of ages and patient populations (Atkinson & Braddick, 1999). VERP tests require the recording to be synchronized with a repetitive visual event, so that brain activity that is time-locked to this event can be extracted from the nonsynchronous background activity of the brain. In this paper we restrict ourselves to discussion of 'steady-state' VERPs, where the relevant stimulus events are repeated sufficiently rapidly (≥ 2 per second) that the brain response becomes a regular rhythm which can be analyzed through frequency analysis. This approach has a number of advantages in analysis (discussed by Atkinson & Braddick, 1999), although clinical electroencephalographers may be more familiar with 'transient' VERP recording, which allows inspection of the individual peaks of a waveform, completed before the next stimulus event comes along.

Table 1 lists some of the visual events that can be used to time-lock VERP recordings, which yield information about different levels of complexity of visual and visuocognitive processing.

Pattern-reversal, using a black and white checkerboard or stripe pattern in which the black and white elements are interchanged, is the stimulus used most commonly in paediatric clinical neurology and neuro-ophthalmology. A response to this stimulus indicates that the visual system is sensitive to contrast between pattern elements of the size used (check size or grating pattern measured as a spatial frequency). Consequently, this method has been widely used to test the

Table 1. Visual event-related potentials associated with different levels of neural processing

Stimulus event	Underlying neural process	Age of onset in typical development
Repeated flash	Light response transmitted to cortex (not necessarily cortical processing)	Preterm
Pattern reversal (checkerboard or grating)	Spatial contrast response transmitted to cortex (not necessarily cortical processing)	Late preterm/term
Orientation reversal (OR-VERP)	Basic cortical pattern processing (area V1 and beyond)	~1–3 months post-term (frequency dependent)
Motion direction reversal (DR-VERP)	Basic cortical processing of motion direction (area V1 and beyond)	~ 2–3 months post-term
Transition between incoherent & coherent global form or global motion	Higher level visual integration – extrastriate cortical areas	3–6 months post-term (motion before form)

visual acuity of infants and children, both in normal development and in visual disorders (see, for example, Harris *et al.*, 1976; Norcia & Tyler, 1985; Sokol, 1978). However, such responses to the black and white contrast in a pattern are initially generated at the level of the retinal ganglion cells and transmitted up the optic nerve and optic radiation. Although the signals picked up from the occipital scalp arise from the region of the visual cortex, they reflect the information that is input to the cortex, possibly postsynaptic events from the geniculostriate synapse in cortical layer IV, rather than cortical processes themselves.

Orientation-selective responses are a property of cortical neurones and not a property of earlier levels of neurones in the visual pathway. The 'orientation-reversal' (OR) sequence (Braddick, 1993; Braddick *et al.*, 1986) measures VERP responses to a stripe pattern that is changing in orientation and is designed to separate the orientation-specific component of this cortical response from the components that are simply a response to local contrast changes when the stripe pattern changes position. These responses have been found to emerge in the first postnatal months, providing part of the evidence that visual cortical processing is normally very immature at birth, and opening the possibility that this test is a sensitive indicator of problems in early cortical development (*e.g.*, see Mercuri *et al.*, 1998).

Direction-selective responses to moving stimuli are another characteristic of neurones in primary visual cortex which are not seen in the input to the cortex. In a similar manner to the orientation-selectivity test described above, a direction-selective VERP stimulus has been devised that isolates this aspect of cortical processing for directional motion (Wattam-Bell, 1991). This also appears in the first postnatal months, but consistently with a few weeks' delay relative to orientation selectivity (Braddick, 1993; Braddick *et al.*, 2005). Direction-selective neurones in V1 represent the first stage in the dorsal processing stream (Livingstone & Hubel, 1988), while orientation selectivity is a key basis for the pattern recognition function of the ventral stream. Thus the relationship between the onset of direction (motion) and orientation (slant) selectivity may provide an indicator of the early developmental foundations of the two major cortical visual streams, the dorsal and ventral streams. Later in this chapter we will outline new work on the origins of these two forms of processing in infancy, comparing OR- and DR-VERPs in healthy infants born prematurely.

The approach of devising VEP stimulus sequences that isolate aspects of cortical processing can be extended beyond the characteristic selective responses of V1. Orientation and motion can be analyzed locally, with the small receptive fields characteristic of V1 neurones.

Extrastriate visual areas contain neurones with much larger receptive fields that can analyze the larger-scale 'global' structure of motion flow fields or of patterns of contour elements. Stimuli alternating between random and coherent global structure are indicated in the bottom row of Table 1, and are able to track the development of this level of visual function (Braddick & Atkinson, 2007). Recently, we have used high-density electrode sensor arrays (using a 'geodesic net' of 126 electrodes placed on the infant's head) to map the spatial distribution of activity connected with this global processing. This method has revealed major reorganization of higher-level visual processes between infancy and adulthood (Wattam-Bell *et al.*, 2010). Findings on the development of global visual processing, and the information it can yield on neurodevelopmental disorders, are discussed below.

Behavioural indicators

Newborn infants show a range of visual behaviours, notably their ability to 'fix and follow', to generate optokinetic eye movements to large field movement, and to show preferential looking, making saccadic eye movements to a conspicuous target in the periphery of their visual field. However, these behaviours can all be accounted for in terms of activity in subcortical visual networks of brain areas, specifically the superior colliculus (SC), which guides orienting eye and head movements, and the nucleus of the optic tract (NOT), which mediates optokinetic nystagmus (OKN). Newborns' acuity can be measured using preferential looking, but the sensitivity to spatial contrast required for measurable acuity can be determined at the level of the retinal ganglion cells, and orienting behaviour elicited by the signals these send to the SC. It follows that in older infants who have been at risk of perinatal cerebral damage, acuity is not a very sensitive predictor of neurocognitive outcome, although low acuity without ocular cause may indicate very severe damage in the cerebral cortex, called 'cerebral visual impairment (CVI)' (see Dutton & Bax, 2010).

However, some aspects of visual behaviour that develop in the early postnatal months do reflect specifically cortical processes which come to modulate and sometimes override subcortical function. One example is seen in using the paradigm of fixation shifts (FS). The ability to shift fixation between two competing targets (described in the accompanying chapter by Atkinson & Braddick, this volume, and in Atkinson *et al.*, 1992) is ascribed to a descending inhibitory pathway from the cortex to the SC which can 'turn off' the reflex–maintained fixation. This FS paradigm offers the possibility of assessing cortical development of attention from a behavioural test. In fact, performance in fixation shifts under competition in the first year has been found to correlate with MRI indicators of perinatal brain injury and to be a predictor of later cognitive outcome, in children born at term with either focal lesions (Mercuri *et al.*, 1996) or more diffuse hypoxic-ischaemic damage (Mercuri *et al.*, 1997, 1999), and in children born very prematurely (Atkinson *et al.*, 2008a).

For the broader functional assessment of vision, from birth through the early years of childhood, we have also applied a battery of age-appropriate tests to children with early brain injury; this test, the Atkinson Battery of Child Development for Examining Functional Vision (ABCDEFV) is described more fully in the accompanying chapter (Atkinson & Braddick, this volume; Atkinson *et al.*, 2002a). Because they are chosen for functional relevance, these tests do not necessarily map directly onto specific cortical systems, although it is possible to suggest the combinations of cortical modules that are engaged by the different tasks, and clearly some tasks involve more processing in the ventral cortical stream and others in the dorsal cortical stream (see the discussion of dorsal and ventral streams below).

Dorsal and ventral cortical streams

The two major streams of visual processing, 'dorsal' and 'ventral', have been referred to above. They have their origins in distinct 'magnocellular' and 'parvocellular' pathways in the optic nerve, and radiation, but become most clearly anatomically separate when these pathways project beyond area V1 (striate cortex) to separate extrastriate cortical areas (Livingstone & Hubel, 1988; Milner & Goodale, 1995). The second section of this chapter introduced the concept of global processing based on the integration of information by large receptive fields in these extrastriate areas. Specifically, neurophysiologic experiments in the macaque monkey show that neurones in area V4 (an early extrastriate ventral stream area) respond to global pattern properties, such as large-scale radial or concentric arrangements of contours (Gallant *et al.*, 1993), while areas V5 (also known as MT) and MST in the dorsal stream integrate motion information to be sensitive to large-scale flow patterns, either coherent motion in a particular direction, radial expansion, or rotary flow about a common centre (Britten *et al.*, 1992; Duffy & Wurtz, 1991). In the human brain, larger networks of areas have been shown to have these two forms of sensitivity to global visual structure, but the network of 'global form' areas seems to be quite independent of the network of 'global motion' areas.

This differential sensitivity to global form and global motion provides the means to test the development of processing in the two streams. This can be done using either VERPs elicited by the onset of coherent organization of random patterns (Braddick & Atkinson, 2007; Wattam-Bell *et al.*, 2010) or by behavioural tests in which coherent structure (*e.g.*, concentrically arranged line segments, or coherent rotation of moving random dots) is mixed with random elements, and the participant tested for the threshold percentage of coherent elements needed to detect the coherent structure. These tasks can be presented as computer games ('find the ball in the grass' for concentric structure, or 'find the road in the snowstorm' for linear coherent motion), which can engage the attention of children as young as 4 years old (Atkinson *et al.*, 1997; Atkinson & Braddick, 2005; Gunn *et al.*, 2002). The advantage of this approach is that the demands of the two tasks in terms of attention and extracting patterns from background 'noise' are closely similar, so any systematic differences of performance in the two tasks across age groups or between groups must reflect differences between the processing of global motion by the dorsal stream and global form by the ventral stream.

Following our demonstration that dorsal stream function was impaired in children with Williams syndrome (Atkinson *et al.*, 1997), these methods have been used widely to compare the function of the two cortical streams in developmental disorders. Table 2 lists the wide variety of genetic and acquired conditions in which global motion thresholds are more impaired, relative to typically developing controls, than are global form thresholds. This pattern of difference has led to the concept of 'dorsal stream vulnerability' as a general feature of impaired brain development (Braddick, Atkinson and Wattam-Bell, 2003). We do not yet know whether this vulnerability is due to the timing of emerging dorsal function during vulnerable periods of brain development, the differential plasticity of different brain systems, or the special demands of achieving the temporal precision required for effective motion processing.

As well as differentially processing motion and spatial information, the dorsal stream is characterized by transmitting the information required for the on-line control of actions, and by including the major sites where visual function is controlled by selective attention (Kastner & Ungerleider, 2000). In the studies of ex-premature babies outlined below, we will refer to evidence that dorsal-stream function is particularly at risk in the perinatal brain injuries found in this group, not only in terms of motion *vs.* form coherence thresholds, but also in visuomotor

Table 2. Evidence for global motion sensitivity more impaired than global form sensitivity ('dorsal stream vulnerability') in developmental disorders

Disorder	Origin of disorder	Reference
Williams syndrome in young children	Genetic: deletion on chromosome 7	Atkinson *et al.*, 1997, 2003
Williams syndrome in adults	See above	Atkinson *et al.*, 2006
Autism in children	Presumed primarily genetic	Spencer *et al.*, 2000; Milne *et al.*, 2005
Hemiplegia in children	Acquired: pre- or perinatal brain injury	Gunn *et al.*, 2002
Developmental dyslexia	Presumed partly genetic	Cornelissen *et al.*, 1995; Hansen *et al.*, 2001; Ridder *et al.*, 2001
Fragile X syndrome	Genetic: mutation of FMR1 gene on X chromosome	Kogan *et al.*, 2004
Early prematurity (< 33 weeks gestation)	Acquired	Atkinson & Braddick, 2007
Congenital cataract	Acquired	Compare Ellemberg *et al.* (2002) with Lewis *et al.* (2002)

behaviour and in visual tasks requiring attentional control. This wider functional involvement of the dorsal stream is explored more fully in the accompanying chapter (Atkinson & Braddick, this volume).

Visual indicators of brain function in infants and children born preterm

Advances in neonatal care have led to greatly increased survival of infants born very preterm (before 33 weeks' gestation and nowadays as young as 24–25 weeks' gestational age). However, the survival of these infants has led to many births of children at risk of severe or more subtle disability (Emsley *et al.*, 1998; Rennie, 2002). Intrauterine infection, which may trigger premature birth, and cerebral anoxia/ischaemia, provide two converging pathologic routes which may lead to white matter abnormality, impaired cerebral development, and cognitive and motor impairment which may be over a wide range of severity (Fig. 1).

Early identification of the degree of potential impairment is important for the management of these children, and early surrogate outcome measures are needed if therapies for neuroprotection or early rehabilitation are to be promptly evaluated. In a series of studies, we have used the assessments of visual function described above to provide measures of developing brain function, and related them to neuroimaging evidence of perinatal brain damage where this has been available.

Early development of cortical selectivity in healthy preterm-born infants

In an early study (Atkinson *et al.*, 2002b) we tested a group of infants at 1 to 3 months post-term age who had been born at 24–32 weeks' gestation. The infants who had no neurologic abnormality detected on ultrasound examination showed no significant difference on the onset of the OR-VERPs, compared to a term-born group matched for gestational age. Results on fixation

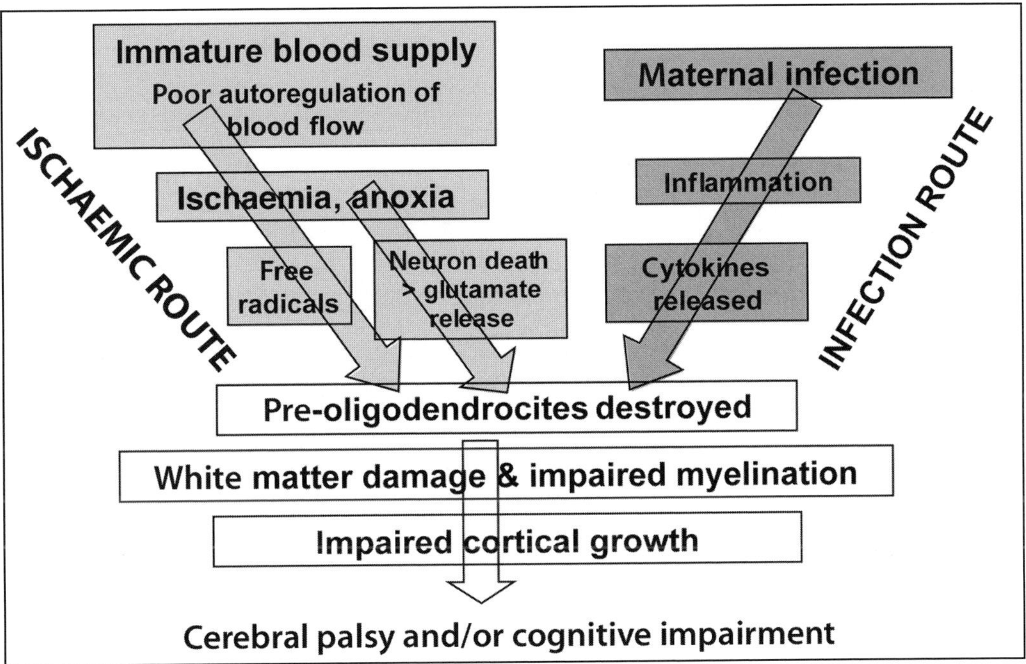

Fig. 1. Potential routes of cerebral damage in children born very preterm (based on review by du Plessis & Volpe, 2002).

shifts were similar. Thus, preterm birth in the absence of neurologic damage does not appear to either delay or accelerate these aspects of early cortical development. However, when the 9 of 20 children in this group who showed minor or major ultrasound abnormalities were included, OR-VERP was significantly delayed in the group taken as a whole, and those with the most severe cases of periventricular leucomalacia never developed the OR-VERP response during the first 4–5 months. These were associated with long-term neurologic problems, including cortical blindness in one case.

Although the study cited found the OR-VERP development was normal in healthy preterm infants, more recently we have found that the development of cortical function is not uniform. Birtles *et al.* (2007), collaborating with neonatalogists at the John Radcliffe Hospital, Oxford, made parallel measurements of the strength (signal-to-noise ratio) of the OR-VERP and DR-VERP in a group of neurologically healthy children born preterm, at post-term ages between 6–20 weeks. In this age range, the OR-VERP showed little change, and results from preterm infants and controls were very similar. However, the DR-VERP is still developing, and the preterms show several weeks' delay in this development (Fig. 2). Thus, the direction-reversal response seems a more sensitive indicator of the impact of prematurity than does the orientation-reversal response, possibly because white matter damage that is not visible on conventional ultrasound (Dyet *et al.*, 2006) may have a greater impact on motion processing, given that motion requires precise neural timing, which may be disrupted if myelination is disordered. Because motion processing is a feature of the dorsal stream, whereas orientation is an elementary property required by the ventral shape-recognition system, this differential impact of prematurity on the two processes can be considered as an early example of dorsal vulnerability. (However, it should be noted that the global motion sensitivity used to characterize this vulnerability in the studies of Table 2 represents a higher level of the system).

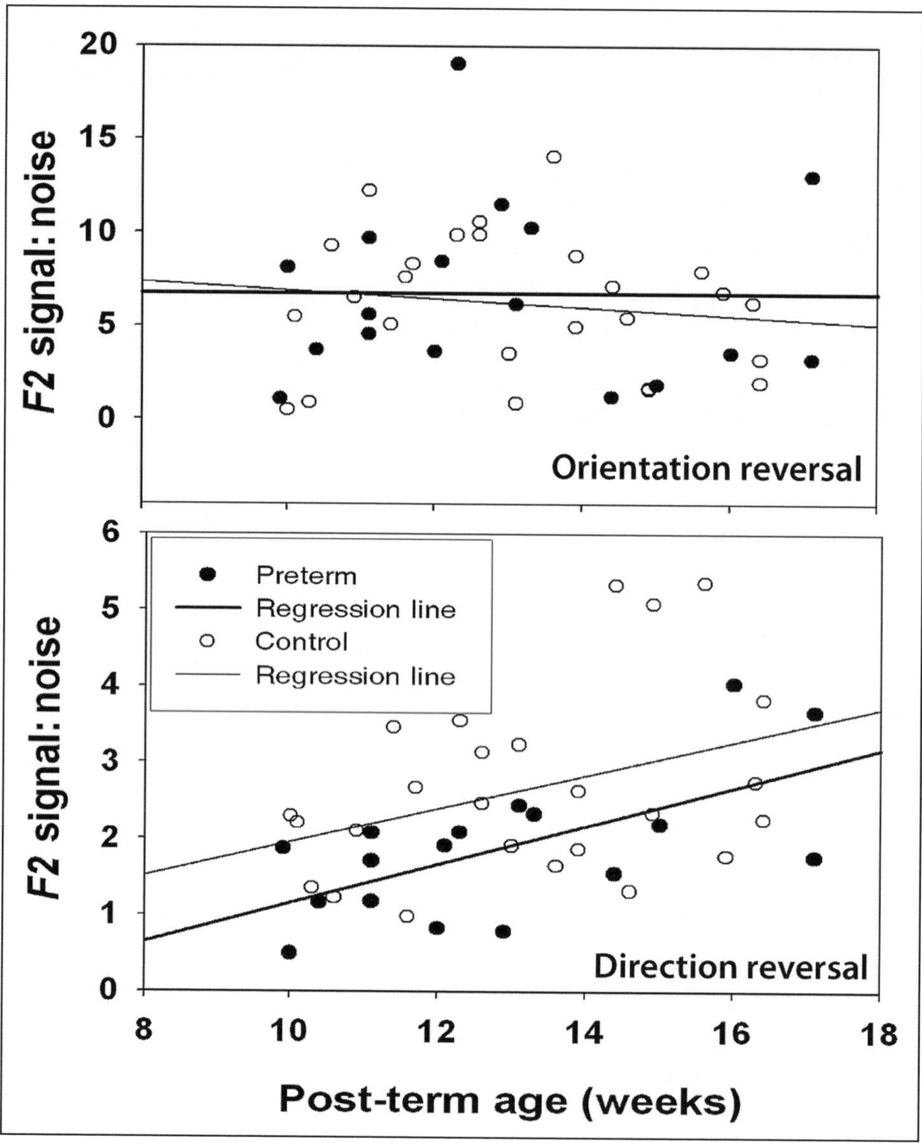

Fig. 2. Orientation-reversal and direction-reversal responses in a group of healthy children born preterm (< 33 weeks' gestation) compared to term-born controls. (From Birtles et al., *2007.)*

Relation of cortical measures in the first year of life to MRI findings in preterm infants

A subsequent collaborative study between the Visual Development Unit (VDU) group and the Hammersmith Hospital team provided the opportunity to assess cortical visual function between 2–7 months in infants born before 33 weeks' gestational age for whom structural brain MRI results at term were available. MRI results were classified on a 3-point scale of severity which took into account white matter abnormality assessed by the presence of diffuse extensive high signal intensity (DEHSI), as well as the presence of frank lesions (Atkinson *et al.*, 2008a). Both the OR-VERP test and the fixation shift test showed that the proportion of these infants reaching a 'passing' criterion for their post-term age progressively decreased with increasingly severe MRI findings. Furthermore, the OR-VERP results and fixation shift results both predicted the infants who would show a developmental quotient < 80 on the 2-year Griffiths assessment, with sensitivity of 86 and 100 per cent, respectively, and specificity of 61 and 65 per cent. Thus these cortical visual measures are associated both with imaging indicators of the state of the brain at term, and with overall neurocognitive development in subsequent years.

Visuocognitive measures with the preterm group between 1 and 5 years

Atkinson and Braddick (2007) report a broader follow-up between 1–5 years, including some of the children who participated in the first-year study outlined above. This follow-up study comprised 'core vision' measures (*e.g.*, visual acuity, visual fields), the age-appropriate visuocognitive tests (*e.g.*, shape matching, overlapping figures, copying block construction) from the ABCDEFV, and the tests mentioned in the third section of this chapter that are designed to assess the development of attentional control ('executive function') (Biro & Russell, 2001; Gerstadt *et al.*, 1994). These tests tap the frontal lobe systems required to inhibit a prepotent response in modes appropriate to different ages between 2–5 years.

Forty-one per cent of the preterm infants failed at least one of the core vision tests, most commonly because of strabismus or limited visual fields. Eighty-one per cent failed at least one of the visuocognitive tests, most commonly shape matching and block constructions (both tests with a significant visuomotor component). Performance on these core vision and visuocognitive tests showed an orderly decline as a function of MRI severity. The executive function tests also showed the preterm infants as a whole to be performing well below age norms; their overall performance was sufficiently low that there was no room for significant variation as a function of MRI severity.

Overall, then, the functional impact of the brain damage seen in neonatal MRI depended on the complexity of the function concerned. For core visual function, deficits are associated with the most severe MRI group. The visuocognitive tests showed poor performance in the 'severe' and 'moderate' groups, but relatively good results for those in the normal/mild group. For the block construction and the frontal executive function tests, especially the latter, even the 'normal/mild' group showed deficits compared to age norms between 1 and 5 years of age. Thus, more complex visuocognitive functions, particularly those involving the frontal lobes, are impaired by the effects of prematurity, even when these are not qualitatively apparent on neonatal and term MRI. This conclusion is reinforced by the follow-up at 6–7 years described below.

Visuocognitive and visuomotor performance of prematurely born children at 6–7 years

A different, larger cohort of ex-preterm children has been studied in collaboration with the Hammersmith team, to gain a fuller picture of the pattern of impairment at 6–7 years, when many areas of competence could be assessed by tests that have been normalized in the population. The tests included in this assessment are listed in Table 3.

Table 3. Tests included in the 6–7 year follow-up of ex-preterm children (Atkinson & Braddick, 2007)

Test	**Designed to assess**	**Reference**
WISC or WPSSI	Verbal and performance intelligence scales	
British Picture Vocabulary Scales (BPVS)	Receptive vocabulary	
ABCDEFV	Core vision tests and block copying scale	Atkinson *et al.* (2002a)
Movement ABC	Standardized assessment of everyday motor competence in three categories: manual dexterity, balance, and ball skills	Henderson & Sugden (1992)
Test of Everyday Attention for Children (TEA-Ch)	Four subtests used: 'Sky Search' (selective attention and visual search task); 'Score' (sustained auditory attention); 'Walk-Don't Walk' (sustained attention and inhibition of an action); 'Opposite Worlds' (switches of attention between two rules and inhibition of a prepotent response)	Manly *et al.* (2001)
Global motion and form coherence thresholds	Functional measures of extrastriate dorsal and ventral streams	Gunn *et al.* (2002)
'Town Square' test	Spatial location memory within different co-ordinate frames (egocentric, allocentric within the room, relative to local landmarks)	Nardini *et al.* (2006)

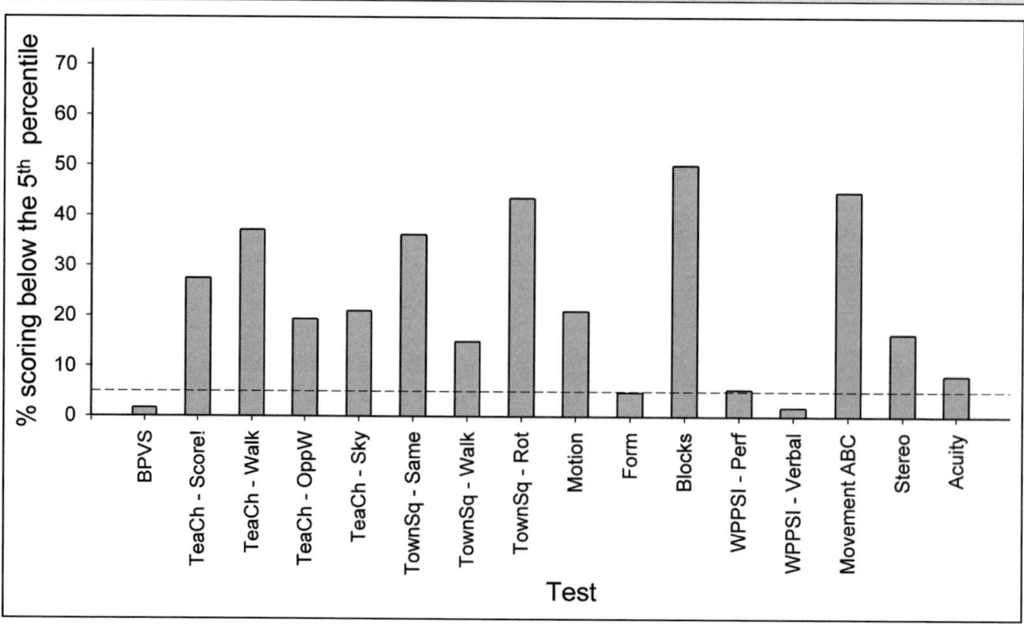

Fig. 3. Proportion of children in the 6–7–year follow-up study of preterm infants who scored below the 5th percentile of population norms on the tests listed in Table 4 (see Atkinson & Braddick, 2007).

Fig. 3 shows the proportion of the overall sample that fell below the 5th percentile for population norms in each test (Atkinson & Braddick, 2007). In some tests, for example, both verbal and performance IQ tests, vocabulary, global form coherence, and visual acuity, the preterm data are consistent with those expected for the normal population. However, on the motor and visuomotor tests of the Movement ABC, all aspects of the TEA-Ch tests of attention (including executive function), block construction, global motion coherence, and stereo vision, a large proportion of the children in this premature cohort fall into this tail of very poor performance.

A similar level of deficit appears in the 'Town Square' spatial memory test (Nardini *et al.*, 2006), which requires the child to locate a hidden toy on a board containing toy buildings as landmarks. The three conditions 'same', 'walk', and 'rotate' require this location memory to be related to different frames of reference (the child's own body, positions and directions in the room, or local landmarks on the board, respectively). These three tasks are progressively more difficult in terms of the typical age of attainment in normal preschool children, but the preterm group show poorer performance on all of them; their impairment appears to be generally in the ability to represent and manipulate spatial information, rather than in any specific operation.

Atkinson and Braddick (2007) discuss the internal structure of these data (how the different scores correlate across the preterm group) and their relationships to perinatal variables. In the latter analysis, some tests show an overall deficit for the group, some correlate with gestational age at birth, and some with the categorization of the structural MRI at term. A number of test scores are not impaired for the group as a whole (*e.g.*, WPPSI/WISC intelligence, and British Picture Vocabulary Scale), but nonetheless show an impact of the brain damage seen on MRI and/or the gestation period. Conversely, other tests, such as the 'Town Square' spatial memory tests are impaired in the group overall, but are not related to MRI findings or gestational age. This suggests that there are some features of brain development that are compromised by premature birth, but that are not reflected in this MRI analysis. It is hoped that future work may identify the structural neural correlates of these effects.

This analysis can be related to factor analysis of the test scores (Atkinson & Braddick, 2007). This shows a general cognitive development factor, loading heavily on both WISC subscales, block construction, and vocabulary, which relates only weakly to MRI results or to overall impairment of the preterm group. A second factor loads most heavily on tests with a component of frontal executive control, such as 'score' and 'opposite worlds' tests of the TEA-Ch, and these scores are the most strongly related to MRI results. This can be contrasted with the results of the younger group, where executive function results showed little variation with MRI category. An interpretation of this is that the effect of perinatal brain damage on frontal function is rather prolonged and becomes more apparent with age.

Looking at the overall pattern of results in Fig. 3, it is striking that the areas of general deficit are related to attention, visuomotor control, processing the spatial layout of the environment, global motion, and stereopsis – all areas associated with processing in the dorsal rather than the ventral stream. The 'dorsal vulnerability' arising from the risk factors of preterm birth is not restricted to the signature task of motion coherence thresholds, but pervades a range of functions in which visual information is used for the control of behaviour and the understanding of spatial relationships.

Global visual processing in infancy

As outlined in Table 1 and in the second section of this chapter, by using a stimulus that alternates between a globally coherent structure (defined in either static form or in motion) and a random arrangement of the same local elements, it is possible to isolate a VERP response that depends on the brain's ability to extract these global structures. Having demonstrated that by 5 months, infants can show responses of both kinds, we have started to use these tools to examine the effect of prematurity on development of these higher visual processing functions, in collaboration again with the Hammersmith group. In this new cohort, MRI results have been categorized according to a more refined system, summarized in Table 4.

Table 4. Outline of the scoring system used for term MRI results in the study of global form and motion processing in 22 infants born at < 33 weeks' gestation[a]

• Neonatal MRI damage scored 0–20 (white matter damage, cysts/lesions, basal ganglia/thalamus damage, cerebellar damage)
• 'Visual network' scored 0–10 (optic radiation, thalami, occipital cortex, dorsal and ventral cortical streams)
• 'Mild/moderate': total score < 6, visual network = 0 (*N* = 12)
• 'Severe': total score = 6–14, visual network = 1–7 (*N* = 10)

[a] Scoring of MRI images was performed by Prof. Mary Rutherford.

The use of a high-density EEG sensor array makes it possible to ask two kinds of question: first, can we record specific responses as evidence of global processing, and second, does the anatomic distribution of these signals differ in infants born preterm from that in term-born controls (Atkinson *et al.*, 2008b)?

Fig. 4 shows data on the first of these questions, indicating the relative strength of VERP responses in preterm-born infants in different MRI categories, and term-born controls, comparing the simple pattern-reversal response and the global responses to motion structure (coherent rotation) and global form (concentric organization). The pattern-reversal response appears unimpaired in the preterm groups, as does the global-form response (although in many infants of all groups, this global form response is only starting to emerge by 5 months of age). The most striking differences are in the global motion response, which is strong in the controls and in those with normal/mild MRI findings, but markedly weaker in the group categorized as 'severe'. Again, the greatest impact of damage is on the dorsal stream function.

If the children with mild or moderate MRI findings after very preterm birth show a similar signal strength to that of controls, does this mean that their global motion processing is the same? It appears not. Our earlier findings (Wattam-Bell *et al.*, 2010) showed that the pattern of activation across the scalp revealed significant reorganization between 5-month-old typically developing infants, and adults. In particular, the response to global motion, which is strongest on the occipital midline in the adult, shows markedly more lateral foci in infant participants. Fig. 5 shows that the pattern of response in children with mild or moderate MRI findings is markedly different from controls of the same post-term age. Specifically, the lateralized foci that occur in the control infants appear even more prominent, and more lateral, in these prematurely born infants. They may represent a more immature configuration in the transition from the infant to adult pattern – a hypothesis that will be testable if data from younger control infants with this paradigm can be recorded.

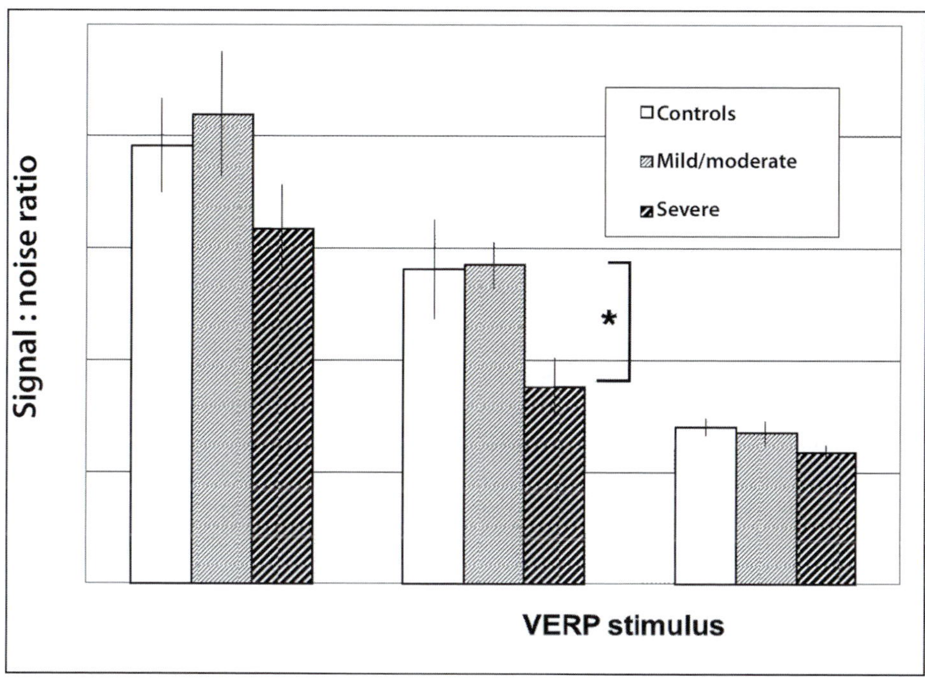

Fig. 4. Maximum signal-to-noise ratio in steady-state VERP recordings for three different stimuli (see Table 1) in prematurely born infants with two different categories of MRI finding at term (see Table 4), compared with term-born controls. All infants were tested around 4–5 months post-term.

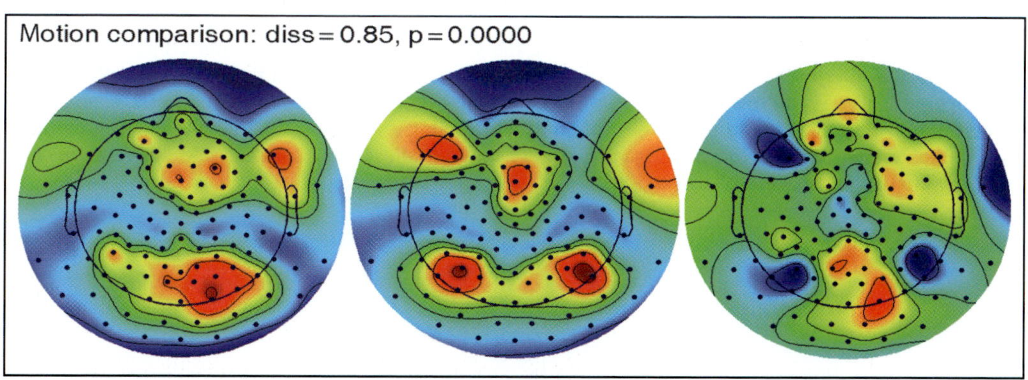

Fig. 5. Scalp distribution of VERP responses to global motion in the preterm-born group with 'mild/moderate' MRI findings (centre) compared with the term-born controls (left). Dots show sensor locations on a flattened representation of the head. The inner circle represents the circumference of the head at its widest point; positions outside this circle are scalp positions outside this line (e.g., *below the inion in the occipital region). The darkness of the shading represents increasing values of T^2_{circ}, a statistic defining the reliability of the steady-state VERP signal at that location (see Wattam-Bell* et al., *2010).*

It is not straightforward to infer the anatomic location of underlying neural sources from data of the kind shown in Fig. 5; ideally this would require individual structural MRIs at the same age as the recording, and data on the electrical properties of infant cranial tissues to model the process by which intracerebral currents generate voltages at the scalp. However, it is tempting to suggest that the isolated lateral foci seen in the centre panel of Fig. 5 represent isolated activity of the motion-sensitive area MT/V5, without the complex network of connected brain areas seen in response to motion coherence in the adult brain (Braddick *et al.*, 2000). Current work in the Visual Development Unit is exploring the hypothesis that the development of global motion responses during infancy and childhood reflects an increasing role of feedback connections between brain areas, including feedback from extrastriate to primary striate cortex. The developmental delay seen in even apparently healthy preterm infants may then be an index of immaturity in these recurrent neural networks.

Conclusions

Behavioural and electrophysiologic measures early in life can provide sensitive measures of overall brain development, which reflect the level of perinatal brain damage and are predictive of later neurocognitive development. Both in early infancy and later in childhood, processes associated with the dorsal stream, going from early integrative motion processing to visuomotor control and spatial cognition, appear to be especially vulnerable – not only to perinatal injury, but also to a wide variety of acquired and genetic neurodevelopmental anomalies. Technical advances are allowing measurements in infancy that are increasingly specific to particular brain systems, and we can hope that advances to come shortly will allow us to map the anatomic and spatiotemporal pattern of activation within the brain with increasing confidence. We believe that the specificity and richness of information gained from visual assessments will enable an increasing contribution to the understanding, and ultimately the therapy, of brain disorders that originate in the pre- and perinatal period.

Acknowledgments: This work was supported by Grants G7908507 and G0601007 from the Medical Research Council. Additionally, this research would not have been possible without the collaboration of John Wattam-Bell and other members of the Visual Development Unit, in particular Dee Birtles, Shirley Anker, and Harriet Hallas. It has also depended on the generous collaboration of our clinical colleagues, notably Mary Rutherford, Frances Cowan, David Edwards, and Leigh Dyet at the Hammersmith Hospital and Imperial College; Andrew Wilkinson of the John Radcliffe Hospital, Oxford; and Janet Rennie, who at the time of the work was at the Rosie Maternity Hospital, Cambridge. Most of all we are grateful to the families of the infants who have participated in these studies; their patience and cooperation have been essential to the success of this work.

References

Atkinson, J. (1984): Human visual development over the first six months of life: a review and a hypothesis. *Hum. Neurobiol.* **3,** 61–74.

Atkinson, J. (2000): *The Developing Visual Brain.* Oxford: Oxford University Press.

Atkinson, J. & Braddick, O. J. (1999): Research methods in infant vision. In: *Vision Research: A Practical Guide to Laboratory Methods*, eds. R.H.S. Carpenter & J.G. Robson, pp. 161–186. Oxford: Oxford University Press.

Atkinson, J. & Braddick, O. (2005): Dorsal stream vulnerability and autistic disorders: the importance of comparative studies of form and motion coherence in typically developing children and children with developmental disorders. *Cah. Psychol. Cognit. (Curr. Psychol. Cognit.)* **23,** 49–58.

Atkinson, J. & Braddick, O. (2007): Visual and visuocognitive development in children born very prematurely. *Prog. Brain Res.* **164,** 123–149.

Atkinson, J. & Braddick, O. (2011): Linked brain development for vision, visual attention, and visual cognition in typical development and in developmental disorders. In: *Brain Lesion Localization and Developmental Functions,* eds. D. Riva, C. Njiokiktjien and S. Bulgheroni. Mariani Foundation Paediatric Neurology Series – XXV. Paris: John Libbey Eurotext (this volume).

Atkinson, J., Hood, B., Wattam-Bell, J. & Braddick, O.J. (1992): Changes in infants' ability to switch visual attention in the first three months of life. *Perception* **21,** 643–653.

Atkinson, J., King, J., Braddick, O., Nokes, L., Anker, S. & Braddick, F. (1997): A specific deficit of dorsal stream function in Williams syndrome. *NeuroReport* **8,** 1919–1922.

Atkinson, J., Anker, S., Rae, S., Hughes, C. & Braddick, O. (2002a): A test battery of child development for examining functional vision (ABCDEFV). *Strabismus* **10,** 245–269.

Atkinson, J., Anker, S., Rae, S., Weeks, F., Braddick, O. & Rennie J. (2002b): Cortical visual evoked potentials in very low birthweight premature infants. *Arch. Dis. Child. Fetal Neonatal Ed.* **86,** F28–F31.

Atkinson, J., Braddick, O., Anker, S., Curran, W. & Andrew, R. (2003): Neurobiological models of visuospatial cognition in children with Williams syndrome: measures of dorsal-stream and frontal function. *Dev. Neuropsychol.* **23,** 141–174.

Atkinson, J., Braddick, O., Rose, F.E., Searcy, Y.M., Wattam-Bell, J. & Bellugi, U. (2006): Dorsal-stream motion processing deficits persist into adulthood in Williams syndrome. *Neuropsychologia* **44,** 828–833.

Atkinson, J., Braddick, O., Anker, S., Nardini, M., Birtles, D., Rutherford, M., *et al.* (2008a): Cortical vision, MRI and developmental outcome in preterm infants. *Arch. Dis. Child. Fetal Neonatal Ed.* **93,** F292–F297.

Atkinson, J., Birtles, D., Anker, S., Braddick, O., Rutherford, M., Cowan, F. & Edwards, D. (2008b): High-density VEP measures of global form and motion processing in infants born very preterm. *J. Vis.* **8,** 422,422a

Biro, S. & Russell, J. (2001): The execution of arbitrary procedures by children with autism. *Dev. Psychopathol.* **13,** 97–110.

Birtles, D., Braddick, O., Wattam-Bell, J., Wilkinson, A. & Atkinson, J. (2007): Orientation and motion-specific visual cortex responses in infants born preterm. *NeuroReport* **18,** 1975–1979.

Braddick, O.J. (1993): Orientation- and motion-selective mechanisms in infants. In: *Early Visual Development: Normal and Abnormal*, ed. K. Simons, pp. 163-177. New York: Oxford University Press.

Braddick, O. & Atkinson, J. (2007): Development of brain mechanisms for visual global processing and object segmentation. In: *From Action to Cognition* (*Progress in Brain Research*, Vol. 164), eds. C. von Hofsten & K. Rosander, pp. 151–168. Amsterdam: Elsevier.

Braddick, O.J., Wattam-Bell, J. & Atkinson, J. (1986): Orientation-specific cortical responses develop in early infancy. *Nature* **320,** 617–619.

Braddick, O.J., O'Brien, J.M.D., Wattam-Bell, J., Atkinson, J. & Turner, R. (2000): Form and motion coherence activate independent, but not dorsal/ventral segregated, networks in the human brain. *Curr. Biol.* **10,** 731–734.

Braddick, O., Atkinson, J. & Wattam-Bell, J. (2003): Normal and anomalous development of visual motion processing: motion coherence and 'dorsal stream vulnerability'. *Neuropsychologia* **41,** 1769–1784.

Braddick, O.J., Birtles, D., Wattam-Bell, J. & Atkinson, J. (2005): Motion- and orientation-specific cortical responses in infancy. *Vis. Res.* **45,** 3169–3179.

Britten, K.H., Shadlen, M.N., Newsome, W.T. & Movshon, J.A. (1992): The analysis of visual motion: a comparison of neuronal and psychophysical performance. *J. Neurosci.* **12,** 4745–4765.

Cornelissen, P., Richardson, A., Mason, A., Fowler, S. & Stein, J. (1995): Contrast sensitivity and coherent motion detection measured at photopic luminance levels in dyslexics and controls. *Vis. Res.* **35,** 1483–1494.

Duffy, C.J. & Wurtz, R.H. (1991): Sensitivity of MST neurons to optic flow stimuli. I. A continuum of response selectivity to large-field stimuli. *J. Neurophysiol.* **65,** 1329–1345.

du Plessis, A.J. & Volpe, J.J. (2002): Perinatal brain injury in the preterm and term newborn. *Curr. Opin. Neurol.* **15,** 151–157.

Dutton, G.N. & Bax, M. (2010): *Visual Impairment in Children Due to Damage to the Brain.* London: MacKeith Press.

Dyet, L.E., Kennea, N., Counsell, S.J., Maalouf, E.F., Ajayi-Obe, M., Duggan, P.J., *et al.* (2006): Natural history of brain lesions in extremely preterm infants studied with serial magnetic resonance imaging from birth and neurodevelopmental assessment. *Pediatrics* **118,** 536–548.

Ellemberg, D., Lewis, T. L., Maurer, D., Brar, S. & Brent, H. P. (2002): Better perception of global motion after monocular than after binocular deprivation. *Vis. Res.* **42,** 169–179.

Emsley, H.C.A., Wardle, S.P., Sims, D.G., Chiswick, M.L. & D'Souza, S.W (1998): Increased survival and deteriorating developmental outcome in 23 to 25 week old gestation infants, 1990–4 compared with 1984–9. *Arch. Dis. Child.* **78,** F99–104.

Gallant, J.L., Braun, J. & Van Essen, D.C. (1993): Selectivity for polar, hyperbolic, and cartesian gratings in macaque visual cortex. *Science* **259,** 100–103.

Gerstadt, C.L., Hong, Y.J. & Diamond, A. (1994): The relationship between cognition and action: performance of children 3 1/2–7 years old on a Stroop-like day-night test. *Cognition* **53,** 129–153.

Gunn, A., Cory, E., Atkinson, J., Braddick, O., Wattam-Bell, J., Guzzetta, A. & Cioni, G. (2002): Dorsal and ventral stream sensitivity in normal development and hemiplegia. *NeuroReport* **13,** 843–847.

Hansen, P.C., Stein, J.F., Orde, S.R., Winter, J.L. & Talcott, J.B. (2001): Are dyslexics' visual deficits limited to measures of dorsal stream function? *NeuroReport* **12,** 1527–1530.

Harris, L., Atkinson, J. & Braddick, O.J. (1976): Visual contrast sensitivity of a 6-month infant measured by the evoked potential. *Nature* **264,** 570–571.

Henderson, S.E. & Sugden, D.A. (1992): *The Movement ABC Manual.* London: The Psychological Corporation.

Hood, B. (1995): Gravity rules for 2-4 year olds. *Cogn. Dev.* **10,** 577–598.

Kastner, S. & Ungerleider, L.G. (2000): Mechanisms of visual attention in the human cortex. *Annu. Rev. Neurosci.* **23,** 315–341.

Kogan, C.S., Boutet, I., Cornish, K., Zangenehpour, S., Mullen, K.T., Holden, J.J.A., *et al.* (2004): Differential impact of the *FMR1* gene on visual processing in fragile X syndrome. *Brain* **127,** 591–601.

Lewis, T.L., Ellemberg, D., Maurer, D., Wilkinson, F., Wilson, H.R., Dirks, M. & Brent, H.P. (2002): Sensitivity to global form in Glass patterns after early visual deprivation in humans. *Vis. Res.* **42,** 939–948.

Livingstone, M. & Hubel, D.H. (1988): Segregation of form, color, movement and depth: anatomy, physiology and perception. *Science* **240,** 740–749.

Manly, T., Nimmo-Smith, I., Watson, P., Anderson, V., Turner, A. & Roberston, I.H. (2001): The differential assessment of children's attention: the test of everyday attention for children (TEA-Ch), normative sample and ADHD performance. *J. Child Psychol. Psychiatry* **42,** 1065–1081.

Mercuri, E., Atkinson, J., Braddick, O., Anker, S., Nokes, L., Cowan, F., *et al.* (1996): Visual function and perinatal focal cerebral infarction. *Arch. Dis. Child.* **75,** F76–F81.

Mercuri, E., Atkinson, J., Braddick, O., Anker, S., Cowan, F., Rutherford, M., *et al.* (1997): Visual function in full-term infants with hypoxic-ischaemic encephalopathy. *Neuropediatrics* **28,** 155–161.

Mercuri, E., Braddick, O., Atkinson, J., Cowan, F., Anker, S., Andrew, R., *et al.* (1998): Orientation-reversal and phase-reversal visual evoked potentials in full-term infants with brain lesions: a longitudinal study. *Neuropediatrics* **29,** 1–6.

Mercuri, E., Haataja, L., Guzzetta, A., Anker, S., Cowan, F., Rutherford, M., *et al.* (1999): Visual function in term infants with hypoxic-ischaemic insults: correlation with neurodevelopment at 2 years of age. *Arch. Dis. Child Fetal Neonatal Ed.* **80,** F99–F104.

Milne, E., Swettenham, J. & Campbell, R. (2005): Motion perception and autistic spectrum disorder: a review. *Cah. Psychol. Cogn./Cur. Psychol. Cognit.* **23,** 3–36.

Milner A.D. & Goodale, M.A. (1995): *The Visual Brain in Action.* Oxford: Oxford University Press.

Mishkin, M., Ungerleider, L. & Macko, K.A. (1983): Object vision and spatial vision: two critical pathways. *Trends Neurosci.* **6,** 414–417.

Nardini, M., Burgess, N., Breckenridge, K. & Atkinson, J. (2006): Differential developmental trajectories for egocentric, environmental and intrinsic frames of reference in spatial memory. *Cognition* **101,** 153–172.

Norcia, A.M. & Tyler, C.W. (1985): Spatial frequency sweep VEP: visual acuity during the first year of life. *Vis. Res.* **25,** 1399–1408.

Rennie, J.M. (2002): A review of the risk of being born too soon. *Fetal Maternal Med. Rev.* **13,** 157–168.

Ridder, W.H., Borsting, E. & Banton, T. (2001): All developmental dyslexic subtypes display an elevated motion coherence threshold. *Optom. Vis. Sci.* **78,** 510–517.

Sokol, S. (1978): Measurement of infant visual acuity from pattern reversal evoked potentials. *Vis. Res.* **18,** 33–41.

Spencer, J., O'Brien, J., Riggs, K., Braddick, O., Atkinson, J. & Wattam-Bell, J. (2000): Motion processing in autism: evidence for a dorsal stream deficiency. *NeuroReport,* **11,** 2765–2767.

Wattam-Bell, J. (1991): The development of motion-specific cortical responses in infants. *Vis. Res.* **31,** 287–297.

Wattam-Bell, J., Birtles, D., Nyström, P., von Hofsten, C., Rosander, K., Anker, S., *et al.* (2010): Reorganization of global form and motion processing during human visual development. *Curr. Biol.* **20,** 411–415.

Brain Lesion Localization and Developmental Functions, D. Riva, C. Njiokiktjien and S. Bulgheroni (eds.)

Chapter 19

Linked brain development for vision, visual attention and visual cognition in typical development and in developmental disorders

Janette Atkinson* and Oliver Braddick°

**Department of Developmental Science, University College, London, United Kingdom;*
°Department of Experimental Psychology, University of Oxford, South Parks Road, Oxford OX1 3UD, United Kingdom
oliver.braddick@psy.ox.ac.uk

Summary

Developing visual neural systems are linked to, and overlap with, systems for controlling visual attention, action, and spatial cognition. These functions are particularly associated with the dorsal stream of cortical visual processing, which is more vulnerable to early brain damage than the ventral cortical stream and is identified in many neurodevelopmental disorders. We review some developmental evidence on (*a*) parietal-frontal modules for the on-line control of visually guided actions (eye movements, reaching, grasping, and locomotion); (*b*) frontal systems for the forward planning of actions; (*c*) visuospatial localization and memory requiring parahippocampal and hippocampal systems. All three are identified in recent work as targets of dorsal stream networks (Kravitz *et al.*, 2011). Visual behaviour therefore involves a wide range of brain functions and systems. We describe the ABCDEFV battery which is designed to provide an assessment across much of this range of functional vision and visuocognitive abilities, in infants and young children.

Attention is believed to comprise separate neural subsystems concerned with spatial selective attention, sustained attention, and attentional control (executive function). We describe the new Early Childhood Attention Battery (ECAB), which is designed to assess individual profiles across these attentional capacities in children of developmental age 3–6 years. We review results of applying this battery, and other work, on the areas of deficit and relative strength in attentional capacities of children with Williams and Down syndromes. These approaches lead to the possibility of identifying, in the individual infant or young child, deficits related to complex interactive functions of processing in the 'multiple dorsal streams'. Such insights will, it is hoped, aid in rehabilitation and support of children with neurodevelopmental disorders.

Introduction

A large proportion of the human brain is involved in processing and analyzing incoming visual signals to provide automatic visual perception and action. The human infant is born with a very immature visual system, but this develops rapidly and provides a key function for children's developing interaction with their physical and social environment. In a number of previous publications we have demonstrated how visual assessments, using standardized brain imaging, electrophysiologic measures such as event-related potentials, and behavioural observational measures, can provide a unique window on the brain in the first months of life, and a sensitive indicator of broader neurocognitive development throughout the pre-school years and early school years (see, for example, Atkinson & Braddick, 2007; Atkinson & van Hof-van Duin, 1993; Atkinson *et al.*, 2008; Hood & Atkinson, 1990; Mercuri *et al.*, 1996, 1997, 1999).

In this chapter we will discuss how developing sensory and perceptual visual subsystems are linked to and overlap with systems for controlling visual attention, actions, and spatial cognition in typical development, and how these brain systems are affected in paediatric developmental disorders. These abnormalities of brain development result from an intricate process of gene expression interacting with a dynamically changing environment, which may be different from the normal environment. At present it is impossible to specify development of these linked subsystems in molecular detail. However, here we describe some aspects of the characteristic phenotype at the behavioural and neural systems level, as it appears in vision, visuomotor actions, and attention.

In this chapter we discuss:
- a model of typical visual brain development in infancy and early childhood;
- the development of the ventral and dorsal cortical streams;
- dorsal stream vulnerability;
- the involvement of the dorsal stream in spatial actions and its links to attentional control;
- the typical development of attention in children, including executive function;
- attention deficits in developmental disorders; and
- the new Early Child Attention Battery (ECAB) for assessment of the components of attention and executive control, giving an attention profile for children of 3–6 years mental age.

Model of typical visual brain development in infancy and early childhood

The model outlined here is described with more detailed evidence in Atkinson (2000) and Atkinson and Braddick (2003).

Neonatal subcortical visual systems

The infant at birth has a working subcortical visual system, giving the newborn infant a crude sense of space. This subcortical system allows the newborn to orient to conspicuous visual stimuli in different parts of a relatively narrow visual field. A functional neonatal subcortical system is also demonstrated in the ability of newborns to show optokinetic nystagmus (OKN), a reflex of stabilizing eye movements, as a response to a large area of pattern, moving horizontally leftwards or rightwards across the field of view.

Functioning in the visual cortex

This starting point of subcortical control is followed in the first few postnatal months by the functional onset of systems in the visual cortex, responding selectively to orientation, motion direction, and binocular disparity, and later to global visual pattern structure, as discussed in the accompanying chapter (Braddick & Atkinson, 2011). These cortical processes start to modulate and control the more automatic reflex subcortical visual responses.

The 'fixation shift' paradigm: shifts of visual attention

The fixation shift paradigm has been developed to assess the ability of infants to make shifts of attention in the first months of life (*e.g.*, Atkinson *et al.*, 1992; Atkinson & Hood, 1997; Hood & Atkinson, 1990, 1993). Newborn infants will orient their head and eyes towards salient stimuli, but cannot readily disengage from a centrally viewed stimulus which has captured their fixation (attention) when a second object appears in the periphery. The ability to make prompt shifts of fixation away from a fixated central target to a second newly appearing target, under conditions of 'competition' (*i.e.*, when both a central and a peripheral target are present together) develops from 3–4 months onwards. This ability, to shift under competition, has been found to be unilaterally absent in infants who, although having intact subcortical visual systems, have had one cerebral hemisphere surgically removed to relieve intractable epilepsy (hemispherectomy). This confirms the cortical basis of this ability to 'disengage' attention and shift to a new target under conditions of competition (Braddick *et al.*, 1992). This 'fixation shift' (FS) paradigm has also been shown to be a sensitive indicator of cerebral injury and predictive of neurocognitive outcome in children with perinatal brain damage such as focal lesions, hypoxic-ischaemic encephalopathy (HIE), or perinatal abnormality of the white matter fibre tracts associated with very preterm birth (*e.g.*, Atkinson & Braddick, 2007; Atkinson *et al.*, 2008; Hood & Atkinson, 1990; Mercuri *et al.*, 1996, 1999). It has also been used successfully to assess attention related to other aspects of cognitive development in children with West syndrome (Guzzetta *et al.*, 2002, 2008) and Williams syndrome (WS) (Atkinson *et al.*, 2003). It is proposed that FS under competition requires the integration of attentional systems in the parietal lobe and frontal eye fields to modulate the subcortical orienting system, which includes areas such as the superior colliculus and oculomotor nuclei (Fig. 1).

Development of the ventral and dorsal cortical streams

In the accompanying chapter (Braddick & Atkinson, 2011), we have outlined the distinction between the ventral and dorsal cortical streams, and their early different development as assessed by VERP and behavioural tests of sensitivity to global static form and global motion.

In addition to these measures, fMRI brain imaging studies with normal adults have shown separate networks of areas sensitive to 'global static form' (ventral) or 'global motion' (dorsal). The two networks appear to be independent and nonoverlapping, and both involve areas in occipital, parietal, and temporal lobes (Braddick *et al.*, 2000). This is a rather different result compared to the classic description derived from work in nonhuman primates, which has placed the dorsal stream primarily in parietal areas and the ventral stream in temporal areas. However, a recent wide-ranging review of anatomic and functional data (Kravitz *et al.*, 2011) proposes that there are multiple branches of the dorsal stream, dividing in the parietal lobe and involving three separate networks underpinning different aspects of spatial processing. We will come back to this idea of multiple dorsal streams below in discussing the neural basis of attention.

Summary of typical development of the dorsal and ventral streams

The sequence of development in early infancy suggests that the initial development of the dorsal stream pathway may be slower than that of the parvocellular or 'ventral' pathway, which specializes in the processing of form (orientation or slant) and colour discrimination (*e.g.*, see Atkinson, 1990). However, the maturation of higher-level aspects of the dorsal stream, which serves the global integration of motion information, proceeds rapidly and at age 5 months is

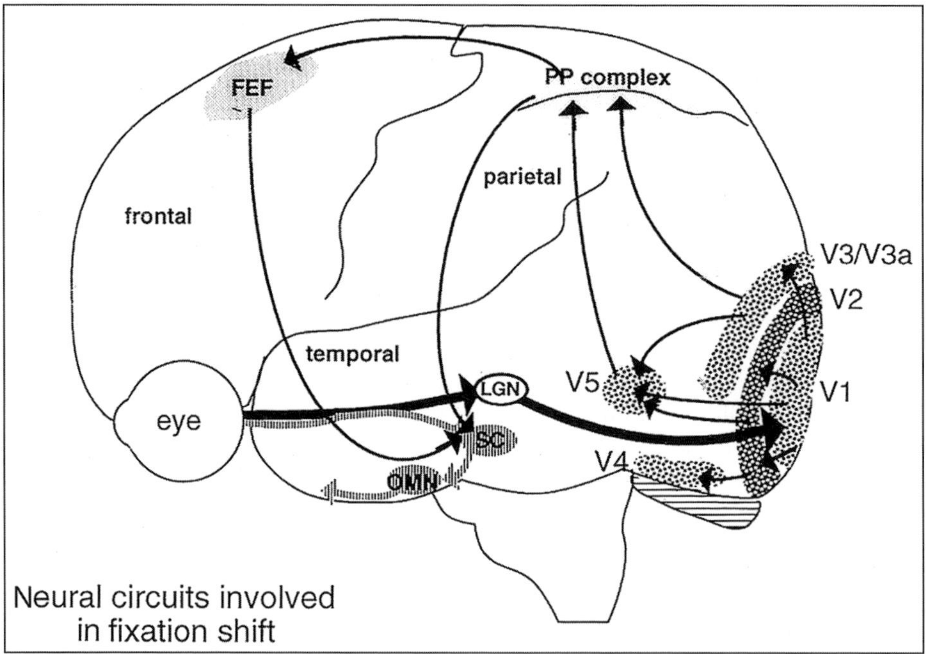

Fig. 1. Simplified diagram of the pathways involved in the control of fixation shifts. The direct route from the retina to the superior colliculus (SC) and oculomotor nuclei (OMN) allows young infants to orient towards a salient stimulus and maintain fixation upon it. The cortical visual network develops (areas V1, V2, V3/V3a, V5 and others not shown) and provides inputs to the posterior parietal (PP) complex and frontal eye fields (FEF), which allow the subcortical pathway to be modulated (e.g., *by inhibition via the caudate nucleus and substantia nigra [not shown]).*

more developmentally advanced than the equivalent response to the global structure of static form (Braddick & Atkinson, 2007; Wattam-Bell *et al.*, 2010). Later, in middle childhood, thresholds for global form and motion structure can be measured and compared in two behavioural tests. Results from these tests indicate that between ages 4 and 10 years, global form processing (ventral) achieves adult levels earlier than does global motion processing (dorsal). The developmental trajectories for ventral and dorsal stream function, therefore, have a complex and changing relationship (Braddick *et al.*, 2003). However, it is not yet known which stages of this developmental relationship are responsible for the differential vulnerability of dorsal stream function in developmental disorders (which will be discussed in the next section) and, of course, in different disorders, different areas within this developing dynamic network may be functionally abnormal or delayed in development.

Dorsal stream vulnerability

Using the computer game tests discussed in the accompanying chapter (Braddick & Atkinson, 2011) we have shown that children and adults with WS perform more poorly on the dorsal stream (motion coherence) task than on the ventral stream task (static form coherence) (Atkinson *et al.*, 1997, 2003, 2006). Table 2 in the accompanying chapter lists the wide range of developmental disorders in which this 'dorsal stream vulnerability' has been identified as a general feature of impaired brain development. It should be noted that the dorsal stream motion task involves identifying a shape defined by motion, so it is possible that the dorsal stream deficit might be specifically in the integration of dorsal motion information into ventral stream processes for shape recognition. However, data from the deficits of children with brain damage consequent to premature birth indicate that a wide range of dorsal stream functions associated with motion, spatial cognition, and visuomotor control are impaired (Atkinson & Braddick, 2007 and 2011), so the vulnerability appears to be more general. This vulnerability may be due to the timing of emerging dorsal function during vulnerable periods of brain development; it could be due to the differential plasticity of different brain systems in recovery from brain damage; or it could be due to the special demands of achieving the temporal precision required for effective motion processing at a relatively low level of visual processing and analysis, with developmental knock-on effects to other domains of dorsal stream function.

Dorsal streams for control of actions, attention, and spatial cognition

As well as differentially processing motion and spatial information, a key characteristic of the dorsal stream is that it transmits the information required for the on-line visual control of actions. It may be more appropriate to speak of 'dorsal streams' rather than 'the dorsal stream'. Different types of visuomotor action appear as paediatric milestones at various points during the first years of life. These actions, such as visual tracking (initially with saccadic eye movements and later smooth-pursuit eye movements), reaching and grasping, and walking and climbing can be considered as functions of specific modules within the dorsal stream, each of which extracts the visual information needed to guide these actions, and translates it into the form required for motor planning and control in that particular task (Rizzolatti *et al.*, 1997). Figure 2 summarizes some of the distinct brain structures and areas that are implicated within the modules for saccadic and smooth-pursuit eye movements, reaching, and grasping (those involved in locomotion are less well understood).

We have already discussed the first action system to develop, that controlling shifts of eye movements to fixate an object of interest, to disengage attention from the current object, and to shift to another object of interest when it appears, as tested by the fixation shift (FS) method. As indicated in Figs. 1 and 2, this involves a network of occipital, parietal, and frontal areas (frontal eye fields [FEF]) to guide the subcortical eye movement system, which then provides the information required for further cognitive analysis.

Development of modules for reaching and grasping

Two of the visuomotor modules shown in Fig. 2 are concerned with the control of visually guided reaching and grasping, respectively. It is controversial how far the crude 'pre-reaches' in the first months of life are visually directed responses, and how far they reflect a nonspecific response to the general direction of attention (see von Hofsten, 1982, 1984, 1991). Typically developing infants usually start to reach and grasp successfully for objects within arm's reach, under visual guidance, between 4 and 6 months of age. This requires the action system to process two kinds of visual information: the direction and distance of the object, and whether its size and shape makes it a suitable target for reaching and grasping.

Visually guided reaching develops at a similar time to binocularity, around 4 months of age, suggesting that binocular disparity information, linked to control of eye convergence, may provide a key input to the visuomotor module for reaching. This is supported by the finding

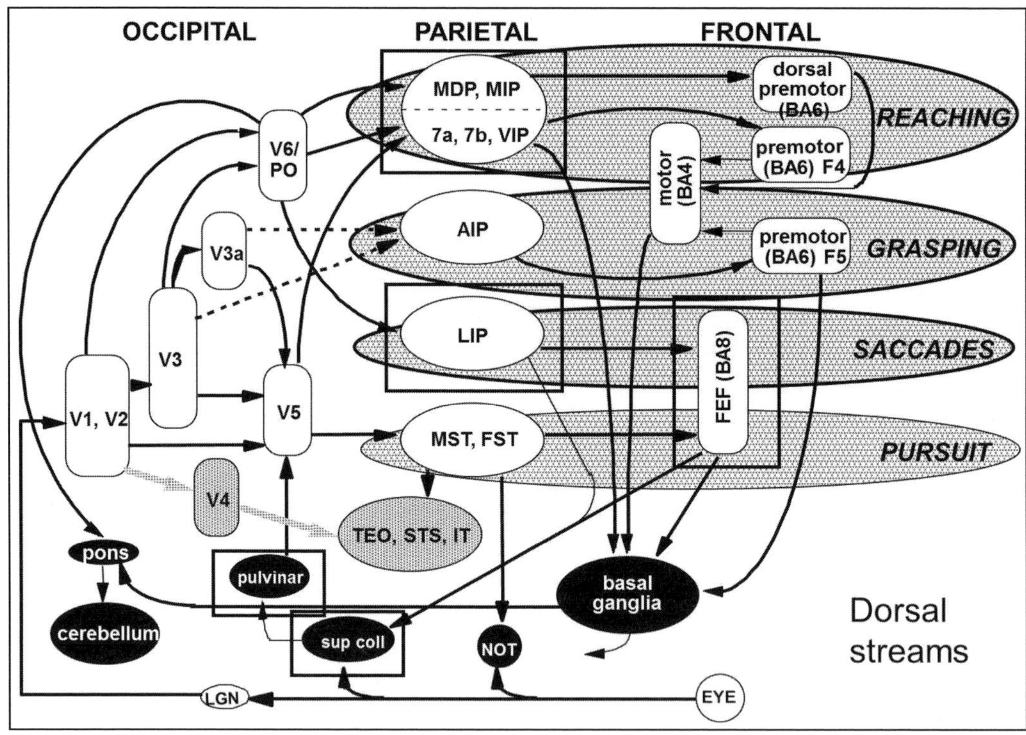

Fig. 2. Schematic summary of action modules within the dorsal stream for visual control of four behaviours: arm movements for reaching, hand movements for grasping, saccadic eye movements, and smooth-pursuit eye movements. Brain areas in white are dorsal stream, shaded areas are ventral stream, and black areas are subcortical structures. Rectangular boxes enclose areas that have been shown to be involved in the spatial direction of attention. Networks shown are based on primate studies and human neuropsychology (data were reviewed by Jeannerod, 1988; Milner & Goodale, 1995; Rizzolatti et al., *1997). Abbreviations for brain areas: V1–5 = visual areas 1–5; PO = parietal-occipital; MDP = medial dorsal parietal; MIP = medial intraparietal; AIP = anterior intraparietal; VIP = ventral intraparietal; LIP = lateral intraparietal; BA6 = Brodmann area 6 (F4, F5 etc are fields within BA6); FEF = frontal eye fields; NOT = nucleus of the optic tract; sup coll = superior colliculus; TEO = a posterior region of inferotemporal cortex; STS = superior temporal sulcus; IT = inferotemporal. (Redrawn and updated from Atkinson & Braddick, 2000.)*

that binocular information is critical in determining the kinematics of infants' reaches (Braddick *et al.*, 1996). This reliance on binocular information extracted in the dorsal stream for guiding reaching shows the developmental synergy between the visual and motor systems.

Infants between 6 and 9 months of age often reach quite compulsively for small objects presented within arm's reach. This behaviour raises the question of the visual information by which an infant determines that an object is graspable and hence a suitable target for reaching. Infants who compulsively reach at this age do not necessarily show the preshaping of the hand, which calibrates grasp aperture during the reach to the object size (McCarty *et al.*, 2001). We have speculated that the computation of 'graspability' is probably a function of the anterior intraparietal area (AIP) in the grasping module, and that this must be connected into the reaching module in determining target selection for this action.

The visuomotor modules used for successful reaching and grasping have been investigated in experiments that combine preferential looking with preferential reaching (Newman *et al.*, 2001). In preferential looking, infants make an orienting response of head and eyes towards the most salient object or region in the visual field. The computation of salience is a function of the cortical modules which contribute to the orienting system through the superior colliculus, or of processing within the superior colliculus itself. When an infant is presented with two solid objects, similar in shape and surface properties, the infant tends to orient to the larger object (King *et al.*, 1996; Newman *et al.*, 2001).

However, reaching is only an appropriate action for objects in the size range that can be grasped. If the infant can visually compute object size, when faced with a pair of objects, one of which is beyond the span of the infant's hand, reaching will be preferentially directed to the smaller, more graspable object of the pair. The form of the action may also be affected by these visual properties. Braddick & Atkinson (2007) examined reaches to a wide range of object sizes (3–46 cm) and found that, at different ages, size determined the incidence of bimanual reaches and of 'nongrasp contact', in which the infants pushed or palpated the surface of large objects. Thus visual size determines not just the initiation of a manual action, but its kinematic form also, with distinct action patterns for 'grasp the object' and 'explore the surface'. Older infants use more subtle visual 'affordances' to determine their actions, such as information about the expected rigidity of an object (Barrett *et al.*, 2008), and how its symmetry will affect grasp stability (Barrett & Needham, 2008).

These specific uses of visual information suggest that the two visuomotor modules – for orienting and for reaching – may be driven by different visual information from the same objects. The studies of King *et al.* (1996) and Newman *et al.* (2001) have shown they interact differently at different ages (Atkinson & Braddick, 2003). When infants first start to reach (up to around 8 months), they do not show a significant reaching preference based on size, but rather their reaching is predominantly directed to the object they initially fixate. We infer that the visual processing of 'graspability' is not yet linked to a visuomotor module for reaching, but that there is a substantial coupling between the systems that control reaching and orienting. Between 8 and 12 months a strong preference emerges for reaching for the smaller, graspable object. Infants at this age show a decoupling of reaching and initial visual orienting – they are more likely than younger or older infants to first fixate one object and then reach for the other if its size is appropriate for grasping. This decoupling can be emphasized by manipulating visual salience: a schematic face on one object increases the visual preference for looking, without altering its 'graspability', and hence without a corresponding increase in the tendency for it to elicit reaching in competition (Newman *et al.*, 2001). After 12 months of age, reaching becomes less selective towards the smaller object (perhaps because the infant's grasp can encompass larger objects), while reaching and initial looking become more congruent again. It appears that the orienting and reaching systems have been integrated into a single piece of goal-directed behaviour.

Action modules for locomotion

Locomotion becomes part of the infant's behavioural repertoire around the end of the first year. It requires information to be registered from distant space. Vision, as well as defining the direction of locomotion towards a target, must also provide the information about the obstacles, surfaces, and gradients that determine whether a chosen route affords locomotion. The classic example of such information comes from the 'visual cliff' studies of Gibson and Walk (1960), which showed that crawling infants avoid a visual depth difference (probably signalled by motion parallax and/or texture perspective). More recent studies have shown sensitivity of infants' locomotor choices to visual information about gaps, obstacles, supports, and slopes (Berger & Adolph, 2007).

Locomotor skills are acquired over a long period of time; for example, stair descent remains immature for several years (partly because the dimensions of the built environment are not adapted to young children). However, it has been shown that the adult ability to use visual information about stair depth to calibrate leg movements even before touching down on the first step (Cowie *et al.*, 2008) is already present, and calibrated to leg length, in children as young as 3 years old (Cowie *et al.*, 2010).

Visual information in action planning: dorsal stream connections with the frontal lobes

The preceding sections have been concerned with systems that use visual information 'on-line' to guide action (for example, to determine the selection of a target for reaching and grasping), and can modulate the form of that action so that it is appropriate to the target. Actions also require planning, such as anticipating the end state (the final position of the limb when the action is completed). For example, an object such as a vertical handle which is to be rotated clockwise with the right hand requires a different orientation of the grasp (thumb-down) from one to be rotated anti-clockwise (thumb up), if the final position of the wrist is to be comfortable (Rosenbaum *et al.*, 1992). Achieving the comfortable end state requires selection between alternative action plans, and perhaps inhibition of an action which may be most directly triggered by the initial visual configuration (for example, a preferred 'thumb-up' grasp of the handle).

Such selection and inhibition is a classic function of frontal lobe systems, which have the most prolonged developmental course in the human brain. Children aged about 4 years tend to follow a strategy in which grasp is determined by the immediate characteristics of the object, but by 7 to 8 years of age move to adult-like end-state planning (Smyth & Mason, 1997). Children with WS, in contrast, continue to use the 'younger' strategy or more stereotyped actions (Newman, 2001). WS is associated with a dorsal stream deficit (Atkinson *et al.*, 1997), but this failure suggests that the interchange of information between dorsal stream and frontal systems is an important aspect of the deficit (Atkinson *et al.*, 2003)

A recent review by Kravitz *et al.* (2011) has provided an extended picture of the dorsal stream and its connections. They present evidence from primate studies and human neuroimaging that the dorsal stream has three distinct targets. One, connecting through parietal areas to premotor cortex, provides the visuomotor modules for the guidance of actions including those outlined for reaching and grasping (Fig. 2). A second connects to frontal eye fields (thus including the saccadic and pursuit systems seen in Fig. 2), but more broadly includes reciprocal connections to prefrontal areas. Although motor planning is not explicitly discussed by Kravitz *et al.* (2011), who focus on the related frontal function of spatial working memory, it is plausible that advance planning based on such things as end-state comfort depends on two-way transmission of information within this pathway. Descending pathways from the frontal lobes must also play a part in many aspects of attention, an area discussed below.

The third pathway, from parietal areas via cingulate cortex to the medial temporal lobe and hippocampus, is, they argue, involved in delivering spatial information and integrating it with the ventral stream for navigation and topographic cognition. Aspects of such navigation and cognition have been found to be part of the pattern of 'dorsal stream deficit' in, for example, the development of prematurely born children (Atkinson & Braddick, 2007).

Figure 3 presents diagrammatically the picture of the multiple dorsal stream pathways offered by Kravitz *et al.* The modules of Fig. 2 are included now as elements within this broader view of dorsal stream processing.

Development of the dorsal stream linked to development of visual attentional subsystems

An important feature of the dorsal stream systems diagrammed in Figs. 2 and 3 is their relationship to attention. Many aspects of attention can be regarded as 'selection for action' (Allport, 1989; Rizzolatti, 1983; Berthoz, 1996). Actions such as reaching, grasping, and locomotion require attentional modulation to select and initiate the appropriate behaviour, to direct it towards a selected goal object, and to inhibit actions that are inappropriate for the current goal. It is therefore not surprising that many of the brain structures that have been identified as part of attention networks (Kastner & Ungerleider, 2000; Posner & Dehaene, 1994; Posner & Petersen, 1990) are within the dorsal streams or closely interconnected with these 'spatial action' networks. A number of these areas are highlighted by rectangular enclosing boxes in Fig. 2. In Kravitz *et al.*'s (2011) broader description of the dorsal stream and its targets, the two-way connections with the frontal lobe, including the frontal eye fields, in the lower third of Fig. 3 are well placed to determine attentional modulation and control of spatial processing. In later sections of this article we provide greater detail about the ways in which functions of attention can be assessed in young children and the impact of neurodevelopmental disorders on these functions.

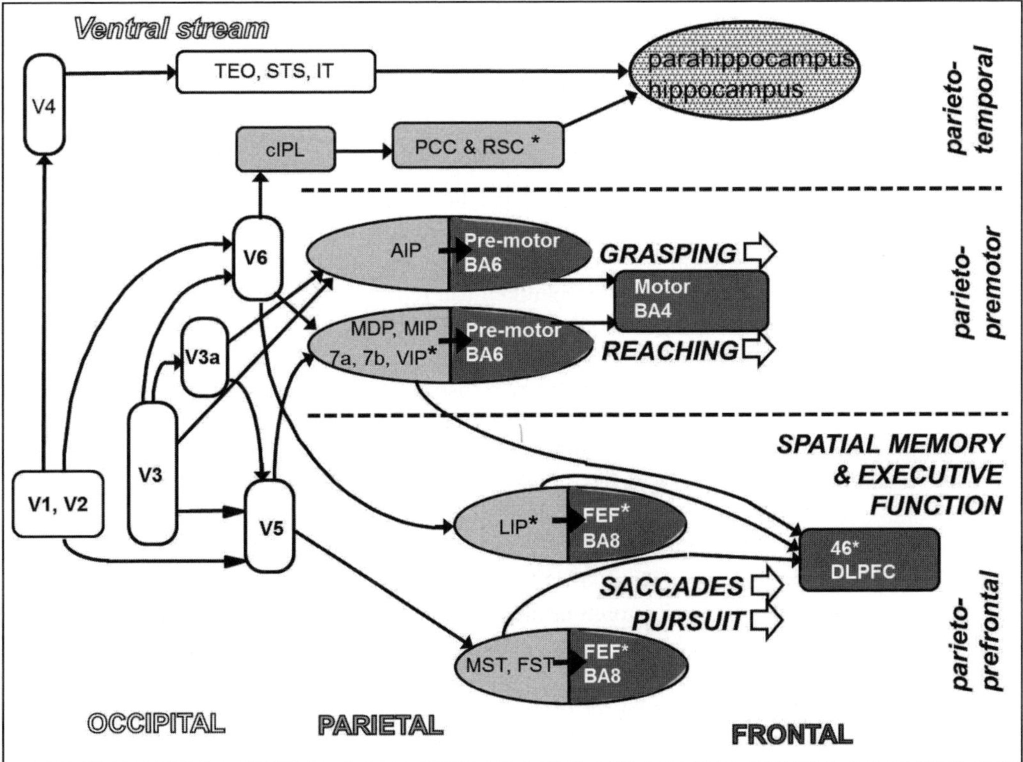

Fig. 3. Schematic summary of the three targets of the dorsal stream and their functional roles, as proposed by Kravitz et al. *(2011). Compare with Fig. 2 for the place of the visuomotor modules in this scheme. Abbreviations as for Fig. 2.*

Development of visuospatial localization and spatial memory

The third dorsal stream network proposed by Kravitz *et al.* (2011) connects spatial processing in the parietal lobe to the parahipppocampal gyrus and hippocampus, structures that are also major targets of ventral stream processing. The established role of the hippocampus in memory for locations in the environment presumably requires both the parietal information about the egocentric layout of space, and the recognition of landmarks and views that is one aspect of ventral stream analysis (Epstein & Kanwisher, 1998). These converging systems allow visual identification of familiar locations in the environment and navigation through that environment and make it possible to tag locations with significant properties that are not themselves visible (spatial memory). The resulting representations of space can be either egocentric (referenced to the individual's body; *e.g.*, ahead of me on the left) or allocentric (referenced to the external environment; *e.g.*, in the northwest corner of the square).

Tests of location memory can serve to identify the visual information used by children at different ages, and the spatial framework that infants use to define the locations. One approach with infants under 1 year of age has been to determine how 'place' is specified in the characteristic A-not-B place error (see, *e.g.*, Bremner, 1994, pp. 150–154). Such studies suggest that infants in this phase search egocentrically defined locations, but that sufficiently prominent landmarks can be enough to define a location in a way that is invariant with respect to the infant's position (Acredolo & Evans, 1980).

Improvements in location memory in mid-childhood follow prefrontal, posterior parietal, and hippocampal maturation (see Klingberg, 2006). Children use different spatial frames of reference to remember visual locations as spatial memory develops in the preschool years. Egocentric representations, using the body as a reference, provide a good basis for immediate action towards objects. More robust representations are provided by encoding where objects are relative to stable landmarks, using an allocentric reference frame. This allows objects to be found even when the viewer changes position. Another way to deal with a change of position is to track where an object is while the observer is moving by 'updating' the egocentric representation as the observer moves. Representations using single external landmarks are reliably used for guiding action by 1–2-year-olds (Huttenlocher *et al.*, 1994). At 16 to 36 months, children can retrieve objects hidden in a sandbox after walking around to the other side (Newcombe *et al.*, 1998), showing coding relative to landmarks and/or spatial updating with self-motion. Nardini *et al.* (2006) compared the ability of 3–6-year-olds to use these different types of representations in a visual location memory task. Across the age range, recall was best when both *body (egocentric)* and *room (external landmarks)* stayed consistent, less accurate when only one of these did, and worst when neither was consistent. In the latter case, successful recall depended on attending to and remembering the relative position of local landmarks. Only children over 5 years of age were successful in this condition where relative spatial position between the landmarks and the hidden object must be encoded. This ability in adults is thought to depend on hippocampal circuitry (King *et al.*, 2002; Burgess *et al.*, 2002). All three versions of this task (depending on egocentric, room-centred, or relative spatial positions) are impaired in children born preterm and tested at 6–7 years (Atkinson & Braddick, 2007). However, children with WS showed a more specific impairment, with particular difficulty using information about position relative to landmarks (Nardini *et al.*, 2008b), indicating that different aspects of spatial representation of the environment can be differentially affected in developmental disorders.

There has been considerable debate over young children's use of different visual cues, such as colour and environmental geometry, to guide their encoding of self-orientation and spatial position. Hermer and Spelke (1994, 1996) found that 18–24-month-olds, disoriented by passive rotation, could use geometric cues (the enclosure shape) to re-establish their orientation and find a hidden toy, but did not use the colour difference between the walls of the enclosure to cue their search. These authors have argued that early reorientation depends on a specialised geometric module and that development of linguistic labels is necessary for successful use of the colour cue (Hermer-Vazquez *et al.*, 1999). While there is evidence against both claims (*e.g.*, Nardini *et al.*, 2008a), the early dominance of room geometry over colour for spatial orientation, when both are available, remains a striking phenomenon which is still not well explained. Young children's neglect of colour may not be specific to disorientation search tasks; children under 2 years of age were found to also be poor at using a colour cue, when combined with a specific action, in a table-top task to locate a toy hidden in one of several boxes (Nardini *et al.*, 2008c). The 'disregard of colour' may be a common developmental phenomenon, arising from an uneven balance and poor integration of dorsal and ventral visual streams in these tasks, which means that colours are less salient relative to actions in guiding behaviour, compared to the balance of this information in adults.

Attention as a component of functional vision testing: the ABCDEFV battery

We have outlined above the close integration of attention into visual development and the interdependence of visuospatial action systems with attentional mechanisms that select, maintain, and switch the targets of these actions. In evaluating the visual capabilities of children at risk of neurodevelopmental disorders, it is not enough to assess simply sensory aspects of vision such as acuity, visual fields, refraction, and binocularity. Rather, we need to gain a picture of the functional implications of vision as a component of the systems we have discussed above, which guide actions, create representations of spatial relationships, and interact with the mechanisms of attention.

Such an integrated view of the assessment of children's visual function is the purpose of the Atkinson Battery of Child Development for Examining Functional Vision (ABCDEFV), which has been devised combining ideas from developmental neuropsychology and paediatric neurology and ophthalmology (Atkinson *et al.*, 2002). Some of the subtests emphasize visual discrimination (*e.g.*, discriminating overlapping animals embedded in a line drawing), which involves primarily ventral stream processing, whereas other subtests involve dorsal stream functions in the planning and execution of visually controlled actions. Other tests in the battery require integration of ventral and dorsal stream processing, such as matching a shape (ventral) and planning an action to place the shape in the appropriately shaped hole (dorsal). Many of the tests involve components of attention which may interact with either dorsal or ventral stream processing or both.

The battery is divided into core vision tests and age-specific tests. The core vision tests are usable throughout the age range since they make minimal demands on manual and cognitive competences. The age-specific tests make more specific demands on these competencies and so each has a minimum age at which it can appropriately be used. Both groups of tests are listed in Tables 1 and 2. Here we highlight some of the tests in which the developmental level of attention is an important component. Among the core vision tests all those marked with an asterisk in Table 1 require brief periods of sustained visual attention and so will be failed by infants and children with very limited attention spans ('fleeting attention', as demonstrated by brief fixations and random eye movements). The test of 'attention over distance' explicitly requires the child to maintain fixation on an observer as they retreat to a distance of 1–2 metres and has proved to be a sensitive indicator of attentional impairment in the first year of life.

Table 1. ABCDEFV: Core vision subtests

Test	Purpose of test
1. Pupil responses	Responsiveness of pupils to light. Failure of pupil constriction in one/both eyes is likely to indicate severe neurologic problems
2. Diffuse light reaction	Responsiveness to light and dark, but not a measure of pattern vision. Only appropriate for very young infants and in cases of suspected total blindness
*3. Lateral tracking	Assessment of eye movements (saccadic and/or smooth pursuit) and visual attention
*4. Peripheral refixation – lateral field testing	Assessment of visual attention (and the extent of visual fields); age norms need to be applied
5. Symmetrical corneal reflections	Alignment of the eyes; measure of strabismus
*6. Convergence of eyes to approaching object	Assessment of convergence of the eyes, dependent on visual binocularity
*7. Attention at distance to retreating silent tester	Assessment of visual attention maintained at moderate distance (up to 2 metres). Age norms apply
8. Defensive blink to object approaching face	Assessment of a visual reflex depending on mechanisms analyzing visual expansion
*9. Visual following of a falling silent toy	Assessment of an early stage in understanding of *object permanence* (*i.e.*, the understanding that an object goes on existing when it disappears from view)
*10. Teller Acuity Cards (optional)	Assessment of visual acuity
11. Optokinetic nystagmus (optional)	Assessment of subcortical reflex eye movement mechanism requiring directional response to large-field motion

Note: Tests marked 'optional' require special equipment which may be unavailable in some test locations.
*Marks tests which make some demands on attention.

Among the 'optional' core tests is the Teller (or Keeler) Acuity Cards Procedure using preferential looking (McDonald *et al.*, 1985). This is intended to measure resolution acuity (the finest grating pattern that can be distinguished from a homogeneous field of matched mean luminance). However, children with neurodevelopmental disorders who fail this acuity test do not necessarily do so because of reduced fineness of vision; failure may be because they do not attend to the task for sufficient time to obtain an acuity measurement or even fail to attend to the region of space where the cards are being presented. An infant's biases in attention between left and right (associated, for instance, with lateralized brain damage and hemiplegia) may also interfere with the determination of acuity by this method. However, such children may use a strategy of searching with head and eye movements to make the target visible to them, but show biases in head posture and in the direction of this scanning, which the tester needs to recognize.

Varying attention over time may also reduce a child's measured acuity. It should also be noted that when a child shows good attention, but has reduced acuity due to refractive or retinal problems, this acuity loss is unlikely to be the reason for failures on other subtests in the battery with more visuocognitive and visuomotor demands since in most cases the acuity level required is quite low.

These more visuocognitive and visuomotor tests are listed in Table 2 and, where marked with an asterisk, indicate significant attentional demands which may involve selective attention rather than simply the ability to sustain attention for the period of the tests. The different components of attention are discussed in a subsequent section.

Table 2. ABCDEFV: age-specific subtests

Test	Minimum age (mo/yr)	Purpose of the test
*11. Batting/ reaching	4 mo	Assessment of visuomotor development
*12. Reaching for and picking up black and white cotton thread	12 mo	Determining fine hand and finger movement (including pincer grasp) and crude test of contrast sensitivity
*13. Retrieval of partially covered object	6 mo	Assessment of later stage of *object permanence* (*i.e.* understanding that an object partially hidden from view still exists)
*14. Retrieval of totally covered object	6 mo	Assessment of later stage of *object permanence* (*i.e.*, understanding that an object fully hidden from view still exists)
*15. Shape matching	18 mo	Shape recognition and manipulation Failure may represent a general delay or specific visual spatial problem
*16. Overlapping figures	2 yr	Assessment of figure-ground segmentation together with shape recognition Requires selective attention to figure in background
*17 Placing letter in envelope	2 yr	Visuocognitive and visuomotor visual abilities: relative orientation matching in space, and planning and control of manual actions
18. Block construction – free play	13 mo	Requires recognition of spatial relations, and use of these for planning and control of manual actions
*19. Copying block constructions	18 mo	A combination of spatial, cognitive, and motor vision Block constructions graded in difficulty for ages 18 months to 5 years ('constructional apraxia')
*20. Lang test of stereopsis (optional)	2 yr	Measurement of stereoscopic vision
*21. Cambridge Crowding Cards (optional)	3 yr	Visual acuity, both for single-letter symbols and 'crowding effects' (effect on acuity of surrounding pattern elements) Requires ability to select central letter and ignore distractors

Note: Tests marked 'optional' require special equipment which may be unavailable in some test locations.

*Marks tests which make some demands on mechanism of attention.

The ABCDEFV has been used to assess functional vision in both dorsal and ventral streams, and visual attention in everyday tasks, in follow-up to 5 years of age in children with marked refractive errors from the Cambridge Videorefractive Screening Programmes (for example, see Atkinson *et al.*, 1984, 1996, 2007), infants and children with WS (*e.g.*, see Atkinson *et al.*, 2003), children at risk of abnormal brain development related to very preterm birth (*e.g.*, see Atkinson & Braddick, 2007; Atkinson *et al.*, 2011) and children born at term with acute perinatal brain injuries (*e.g.*, see Atkinson & van Hof-van Duin, 1993; Mercuri *et al.*, 1996, 1997).

Component subsystems of attention: typical development

It is widely accepted that attention has a number of distinct components based on separate neural subsystems. Above, we have suggested that young infants have a subcortical orienting system, which comes under cortical attentional control a few months after birth (Atkinson,

1984, 2000; Atkinson & Braddick, 2003; Atkinson & Hood, 1997). The inability to shift attention under competition (in the fixation shift paradigm) has been found to a useful indicator of early attentional problems in children with perinatal cerebral damage, and can be used to predict future neurologic status in cognitive tasks (*e.g.*, see Braddick *et al.*, 1992; Hood & Atkinson, 1990; Mercuri *et al.*, 1996, 1997, 1999). These early attentional cortical networks overlap strongly with dorsal stream networks controlling and planning visuocognitive spatial actions, as discussed above.

On the basis of neuropsychological evidence from adult patients with specific brain damage, and from functional neuroimaging (*e.g.*, Fan *et al.*, 2005), it has been proposed that the mature brain contains three distinct subsystems for attention (Posner & Petersen, 1990). These are (1) an orienting subsystem, whose activity is reflected in spatial selective attention; (2) a second subsystem for sustaining attention; and (3) a third subsystem for top-down attentional control of cognitive processing (often called 'executive function'). This work has provided a framework for subsequent models of attention based on these three subsystems, tested by examining individual differences in performance across a range of attention tasks for the same individuals, and using factor analysis to establish whether factor loadings support the proposed differentiation of attention functions. This approach has provided evidence for attentional subsystems in adults (*e.g.*, Mirsky *et al.*, 1991; Robertson *et al.*, 1996).

However, such a structure is the end point of a dynamic developmental process. The developmental course over childhood of these types of performance needs to be examined, with the question of whether they develop independently and can be considered distinct at early stages.

Many studies have measured individual elements of attention during childhood, providing evidence for age-related improvements in selective attention (*e.g.*, Scerif *et al.*, 2004; Trick & Enns, 1998), sustained attention (*e.g.*, Aylward *et al.*, 2002; Levy, 1980; Lin *et al.*, 1999), and in the ability to switch attention flexibly between rules and inhibit prepotent responses, which are key components of attentional control (*e.g.*, Gerstadt *et al.*, 1994; Jacques & Zelazo, 2001; Jones *et al.*, 1998; Kirkham *et al.*, 2003). Evidence for differences in developmental trajectories between different attention subsystems have also been put forward (*e.g.*, Kelly, 2000; McKay *et al.*, 1994; Rueda *et al.*, 2004). In a number of studies, data sets from typically-developing school-age children have provided support for an attention system in which distinct functions of selective/focused attention, sustained attention, and executive aspects of attention can be identified (*e.g.*, Kelly, 2000; Manly *et al.*, 2001; Mirsky *et al.*, 1991). Although there are some inconsistencies, these studies have provided support for attention as a multi-dimensional construct even in childhood.

Attention deficits in neurodevelopmental disorders

Many children with developmental disorders have been reported to have attentional deficits which resemble those described for adult patients with frontal lobe lesions. These include distractibility, impulsivity, and difficulty in grasping the global aspects of a complex task or situation and in mastering new tasks. The frontal lobes in adults have been considered as a complex of systems involved in the executive control of behaviour, including spatial planning, working memory, maintaining attention on the task in hand, cognitive flexibility in switching between tasks when necessary, and inhibiting well-learned responses that are inappropriate to the present situation (see, for example, Duncan *et al.*, 1996; Goldman-Rakic, 1996; Robbins, 1996). These functions are embraced in the concept of 'attentional control' (executive function), one of the three components of attention within the framework outlined above. Duncan (2010) argues that this system in the frontal lobes can be characterized as a network that enables the human brain to deal with multiple demands and is closely associated with psychometric 'fluid intelligence'.

For example, a number of studies have been carried out with children with WS, a disorder identified from a genetic marker test (FISH) showing a deletion of around 30 genes on one arm of chromosome 7. WS individuals have a characteristic and unusual cognitive profile (*e.g.*, see Bellugi *et al.*, 1988, 1999). They typically combine 'hypersocial' behaviour with a degree of mental retardation, but within this there is a very uneven profile of abilities. Language, particularly productive language, although atypical (Karmiloff-Smith *et al.*, 1998), is at a relatively high level, but visuospatial and visuomotor abilities are severely impaired, typically not progressing beyond the 4–5-year-old level. WS individuals are often reported to have attentional deficits. They have difficulties switching from one task to another and show perseverative behaviour.

Persons with WS have difficulty with tasks of selective spatial attention. Young WS children (under 6 years of age) show a deficit in the fixation-shift task, in disengaging attention from a centrally fixated target to fixate on a newly appearing peripheral target. In this condition ('fixation shifts under competition') they show very long latencies to shift fixation compared to those of typically developing children (Atkinson *et al.*, 2003). A more advanced form of inhibitory control has been examined *via* the 'pointing/counterpointing' task (Atkinson *et al.*, 2003). This is an adaptation of the anti-saccade task (*e.g.*, Pierrot-Deseilligny *et al.*, 1991), in which after the appearance of a central target, another target appears in a lateral position to the left or right. In the pointing task, the participant simply has to point to the appearing target as rapidly as he or she can; in the counterpointing task, the child is required to point to the blank side of the screen opposite the newly appearing target. WS children showed severe difficulties with this task, both in latencies and error rates (Atkinson *et al.*, 2003), indicative of poor inhibitory control in WS.

Children with WS have been tested on a number of other attention tasks requiring the inhibitory control of prepotent responses (Atkinson *et al.*, 2003). In the 'day-night' task (Gerstadt *et al.*, 1994) the response is verbal: the participant has to name a daylight scene, showing a sun, as 'night' and a night-sky scene, showing a moon, as 'day'. WS participants performed relatively well on this task, in line with or often better than their overall verbal mental age. In contrast, in the 'detour box' task (Biro & Russell, 2001; Hughes & Russell, 1993), the same group showed a marked deficit, whether considered in terms of chronological age or verbal developmental age. This test requires the child to inhibit direct reaching for a ball and instead to retrieve it by an indirect operation. As a function of verbal developmental age (assessed with the British Picture Vocabulary Scale [BPVS]) the WS group showed a progressive mastery of the task with age, but this occurred with a sharp improvement at developmental equivalent age around 7 years rather than the 3.5 years seen in typical development.

Overall these results show that WS children have deficits in executive control processes, and the intercorrelations between the three tests (day-night, detour box, and counterpointing) indicated a general 'frontal' factor in individuals' scores, even when the overall level of cognitive development indexed by the BPVS was partialled out. However, the more striking result is the variation between tasks: a severe difficulty in inhibiting a prepotent response in spatial/motor domains (counterpointing and detour box) contrasting with the near-normal ability to inhibit a verbal response (day/night). A neuroimaging study (Mobbs *et al.*, 2007) has shown that frontostriatal systems are underactivated by a response inhibition ('go/no-go') task in WS individuals compared to controls, but the test used did not differentiate between spatial and nonspatial inhibitory control. There is some evidence for segregated subsystems within prefrontal cortex involved in the control of spatial as opposed to nonspatial behaviours (Goldman-Rakic, 1996), although this is controversial (Owen *et al.*, 1998). The pattern of deficit in WS may reflect either a deficit in the information transmitted to such systems or differential processing capacities within them (perhaps as a developmental consequence of these prefrontal networks receiving limited or disorganized input through the dorsal stream). The fact that these attentional deficits are particularly pronounced in tasks involving visuospatial actions supports the idea that networks involved in control of attention are linked to those within the dorsal stream for controlling actions.

Studies by Brown *et al.* (2003) and Cornish *et al.* (2007) provide other examples suggesting early difficulties for WS children in the selection of targets for visual attention. Targets are typically specified by some sensory properties (size, colour, *etc.*), but the ability to find them efficiently depends on a strategy of moving the focus of attention systematically around the array. Difficulties of selective attention have been observed with WS toddlers in a visual search task (Scerif *et al.*, 2004), in which they made significantly more errors than did matched controls. Specifically, errors tended to be erroneous responses to distractors, rather than repetitions on found targets, suggesting a problem with limiting selection and response to targets. There was an interesting contrast with children with Fragile X syndrome (FXS), who made more perseveration errors on found targets, suggesting that in this condition performance is limited by a problem with inhibitory control.

The Test of Everyday Attention in Children (TEA-Ch) (Manly *et al.*, 1999, 2001) contains subtests of selective attention, sustained attention, and executive control. Older children with WS show deficits in selective attention, sustained attention, and visuospatial inhibition tasks, but not verbal inhibition, compared to typically developing children matched for mental age in the control group (Breckenridge, 2007). However, this study raised issues regarding the impact of the nonattentional demands in some of these TEA-Ch subtests (particularly counting as a component in the sustained attention task); some data using a test battery designed to be more appropriate in its nonattentional demands is discussed below.

The TEA-Ch has also been included in an extensive follow-up study of children born very preterm (before 33 weeks' gestation), tested between 6 and 7 years of age. Overall performance of the group showed a range of deficits (Atkinson & Braddick, 2007), including global motion coherence sensitivity, performance on fine and gross visuomotor tests (Henderson & Sugden, 1992), subtests of TEA-Ch, and spatial memory (Nardini *et al.*, 2006). In contrast, the IQ scores and language (vocabulary) tests of the group were overall in the normal range. As discussed above, deficits of spatial processing, attention, and visual control of actions are those primarily associated with processes in the dorsal stream. Factor analysis has shown that the different test results also show differential patterns of association with MRI findings of perinatal brain damage, gestational age at birth, and impairment in the group as a whole (see Atkinson & Braddick, 2007).

The Early Childhood Attention Battery

The requirement to understand relatively complex tasks, and the quite long testing duration, make test batteries such as the TEA-Ch and other standardized tests of attention inappropriate for most typically developing children under 6 years of age, or indeed for children who are below this mental age because of neurodevelopmental delays. The Early Childhood Attention Battery (ECAB) (Breckenridge, 2007; submitted for publication, a) is designed to overcome these problems and to be suitable for use with children with mental ages between 3 and 6 years. From extensive piloting of a range of tests in a large group of typically developing children aged between $2^1/_2$ and 6 years, eight subtest measures have been selected for the ECAB to correspond as closely as possible to the tests of proven use with older children, whilst maximizing developmental sensitivity and age-appropriateness, and minimizing nonattentional confounding variables. Table 3 lists these component subtests. Their validity, in allowing existing measures to be extended to younger ages, has been supported by a strong correlation with TEA-Ch scores in a subgroup of children (aged 6:1 to 7:1 years) who were tested with the TEA-Ch 7 to 15 months after the ECAB test.

Table 3. Component subtests of the ECAB (Early Childhood Attention Battery) and proposed attentional underpinnings

Subtest	Attention component tested	Task requirements
Visual search	Selective attention	Identify target items from an array; conjunction task
Flanker task	Selective attention	Respond selectively to a central item, ignoring distractors
Visual sustained	Sustained attention	Maintain attention on visual stimuli to identify rare targets (5-min duration)
Auditory sustained	Sustained attention	Maintain attention on auditory stimuli to identify rare targets (5-min duration)
Dual sustained	Sustained attention	Monitor both visual and auditory stimuli to detect targets (2.5-min duration)
Verbal opposites	Attentional control	Respond to cat and dog pictures by giving the incorrect, opposite name
Counterpointing	Attentional control	Point to the opposite side of screen to where a target appears
Balloon sorting	Attentional control	Sort balloons according to hidden changing rules (*e.g.*, colour, shape)

Exploratory factor analysis on the normalization data for the ECAB revealed that for the younger children (*i.e.*, those aged 3 to $4^1/_2$ years) there were two attentional components with substantial overlap between them, whilst data from the older children (*i.e.*, from $4^1/_2$ to 6 years) indicated three components, very similar to those identified in adults and older children, corresponding to selective attention, sustained attention, and executive control. Thus the established structure of attentional components appears to emerge over this age range. It is not yet known whether this is a true differentiation of functional networks, or whether these networks are present in the younger group, but that performance involving each is limited by some common constraint or constraints. In any case, these normative data allow percentiles for each age group to be established for each age group and to provide the means for a norm-based profile of performance across the different components to be defined for individual children and for groups with specific developmental disorders.

However, it should not be assumed that there is complete equivalence between scores from typically developing children and those with developmental disorders It is quite possible that the strategies used may vary across syndromes and that the developmental trajectories also vary with age across each specific syndrome.

Components of attention in children with Williams syndrome and Down syndrome assessed using the ECAB

The normative data from typically developing children, outlined above, served as the basis for examining attentional profiles in a study of two groups of children with developmental disorders – WS and Down syndrome (DS). Given the overall developmental delay in these groups, the ECAB allows comparative measures which are developmentally appropriate for children aged 5 to 15 years with these conditions and to define the characteristic profile of these groups across component functions of the attention domain. Previous reports, some cited above, have indicated considerable attention problems in both of these groups. Children with WS or DS are frequently reported by parents and teachers to be more inattentive, distractible, and hyperactive than are their typically-developing peers (*e.g.*, see Cuskelly & Dadds, 1992; Greer *et al.*, 1997; Pagon *et al.*, 1987; Pueschel, 1990).

A study by Breckenridge *et al.* (submitted for publication, b) compared a group of children with WS and a group of children with DS with each other and with norms from typically developing children, matched overall in terms of mental age (MA) from selected subtests of the Wechsler Preschool and Primary Scale of Intelligence (WPPSI) and in chronological age (range 5–15 years; mental age range 3–6 years). For each child, mental age was used to derive age-scaled scores on each of the ECAB subtests, so that attention performance could be considered relative to the children's overall cognitive level. This study found that sustained attention was a relative strength for both WS and DS children, with performance at or above MA level on all subtests designed to measure this function. Auditory sustained attention was a particular strength for the DS group, with performance significantly better than in the WS group, and better than expected for their mental age. Although this will still generally represent a delay relative to chronological age, it was an area of particular proficiency relative to other skills. Auditory sustained attention was somewhat better than visual sustained attention in both groups. One possible explanation is that maintaining visual attention requires the participant to fix attention on a particular spatial location; this control was apparently a potential problem for both groups, and may be an aspect that relates to dorsal stream deficits.

Visual search, response inhibition (counterpointing and verbal opposites) and task switching (balloon sorting) were significantly below MA level for both groups. Visuospatial response control in the counterpointing task was a particular weakness for the WS group, consistent with the earlier findings of Atkinson *et al.* (2003), with performance significantly worse than in the DS group. Both groups also showed significant deficits on the set-shifting task (balloon sorting), indicating problems of perseveration, consistent with impairments on the Wisconsin Card Sorting Task (WCST) in DS adults (Cornish *et al.*, 2001). Figure 4 shows the profiles of ECAB performance for the two groups, illustrating the kind of detailed characterization of components that is possible with this approach.

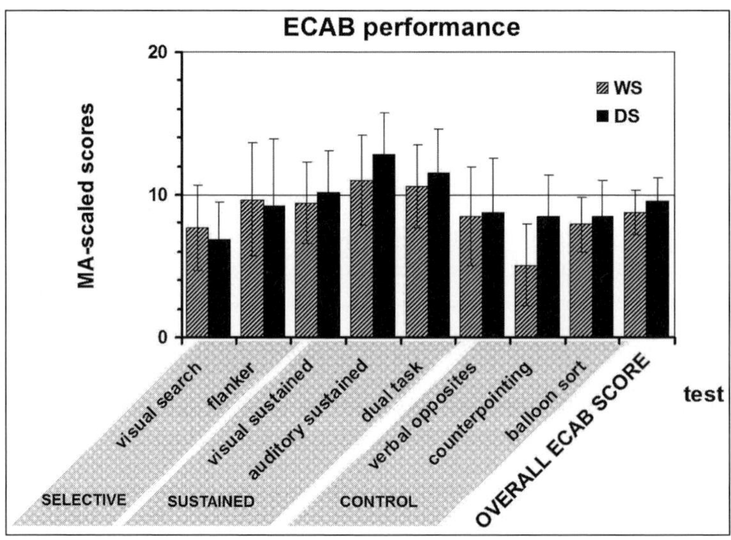

Fig. 4. Scores of WS and DS groups on individual subtests of the Early Childhood Attention Battery (ECAB). The overall score across all subtests is shown in the far right column. Scores are scaled for mental age norms so that a score of 10 represents the expected mean score for mental age. Error bars show standard error (N = 32 in each group).

Conclusions

In summary, this article has covered a number of areas in discussing how visual brain mechanisms are linked to the broader development of brain systems for cognition, attention and actions:

• *Visual brain models:* We presented a brief summary of development of the visual brain in typically developing infants. This model allows us to establish developmental milestones for the normal onset of functions in the visual cortex (striate cortex – V1 – and beyond) and in particular to identify critical stages of development for the ventral and dorsal stream (more details can be found in Atkinson, 2000 and in Atkinson & Braddick, 2003, 2011).

• *Dorsal and ventral streams and dorsal stream vulnerability:* Specially designed visual stimuli for measuring global coherence thresholds for directional motion and static form can provide signatures of the level of functioning in the dorsal and ventral streams. We and others have used these to identify a common theme of visual dorsal stream deficits or 'dorsal stream vulnerability' in children with a range of developmental disorders including WS, autism, and perinatal brain anomalies, such as those related to preterm birth. Visual event-related potentials from high-density arrays have allowed us to identify different spatial distributions of activated extrastriate brain areas in these dorsal and ventral systems, showing reorganization of these systems during development and identifying delays in motion coherence development for very preterm-born infants (Atkinson & Braddick, 2011; Wattam-Bell *et al.*, 2010).

• *Links in the dorsal stream between vision, spatial actions, and attention:* This dorsal stream vulnerability is not limited to the striate and extrastriate visual cortical areas. In addition, we have discussed the overlap between dorsal stream brain networks, which underpin visuomotor spatial tasks and brain networks for controlling visual attention. A new neuroanatomic model of the targets of the dorsal stream, in parietal, frontal, and temporal areas (Kravitz *et al.*, 2011) provides a framework for the development and disorders of (*a*) visuomanual systems (parietal); (*b*) oculomotor control and attentional feedback circuits and motor planning (frontal), including the performance of attention switching tapped by the fixation shift task; and (*c*) integration with ventral stream information in medial temporal areas including the hippocampus for spatial cognition and navigation – aspects of which form part of the pattern of 'dorsal stream deficit' in, for example, the development of prematurely born children (Atkinson & Braddick, 2007).

• *Infant attention measures:* Fixation shifts (FS) provide the earliest behavioural test to gauge infants' links between visual spatial processing and selective attention. Responses to competition between two visual targets can indicate deficits in in the first few months of life in parieto-frontal networks, which control selection of targets and disengagement processes to switch attention between objects. Such deficits in the first year of life can predict later neurocognitive status related to perinatal brain injury.

• *Attention measures using the ABCDEFV:* The FS paradigm and electrophysiologic measures such as VERPs require specific technology and trained personnel. The ABCDEFV battery, described briefly here (see also Atkinson & Braddick, 2011), can be used to pinpoint visual and attentional dysfunction in settings without such specialist equipment, although, of course, training and aptitude for testing infants and young children is still required. The battery aims to assess the functional implications of the child's visual abilities, including both ventral stream shape discrimination, dorsal stream visuomotor and attentional functions, and tasks requiring integration of these systems.

• *Paediatric attention batteries – TEA-Ch and ECAB:* We have argued that attention is not unitary: it has distinct subcomponents, including the ability to select the current object of attention, the ability to maintain sustained processing for a specific goal, and executive control, which includes relating behaviour to current goals, ignoring distractions, switching tasks when necessary, and inhibiting prepotent but irrelevant responses. We have discussed in this article data on the development in childhood of these three major components of attention. The ECAB, a new battery for typical 3- to 6-year-olds described here, builds on previous work on older children with the TEA-Ch battery to show that the three major components of attention can be successfully separated to provide a profile of the attentional abilities of individual children.

• *Attention deficits in developmental disorders:* Our results with these attention batteries show that in developmental disorders (for example, in Williams and Down syndromes) strengths and weaknesses may be identified beyond those anticipated from the individual's overall performance on standard intelligence tests. The profiles of attention deficit we have identified in our studies with the ECAB are to some extent specific to particular syndromes, and are linked to aspects of the cognitive profile outside the attentional domain (*e.g.*, differential competence with linguistic versus spatial information). This relates to our discussion of the links between attentional deficits and other dorsal stream functions described in this paper in the visuomotor and spatial domains.

• *Goals for the future:* Given that we now have tools to identify in the individual infant and child, at an early age, a range of specific deficits related to complex interactive function of processing in multiple dorsal streams, the goal of such work should be two-fold. First, we need to maintain the goal of better understanding of developing human function in infancy and childhood. We need to disseminate information about current theoretical and applied knowledge on these tests, the rationale for using them in appropriate settings, and the adequate training of the staff who care for and advise families with children with neurodevelopmental disorders. Second, we should aim to help individuals by characterizing their patterns of strengths and deficits in greater detail. Such insights will hopefully aid in devising programmes of rehabilitation and support that reflect these insights.

Acknowledgments: This work was supported by Grants G7908507 and G0601007 from the Medical Research Council and grants from the Economic and Social Research Council. We thank the Williams Syndrome Foundation for grants to the Visual Development Unit to fund part of the research in persons with WS. In addition, this work would not have been possible without the collaboration of many members, past and present, of the Visual Development Unit, in particular John Wattam-Bell, Shirley Anker, Dee Birtles, and Kate Breckenridge. The work on development of the ECAB and its use was carried out as Kate Breckenridge's doctoral thesis and postdoctoral research. A number of the studies described have also depended on the generous collaboration of our clinical colleagues, notably Mary Rutherford, Frances Cowan, David Edwards, and Leigh Dyet at the Hammersmith Hospital and Imperial College. Most of all, we are grateful for the patience and cooperation of the families of the infants and children who have participated in these studies.

References

Acredolo, L.P. & Evans, D. (1980): Developmental changes in the effects of landmarks on infant spatial behaviour. *Dev. Psychol.* **16,** 312–318.

Allport, A. (1989): Visual attention. In: *Foundations of Cognitive Science*, ed. M. I. Posner. Cambridge, MA: MIT Press.

Atkinson, J. (1984): Human visual development over the first six months of life: a review and a hypothesis. *Hum. Neurobiol.* **3,** 61–74.

Atkinson, J. (1990): Development of precortical and cortical visual pathways in human infants. In: *Visual Perception: The Neurophysiological Foundations*, eds. L. Spillman & J.S. Werner, pp. 359–365. San Diego, CA: Academic Press.

Atkinson, J. (2000): *The Developing Visual Brain.* Oxford: Oxford University Press.

Atkinson, J. & Braddick, O. (2003): Neurobiological models of normal and abnormal visual development. In: *The Cognitive Neuroscience of Development*, eds. M. De Haan & M.H. Johnson, pp. 43–71. Hove, Sussex: Psychology Press.

Atkinson, J. & Braddick, O. (2005): Dorsal stream vulnerability and autistic disorders: the importance of comparative studies of form and motion coherence in typically developing children and children with developmental disorders. *Cah. Psychol. Cognit. Curr. Psychol. Cognit.* **23,** 49–58.

Atkinson, J. & Braddick, O. (2007): Visual and visuocognitive development in children born very prematurely. *Progr. Brain Res.* **164,** 123–149.

Atkinson, J. & Braddick, O. (2011): Neurophysiological and behavioural aspects of visual assessment: correlation with neuro-imaging. In: *New Diagnostic and Therapeutic Tools in Child Neurology*, eds. E. Mercuri, E. Fedrizzi and G. Cioni. Mariani Foundation Paediatric Neurology Series-XXIV. Paris: John Libbey Eurotext.

Atkinson, J. & Braddick, O. (in press): Visual and visuocognitive development of children born very prematurely. In: *Handbook of Growth and Growth Monitoring in Health and Disease*, ed. V.R. Preedy. New York: Springer.

Atkinson, J. & Hood, B. (1997): Development of visual attention. In: *Attention, Development, and Psychopathology*, eds. J.A. Burack & J.T. Enns, pp. 31–54. New York: Guilford Press.

Atkinson, J. & Van Hof-van-Duin, J. (1993): Visual assessment during the first years of life. In: *Management of Visual Impairment in Childhood: Clinics in Developmental Medicine*, eds. A. Fielder & M. Bax, vol. 128, pp. 9–29. London: MacKeith Press.

Atkinson, J., Braddick, O.J., Durden, K., Watson, P.G. & Atkinson, S. (1984). Screening for refractive errors in 6–9–month old infants by photorefraction. *Br. J. Ophthalmol.* **68,** 105–112.

Atkinson, J., Hood, B., Wattam-Bell, J. & Braddick, O.J. (1992): Changes in infants' ability to switch visual attention in the first three months of life. *Perception* **21,** 643–653.

Atkinson, J., Braddick, O., Bobier, B., Anker, S., Ehrlich, D., King, J., Watson. P. & Moore, A. (1996): Two infant vision screening programmes: prediction and prevention of strabismus and amblyopia from photo- and videorefractive screening. *Eye* **10,** 189–198.

Atkinson, J., King, J., Braddick, O., Nokes, L., Anker, S. & Braddick, F. (1997): A specific deficit of dorsal stream function in Williams syndrome. *NeuroReport* **8,** 1919–1922.

Atkinson, J., Anker, S., Rae, S., Hughes, C. & Braddick, O. (2002): A test battery of child development for examining functional vision (ABCDEFV). *Strabismus* **10,** 245–269.

Atkinson, J., Braddick, O., Anker, S., Curran, W. & Andrew, R. (2003): Neurobiological models of visuospatial cognition in children with Williams syndrome: measures of dorsal-stream and frontal function. *Dev. Neuropsychol.* **23,** 141–174.

Atkinson, J., Braddick, O., Rose, F.E., Searcy, Y.M., Wattam-Bell, J. & Bellugi, U. (2006): Dorsal-stream motion processing deficits persist into adulthood in Williams syndrome. *Neuropsychologia* **44,** 828–833.

Atkinson, J., Braddick, O., Nardini, M. & Anker, S. (2007): Infant hyperopia: detection, distribution, changes and correlates: outcomes from the Cambridge Infant Screening Programs. *Optom. Vis. Sci.* **84,** 84–96.

Atkinson, J., Braddick, O., Anker, S., Nardini, M., Birtles, D., Rutherford, M., *et al.* (2008): Cortical vision, MRI and developmental outcome in preterm infants. *Arch. Dis. Child: Fetal Neonatal Ed.* **93,** F292–F297.

Aylward, G.P., Brager, P. & Harper, D.C. (2002): Relations between visual and auditory continuous performance tests in a clinical population: a descriptive study. *Dev. Neuropsychol.* **21,** 285–303.

Barrett, T.M. & Needham, A. (2008): Developmental differences in infants' use of an object's shape to grasp it securely. *Dev. Psychobiol.* **50,** 97–106.

Barrett, T.M., Traupman, E. & Needham, A. (2008): Infants' visual anticipation of object structure in grasp planning. *Infant Behav. Dev.* **31,** 1–9.

Bellugi, U., Sabo, H. & Vaid, J. (1988): Spatial deficits in children with Williams syndrome. In: *Spatial Cognition: Brain Bases and Development*, Eds. J. Stiles-Davis, M. Kritchevsky & U. Bellugi. Hillsdale, NJ: Lawrence Erlbaum.

Bellugi, U., Lichtenberger, L., Mills, D., Galaburda, A. & Korenberg, J.R. (1999): Bridging cognition, the brain, and molecular genetics: evidence from Williams syndrome. *Trends Neurosci.* **22,** 197–207.

Berger, S.E. & Adolph, K.E. (2007): Learning and development in infant locomotion. *Progr. Brain Res.* **164,** 237–55.

Berthoz, A. (1996): Neural basis of decision in perception and the control of movement. In: *Neurobiology of Decision Making*, eds. A.R. Damasio, H. Damasio & Y. Christen. Berlin: Springer.

Biro, S. & Russell, J. (2001): The execution of arbitrary procedures by children with autism. *Dev. Psychopathol.* **13,** 97–110.

Braddick, O. & Atkinson, J. (2007): Development of brain mechanisms for visual global processing and object segmentation. In: *From Action to Cognition,* eds. C. von Hofsten & K. Rosander, vol. 164, pp. 151–168 of *Progress in Brain Research.* Amsterdam: Elsevier.

Braddick, O. & Atkinson, J. (2011): Neurophysiological and behavioural aspects of visual assessment: correlation with neuro-imaging. In: *Brain Lesion Localization and Developmental Functions*, eds. D. Riva, C. Njiokiktjien and S. Bulgheroni. Mariani Foundation Paediatric Neurology Series-XXV. Paris: John Libbey Eurotext (this book).

Braddick, O., Atkinson, J., Hood, B., Harkness, W., Jackson, G. & Vargha-Khadem, F. (1992): Possible blindsight in infants lacking one cerebral hemisphere. *Nature* **360,** 461–463.

Braddick, O.J., Atkinson, J. & Hood, B. (1996): Monocular *vs* binocular control of infants' reaching. *Invest. Ophthalmol. Vis. Sci.* **37,** S290.

Braddick, O.J., O'Brien, J.M.D., Wattam-Bell, J., Atkinson, J. & Turner, R. (2000): Form and motion coherence activate independent, but not dorsal/ventral segregated, networks in the human brain. *Curr. Biol.* **10,** 731–734.

Braddick, O., Atkinson, J. & Wattam-Bell, J. (2003): Normal and anomalous development of visual motion processing: motion coherence and 'dorsal stream vulnerability'. *Neuropsychologia* **41,** 1769–1784.

Braddick, O.J., Birtles, D., Wattam-Bell, J. & Atkinson, J. (2005): Motion- and orientation-specific cortical responses in infancy. *Vis. Res.* **45,** 3169–3179.

Breckenridge, K. (2007): *The Structure and Function of Attention in Typical and Atypical Development*, Ph.D. thesis, University of London.

Breckenridge, K., Braddick, O. & Atkinson, J. (submitted for publication, *a*): The organisation of attention in typical development: A new preschool attention test battery.

Breckenridge, K., Braddick, O., Anker, S., Woodhouse, M. & Atkinson, J. (submitted for publication, *b*): Attention in Williams syndrome and Down's syndrome: performance on the new Early Childhood Attention Battery (ECAB).

Bremner, J.G. (1994): *Infancy*, 2nd ed. Oxford: Blackwell.

Britten, K.H., Shadlen, M.N., Newsome, W.T. & Movshon J.A. (1992): The analysis of visual motion: a comparison of neuronal and psychophysical performance. *J. Neurosci.* **12,** 4745–4765.

Brown, J.H., Johnson, M.H., Paterson, S.J., Gilmore, R., Longhi, E. & Karmiloff-Smith, A. (2003): Spatial representation and attention in toddlers with Williams syndrome and Down syndrome. *Neuropsychologia* **41,** 1037–1046.

Burgess, N., Maguire, E.A. & O'Keefe, J. (2002): The human hippocampus and spatial and episodic memory. *Neuron* **35,** 625–641.

Cornish, K.M., Munir, F. & Cross, G. (2001): Differential impact of the FMR-1 full mutation on memory and attention functioning: a neuropsychological perspective. *J. Cognit. Neurosci.* **13,** 144–150.

Cornish, K., Scerif, G. & Karmiloff-Smith, A. (2007): Tracing syndrome-specific trajectories of attention across the lifespan. *Cortex* **43,** 672–685.

Cowie, D., Braddick, O. & Atkinson, J. (2008): Visual control of action in step descent. *Exp. Brain Res.* **186,** 343–348.

Cowie, D., Atkinson, J. & Braddick, O. (2010): Development of visual control in stepping down. *Exp. Brain Res.* **202,** 181–188.

Cuskelly, M. & Dadds, M. (1992): Behavioral problems in children with Down's syndrome and their siblings. *J. Child Psychol. Psychiatry* **33,** 749–761.

Duffy, C.J. & Wurtz, R.H. (1991): Sensitivity of MST neurons to optic flow stimuli. I. A continuum of response selectivity to large-field stimuli. *J. Neurophysiol.* **65,** 1329–1345.

Duncan, J. (2010): The multiple-demand (MD) system of the primate brain: mental programs for intelligent behaviour. *Trends Cognit. Sci.* **14,** 172–179.

Duncan, J., Emslie, H., Williams, P., Johnson, R. & Freer, C. (1996): Intelligence and the frontal lobe: The organization of goal-directed behavior. *Cognit. Psychol.* **30,** 257–303.

Epstein, R. & Kanwisher, N. (1998): A cortical representation of the local visual environment. *Nature* **392,** 598–601.

Fan, J., McCandliss, B.D., Fossella, J., Flombaum, J.I. & Posner, M.I. (2005): The activation of attentional networks. *NeuroImage* **26,** 471–479.

Gallant, J.L., Braun, J. & Van Essen, D.C. (1993): Selectivity for polar, hyperbolic, and cartesian gratings in macaque visual cortex. *Science* **259,** 100–103.

Gerstadt, C.L., Hong, Y.J. & Diamond, A. (1994): The relationship between cognition and action: performance of children 3 1/2–7 years old on a Stroop-like day-night test. *Cognition* **53,** 129–153.

Gibson, E.J. & Walk, R.D. (1960): The 'visual cliff'. *Sci. Am.* **202,** 67–71.

Goldman-Rakic, P.S. (1996): The prefrontal landscape: implications of functional architecture for understanding human mentation and the central executive. *Phil. Trans. Roy. Soc. London B*, **351,** 1445–1453.

Greer, M.K., Brown, F.R., Pai, G.S., Choudry, S.H. & Klein, A.J. (1997): Cognitive, adaptive, and behavioral characteristics of Williams syndrome. *Am. J. Med. Genet. 74,* 521–525.

Gunn, A., Cory, E., Atkinson, J., Braddick, O., Wattam-Bell, J., Guzzetta, A. & Cioni, G. (2002): Dorsal and ventral stream sensitivity in normal development and hemiplegia. *NeuroReport* **13,** 843–847.

Guzzetta, F., Frisone, M.F., Ricci, D., Randò, T. & Guzzetta, A. (2002): Development of visual attention in West syndrome. *Epilepsia* **43,** 757–763.

Guzzetta, F., Cioni, G., Mercuri, E., Fazzi, E., Biagioni, E., Veggiotti, P., *et al.* (2008): Neurodevelopmental evolution of West syndrome: a 2-year prospective study. *Eur. J. Paediatr. Neurol.* **12,** 387–397.

Henderson, S.E. & Sugden, D.A. (1992): *The Movement ABC Manual.* London: The Psychological Corporation.

Hermer, L. & Spelke, E. (1994): A geometric process for spatial reorientation in young children. *Nature* **370,** 57–59.

Hermer, L. & Spelke, E. (1996): Modularity and development: the case of spatial reorientation. *Cognition* **61,** 195–232.

Hermer-Vazquez, L., Spelke, E.S. & Katsnelson, A.S. (1999): Sources of flexibility in human cognition: dual task studies of space and language. *Cognit. Psychol.* **39,** 3–36.

Hood, B. & Atkinson, J. (1990): Sensory visual loss and cognitive deficits in the selective attentional system of normal infants and neurologically impaired children. *Dev. Med. Child Neurol.* **32,** 1067–1077.

Hood, B. & Atkinson, J. (1993). Disengaging visual attention in the infant and adult. *Infant Behav. Devel.* **16,** 405–422.

Hughes, C. & Russell, J. (1993): Autistic children's difficulty with mental disengagement from an object: its implications for theories of autism. *Dev. Psychol.* **29,** 498–510.

Huttenlocher, J., Newcombe, N. & Sandberg, E. (1994): The coding of spatial location in young children. *Cognit. Psychol.* **27,** 115–147.

Jacques, S. & Zelazo, P.D. (2001): The Flexible Item Selection Task (FIST): a measure of executive function in preschoolers. *Dev. Neuropsychol.* **20,** 573–591.

Jeannerod, M. (1997): *The Cognitive Neuroscience of Action.* Oxford: Blackwell.

Jones, B.L., Rothbart, M.K. & Posner, M.I. (2003): Development of executive attention in preschool children. *Dev. Sci.* **6,** 498–504.

Karmiloff-Smith, A. (1998): Development itself is the key to understanding developmental disorders. *Trends Cognit. Sci.* **2,** 389–398.

Kastner, S. & Ungerleider, L.G. (2000): Mechanisms of visual attention in the human cortex. *Annu. Rev. Neurosci.* **23,** 315–341.

Kelly, T.P. (2000): The clinical neuropsychology of attention in school-aged children. *Child Neuropsychol.* **6,** 24–36.

King, J.A., Atkinson, J., Braddick, O.J., Nokes, L. & Braddick, F. (1996): Target preference and movement kinematics reflect development of visuomotor modules in the reaching of human infants. *Invest. Ophthal. Vis. Sci.* **37,** S526.

King, J.A., Burgess, N., Hartley, T., Vargha-Khadem, F. & O'Keefe J. (2002): Human hippocampus and viewpoint dependence in spatial memory. *Hippocampus* **12,** 811–820.

Kirkham, N.Z., Cruess, L. & Diamond, A. (2003): Helping children apply their knowledge to their behavior on a dimension-switching task. *Dev. Sci.* **6,** 449–476.

Klingberg, T. (2006): Development of a superior frontal-intraparietal network for visuo-spatial working memory. *Neuropsychologia* **44,** 2171–2177.

Kravitz, D.J., Saleem, K.S., Baker, C.I. & Mishkin, M. (2011): A new neural framework for visuospatial processing. *Nature Rev. Neurosci.* **12,** 217–230.

Levy, F. (1980): The development of sustained attention (vigilance) and inhibition in children: some normative data. *J. Child Psychol. Psychiatry* **21,** 77–84.

Lin, C.C.H., Hsiao, C.K. & Chen, W.J. (1999): Development of sustained attention assessed using the Continuous Performance Test among children 6–15 years of age. *J. Abnorm. Child Psychol.* **27,** 403–412.

Livingstone, M. & Hubel, D.H. (1988): Segregation of form, color, movement and depth: anatomy, physiology and perception. *Science* **240,** 740–749.

Manly, T., Roberston, I.H., Anderson, V. & Nimmo-Smith, I. (1999): *The Test of Everyday Attention for Children: TEA-Ch.* Bury St Edmunds: Thames Valley Test Company.

Manly, T., Nimmo-Smith, I., Watson, P., Anderson, V., Turner, A. & Roberston, I.H. (2001): The differential assessment of children's attention: the Test of Everyday Attention for Children (TEA-Ch), normative sample and ADHD performance. *J. Child Psychol. Psychiatry* **42,** 1065–1081.

Mason, A.J.S., Braddick, O. & Wattam-Bell, J. (2003): Motion coherence thresholds in infants: different tasks identify at least two distinct motion systems. *Vis. Res.* **43,** 1149–1157.

McCarty, M.E., Clifton, R.K., Ashmead, D.H., Lee, P. & Goubet, N. (2001): How infants use vision for grasping objects. *Child Dev.* **72,** 973–987.

McDonald, M.A., Dobson, V., Sebris, S.L., Baitch, L., Varner, D. & Teller, D.Y. (1985): The acuity card procedure: a rapid test of infant acuity. *Invest. Ophthalmol. Vis. Sci.* **26,** 1158–1162.

McKay, K.E., Halperin, J.M., Schwartz, S.T. & Sharma, V. (1994): Developmental analysis of three aspects of information processing: sustained attention, selective attention, and response organization. *Dev. Neuropsychol.* **10,** 121–132.

Mercuri, E., Atkinson, J., Braddick, O., Anker, S., Nokes, L., Cowan, F., *et al.* (1996): Visual function and perinatal focal cerebral infarction. *Arch. Dis. Child.* **75,** F76–F81.

Mercuri, E., Atkinson, J., Braddick, O., Anker, S., Cowan, F., Rutherford, M., *et al.* (1997): Visual function in full-term infants with hypoxic-ischaemic encephalopathy. *Neuropediatrics* **28,** 155–161.

Mercuri, E., Haataja, L., Guzzetta, A., Anker, S., Cowan, F., Rutherford, M., *et al.* (1999): Visual function in term infants with hypoxic-ischaemic insults: correlation with neurodevelopment at 2 years of age. *Arch. Dis. Child.: Fetal Neonatal Ed.* **80,** F99–F104.

Milner, A.D. & Goodale, M.A. (1995): *The Visual Brain in Action*. Oxford: Oxford University Press.

Mirsky, A.F., Anthony, B.J., Duncan, C.C., Ahearn, M.B. & Kellam, S.G. (1991): Analysis of the elements of attention: a neuropsychological approach. *Neuropsychol. Rev.* **2,** 109–145.

Mishkin, M., Ungerleider, L. & Macko, K.A. (1983): Object vision and spatial vision: two critical pathways. *Trends Neurosci.* **6,** 414–417.

Mobbs, D., Eckert, M.A., Mills, D., Korenberg, J., Bellugi, U., Galaburda, A.M. & Reiss, A.L. (2007): Frontostriatal dysfunction during response inhibition in Williams syndrome. *Biol. Psychiatry* **62,** 256–261.

Nardini, M., Burgess, N., Breckenridge, K. & Atkinson, J. (2006): Differential developmental trajectories for egocentric, environmental and intrinsic frames of reference in spatial memory. *Cognition* **101,** 153–172.

Nardini, M., Atkinson, J. & Burgess, N. (2008a): Children reorient using the left/right sense of coloured landmarks at 18–24 months. *Cognition* **106,** 519–527.

Nardini, M., Atkinson, J., Braddick, O. & Burgess N. (2008b): Developmental trajectories for spatial frames of reference in Williams syndrome. *Dev. Sci.* **11,** 583–595.

Nardini, M., Braddick, O., Atkinson, J., Cowie, D.A, Ahmed, T. & Reidy, H. (2008c): Uneven integration for perception and action cues in children's working memory. *Cognit. Neuropsychol.* **25,** 968–984.

Newcombe, N., Huttenlocher, J., Bullock Drummey, A. & Wiley, J.G. (1998): The development of spatial location coding: place learning and dead reckoning in the second and third years. *Cognit. Dev.* **13,** 185–200.

Newman, C. (2001): *The Planning and Control of Action in Normal Infants and Children with Williams Syndrome,* Ph.D. thesis, University of London.

Newman, C., Atkinson, J. & Braddick, O. (2001): The development of reaching and looking preferences in infants to objects of different sizes. *Dev. Psychol.* **37,** 561–572.

Owen, A.M., Stern, C.E., Look, R.B., Tracey, I., Rosen, B.R. & Petrides, M. (1998): Functional organization of spatial and nonspatial working memory processing within the human lateral frontal cortex. *Proc. Nat. Acad. Sci. USA* **95,** 7721–7726.

Pagon, R.A., Bennett, F.C., Laveck, B., Stewart, K.B. & Johnson, J. (1987): Williams syndrome: features in late childhood and adolescence. *Pediatrics* **80,** 85–91.

Pierrot-Deseilligny, C., Rivaud, S., Gaymard, B. & Agid, Y. (1991): Cortical control of reflexive visually-guided saccades. *Brain* **114,** 1473–1485.

Posner, M.I. & Dehaene, S. (1994): Attentional networks. *Trends Neurosci.* **17,** 75–79.

Posner, M.I. & Petersen, S.E. (1990): The attention system of the human brain. *Annu. Rev. Neurosci.* **13,** 25–42.

Pueschel, S.M. (1990). Clinical aspects of Down syndrome from infancy to adulthood. *Am. J. Med. Genet.* Suppl **7,** 52–56.

Rizzolatti, G. (1983): Mechanisms of selective attention in mammals. In: *Advances in Vertebrate Neuroethology*, eds. J.P. Ewert, R.R. Capranica & D.J. Ingle, pp. 261–297. Amsterdam: Elsevier.

Rizzolatti, G., Fogassi, L. & Gallese, V. (1997): Parietal cortex: from sight to action. *Curr. Opin. Neurobiol.* **7,** 562–567.

Robbins, T.W. (1996): Dissociating executive functions of the prefrontal cortex. *Phil. Trans. Roy. Soc. London B,* **351,** 1463–1471.

Robertson, I.H., Ward, T., Ridgeway, V. & Nimmo-Smith, I. (1996): The structure of normal human attention: the Test of Everyday Attention. *J. Int. Neuropsychol. Soc.* **2,** 525–534.

Rosenbaum, D.A., Vaughan, J., Barnes, H.J. & Jorgensen, M.J. (1992): Time course of movement planning: selection of handgrips for object manipulation. *J. Exp. Psychol.: Learn. Mem. Cognition* **18,** 1058–1073.

Rueda, M.R., Fan, J., McCandliss, B.D., Halparin, J.D., Gruber, D.B., Lercari, L.P., *et al.* (2004): Development of attentional networks in childhood. *Neuropsychologia* **42,** 1029–1040.

Scerif, G., Cornish, K., Wilding, J., Driver, J. & Karmiloff-Smith, A. (2004): Visual search in typically developing toddlers and toddlers with Fragile X or Williams syndrome. *Dev. Sci.* **7,** 116–130.

Smyth, M.F. & Mason, U.C. (1997): Planning and execution of action in children with and without developmental coordination disorder. *J. Child Psychol. Psychiatry* **38,** 1023–1037.

Trick, L.M. & Enns, J.T. (1998): Lifespan changes in attention: the visual search task. *Cogn. Dev.* **13,** 369–386.

von Hofsten, C. (1982): Eye-hand coordination in newborns. *Dev. Psychol.* **18,** 450–461.

von Hofsten, C. (1984): Developmental changes in the organization of pre-reaching movements. *Dev. Psychol.* **20,** 378–388.

von Hofsten, C. (1991): Structuring of early reaching movements: a longitudinal study. *J. Motor Behav.* **23,** 280–292.

Wattam-Bell, J. (1994): Coherence thresholds for discrimination of motion direction in infants *Vis. Res.* **34,** 877–883.

Wattam-Bell, J., Birtles, D., Nyström, P., von Hofsten, C., Rosander, K., Anker, S., *et al.* (2010): Reorganization of global form and motion processing during human visual development. *Curr. Biol.* **20,** 411–415.

Brain Lesion Localization and Developmental Functions, D. Riva, C. Njiokiktjien and S. Bulgheroni (eds.)

Chapter 20

Visuocognitive and visual disorders in children born preterm

Sara Bulgheroni*, Chiara Treccani*, Daria Riva*, Giovanni Cioni[°,#] and Francesca Tinelli[°,§]

**Developmental Neurology Division, Fondazione IRCCS Istituto Neurologico 'C. Besta', via Celoria 11, 20133 Milan, Italy;*
[°]Department of Developmental Neuroscience, Stella Maris Scientific Institute, Pisa, Italy;
[#]Division of Child Neurology and Psychiatry, University of Pisa, Pisa, Italy;
[§]Department of Psychology, University of Florence, Florence, Italy
neuropsicologia@istituto-besta.it

Summary

Advances in medical care over the last few decades have increased the survival rates for children born prematurely, even for those born extremely prematurely. Many such children develop no major sequelae such as cerebral palsy or mental retardation, but despite a 'typical' development and no brain lesions, they may still develop cognitive impairments, delays in acquiring language skills, visuospatial or perceptual problems, behavioural disorders, and learning difficulties as they grow older. Little is known about the related visuocognitive and visual disorders, however. Children born preterm with brain lesions have problems in the visual and visuocognitive components, depending on the site affected by the lesions typical of the premature (*e.g.*, periventricular leucomalacia), involving both the ventral and the dorsal pathways; it is not clear whether similar impairments in these skills are also found in subjects born preterm without brain lesions. Preterm birth places infants in a visual environment at a time when the visual system is extremely immature, and this probably affects the set-up of their visual neural architecture, which will be refined by later experience. This chapter contains a review of the literature focusing on these issues, particularly regarding possible correlations with dorsal and ventral stream vulnerability.

Introduction

Around 5–10 per cent of all births in resource-rich countries are born preterm, but in recent years the incidence seems to have risen in some countries, particularly in the USA, where the rate reached 12–13 per cent in 2007 with survival rates of 81 per cent (Goldenberg *et al.*, 2008). Buitendijk *et al.* (2003) found that 1.1–1.6 per cent of live births in European countries are very preterm, that is, before 33 weeks of gestational age (GA). The number of newborn infants surviving very preterm birth has gradually increased thanks to progress in therapy and quality of care, but this increasing survival has raised issues about the rising rate of adverse developmental outcomes. Most studies have focused on severe sequelae, such as cerebral palsy, with or without associated mental retardation, deficits in cognitive performance, delayed language skills, visuospatial or perceptual problems, behavioural difficulties, and learning difficulties in school age.

In this chapter, we focus on the visuocognitive and visual disorders in this setting, for these disorders occur even in children born preterm without focal retinal problems or brain lesions.

Review of the topic

Visual cognition disorders

The follow-up of preterm (PT) children has always focused on monitoring the development of their major motor and sensory functions. It is only since the end of the 1980s and, more systematically, since the 1990s, that clinicians and researchers have shown a growing interest in assessing their perceptive and visuomotor aspects.

As early as 1964 Abercrombie spoke of perceptual and visuomotor disorders in cerebral palsy, but Fedrizzi *et al.* (1993; 1996) were among the first to systematically study the neurocognitive outcome in PT children, providing evidence of lesions on MRI and describing pictures of spastic diplegia. They highlighted a typical cognitive pattern characterized by impairments mainly in visuoperceptual and visuoconstructive abilities, while the verbal skills are relatively spared. This was an early neuropsychological marker, already evident in early infancy. The nonverbal abilities, assessed by the Performance IQ of Wechsler scales or the Performance subquotient of the Griffiths Mental Development Scales, correlated significantly with the features of periventricular leucomalacia (PVL) on MRI, including the severity of ventricular dilation, the degree and extent of white matter reduction, involvement of the optic radiation, and thinning of the posterior corpus callosum (Fedrizzi *et al.*, 1996). The neuropsychological pattern characterized by a more deficient Performance IQ was confirmed by Pagliano *et al.* (2007) in a study conducted on 15 PT children and 9 children born full-term with spastic diplegia. Cognitive performance was substantially similar in the two groups, but the overall scores in the Developmental Test of Visual Perception (DTVP) were below normal range in the PT children and normal in the term-born children. The PT children's visuoperceptual abilities were also affected differently, their visuomotor abilities being more severely impaired than their non-motor visuoperceptual skills. These children had much the same cognitive performance and MRI findings, so the worse visuoperceptual impairment in the PT group points to a specific role of prematurity, which may have adversely influenced the reorganization of the visual centers and pathways after the initial developmental insult. There is a far from negligible strabismus in the vast majority of PT children, which usually correlates with abnormal stereopsis. This finding suggests that it is important not only to consider the type and extent of cerebral damage, but also to check for the presence and severity of ophthalmologic impairments when studying the effects of prematurity *per se* on visuoperceptual and visuomotor outcomes.

The PT group's profile emerging from the DTVP confirms the results previously obtained by Fazzi *et al.* (2004), who found visuomotor integration disorders and constructional dyspraxia, suggesting a malfunctioning of the occipital–parietal pathway, that is, the dorsal stream. This hypothesis is reinforced by the emergence of a significant correlation between neuroradiologic findings and impairments in visually-guided movements. The perceptual skills were relatively spared, apart from the Closure subtest (identifying whole figures from incomplete visual information).

A more recent study conducted by the same group identified widespread involvement of the higher visual processing system, with involvement of both the ventral and the dorsal streams in PT children with PVL (Fazzi *et al.*, 2009). This supports the idea of a profound integration between the two pathways, as suggested by clinical, neurophysiologic, and functional studies (Atkinson & Braddick, 2007; Goodale & Westwood, 2004).

A deficiency in the perceptual area is confirmed by a number of works by Stiers, who developed the L94 battery for his doctoral thesis in 1998; this battery comprises six object-recognition and two visuoconstructive tasks (Stiers, 1998). In 5-year-old children with early brain injury, Stiers *et al.* (2001) found a significant decline in all the test results, not only for the visuomotor skills. Visuoperceptual impairment was prevalent in the subpopulations of PT children with PVL, while those with right-sided parenchymal haemorrhages appeared to have better performance (Van den Hout *et al.*, 2000). Good motor and cognitive skills and a preserved volume of right optic radiation and of the splenium of the corpus callosum seem to be specific factors protecting against visuoperceptual impairment (van den Hout *et al.*, 2004).

Atkinson & Braddick (2007) reviewed the literature and their works on visual and visuocognitive development in children born very preterm, and proposed a model suggesting that the cluster of deficits seen in this population may be related to networks involving the cortical dorsal stream and its connections to parietal, frontal, and hippocampal areas for processing attention and memory (for details, see the chapter by Atkinson and Braddick in this volume).

In the last 15 years, an increasing number of works has been published on the outcome of typically developing children born preterm. This is an extremely interesting population because it gives us the opportunity to assess the effect of prematurity in subjects with no neurologic, motor, or neurophthalmologic sequelae. Below, we provide a critical account of the main studies conducted on the visual functioning and visual cognition in this population.

In 16 six-year-old PT children (born at 27–32 weeks), Foreman and colleagues (1997) found impaired visual search skills but a well preserved perception. The methodologic limitation of their study lies in the absence of any cognitive and neuroradiologic assessment (not even brain ultrasound), the definition of normality in their sample being based on clinical examination alone.

Goyen *et al.* (1998) studied 83 five-year-old PT children and found that 17 per cent fared poorly in the Developmental Test of Visual-motor Integration, 11 per cent in the Motor-free Visual Perception Test, and 73 per cent on the Peabody Developmental Fine Motor Scale. Not having recruited a control group, they defined as deficient any performance that came below 1 standard deviation with respect to the normative data. The higher incidence of impairments correlated significantly with the clinical variables, that is, GA less than 28 weeks, respiratory distress, and need for ventilation persisting for more than 8 days. The perinatal clinical history of this sample goes to show the methodologic weakness deriving from the absence of neuroradiologic exam: very premature birth and birth complications are risk factors for neurologic and cognitive development and could have minor functional and lesional sequelae even in the absence of definite clinical signs.

In even younger children, aged 3-4 years, Caravale *et al.* (2005) also found deficit in DTVP, position recall, and sustained attention tests even after adjusting for IQ, but an unexpected preservation of visuomotor abilities and visuoconstructive praxia.

Finally, Luoma *et al.* (1998) administered the Wechsler scales to 46 five-year-old PT children with no neuroradiologic damage born at 32 weeks or earlier, obtaining Full IQ within normal range and no significant difference between Performance and Verbal IQ. The absence of asymmetric VIQ–PIQ patterns was confirmed by the successive study by Torrioli *et al.* (2000), which found in 36 children aged 4-6 years a worse performance in the visuomotor tasks (Movement-ABC and Developmental Test of Visuomotor Integration) and selective visual attention test (Bell test) in the 17 children with anomalous stereopsis.

The most recent studies are characterized by a more rigorous methodologic approach to selecting the sample of healthy PT children, that is, those with normal MRI findings and neurophthalmologic functioning.

Using hierarchical stimuli, Santos *et al.* (2009b) found an atypical performance pattern in PT children compared with controls born full-term, but only in the dorsal-drawing task. The visuoperceptual task included eight stimuli, and each trial consisted of a target figure with two comparison figures presented below, one of which had the same overall shape as the target but consisted of different local shapes, while the other contained the same local shapes as the target, but formed a different overall shape. For instance, if the target was an 'H' composed of 's', the local comparison figure was an 'S' made up of 's' and the overall comparison figure was an 'H' made up of 'h'. The PT children relied on the overall information to the same extent as the controls born at term, that is, between the two comparison figures they chose the 'H'. Differences emerged, however, in the visuoconstructive task, in which the children were asked to copy the object: the PT children were good at reproducing the local shapes (*i.e.*, they drew the small 's' well), but not the overall shape of the 'H', and their performance was correlated with low birth weight and GA. It therefore seems that the local level is preserved while the global level is impaired, confirming a greater vulnerability of the dorsal stream responsible for processing motion and space. The PT children had an atypical pattern of performance in configural processing, however, showing a significant bias towards local information under experimental conditions in which the comparison figures either corresponded to the target's configural features (same relationships between different elements) or matched in terms of local features (different spatial relationships between the same elements) (Santos *et al.*, 2009a). A fMRI study on face processing found evidence of a dual-code route, where configural and local information is processed by different pathways which coincide with the ventral and dorsal streams (Lobmaier *et al.*, 2008). Indeed, the greater vulnerability of the dorsal than the ventral functions is confirmed both on the global level in visuoconstructive tasks and on the configural level in perceptual tasks, in which the processing of spatial changes in the relative position of elements constituting a visual stimulus prevails.

Both clinical studies as well as evidence from neuroimaging studies such as diffusion tensor imaging (DTI) seem to support a dysfunction (albeit mild) in healthy preterm children. Just as Fedrizzi *et al.* (1996) reported a correlation between Performance IQ and severity of leucomalacia in PT children with cerebral palsy, Counsell *et al.* (2008) found an abnormal white matter microstructure [fractional anisotropy (FA)] in 33 healthy infants born preterm (at 2 years of corrected age; GA: 24–32 weeks; GQ $\geq$ 80). GQ correlated linearly with FA values in parts of the corpus callosum, while Performance subQ correlated with FA in the corpus callosum and cingulum, and eye–hand coordination subQ correlated with FA in the cingulum, fornix, anterior commissure, corpus callosum, and right uncinate fasciculum. In short, specific neurodevelopmental impairments are related to microstructural abnormalities in particular regions of the cerebral white matter, which are consistent among individuals, even in the absence of brain alterations on structural MR.

We conclude with a reported finding that goes against the trend, coming from recent work by O'Reilly *et al.* (2010). From a cohort of 90 PT children, the authors selected approximately 50 who were administered a very extensive battery of tests, which included neuromotor function assessment, ophthalmologic tests, electrophysiologic parameters (pattern-reversal visual evoked potentials) and MRI measures (structural MR, VBM, and DTI). These authors discussed the results only for 12 children who completed the protocol, concluding that healthy PT born children did not differ significantly from those born at full term in the majority of the tests (they had mild anomalies in the electrophysiologic measurements), although their mean performance was lower and less consistent (*i.e.*, the standard deviations were higher). These preliminary findings would seem to suggest that chronic deficits of visuoperceptual and visuomotor functions are not systematically associated with preterm birth in children with a normal neurologic status. Further studies on larger samples will be needed to confirm this unexpected finding.

Visual disorders

It is now clear that the normal development of visual function depends on the integrity of a network that includes not only optic radiations and the primary visual cortex, but also other cortical and subcortical areas, such as the frontal or temporal lobes, or basal ganglia (Ramenghi *et al.*, 2010).

In recent years, great interest has focused on the correlation between basic visual functions and the development of white matter in the optic radiations in children born preterm once they reached term-equivalent age. Bassi *et al.* (2008) studied 37 PT infants born at a median 28^{+4} (range 24^{+1}–32^{+3}) weeks GA and at a post-menstrual age of 42 (39^{+6}–43) weeks, including ten infants with cerebral lesions on conventional MRI. All cases were studied with 3 Tesla MRI and DTI, and visual assessment was performed using a battery of nine items assessing different visual abilities (see Ricci *et al.*, 2008). On multiple regression analysis, the authors found that the children's visual assessment scores correlated independently with their FA values, whereas no correlation emerged with GA.

Similar results were reported by Berman *et al.* (2009), who studied the correlation between quantitative fibre tracking of the optic radiation and visual performance in children born preterm (less than 34 weeks) assessed at ages from 29 to 41 weeks. These researchers also confirmed the significant correlation between optic FA and scores in visual fixation tracking assessments, and they showed that FA of the optic radiation increased with GA and that the anterior segment on the optic radiation is the one with the higher FA. The same group (Glass *et al.*, 2010) was able to identify an important correlation with electrophysiologic measurements such as visual evoked potentials. They studied nine children born before 34 weeks, measuring their visual evoked response amplitudes as a function of spatial frequency, contrast, and vernier offset size with sVEP 6–20 months after birth. They found that the microstructure of the optic radiations measured shortly after birth was associated with quantitatively measured responses elicited by moderate- to high-contrast spatiotemporal gratings in infancy. These results confirm the important role of early visual assessment, a simple behavioural test that can give highly relevant information on an infant's normal/abnormal development.

An abundance of evidence has accumulated on visual disorders in PT children with brain lesions such as PVL, involving their visual acuity, ocular movements, visual fields, contrast sensitivity (see Cioni *et al.*, 2000; Fedrizzi *et al.*, 1998; Jacobson, 1999; Jacobson & Dutton, 2000), and high-level visual functions (MacKay *et al.*, 2005; Taylor *et al.*, 2009) such as object and form recognition, and motion perception, due to the involvement of the ventral and dorsal pathways, respectively.

Less is known about the development of basic and high-level visual functions in children born preterm without major brain lesions. Only a few studies have been published on the development of basic visual function in 'healthy' PT babies once they reach term age. Ricci *et al.* (2010) confirmed that infants born at 36 and 40 weeks are able to fix on a black and white circular target and track it horizontally and vertically. Preterm infants examined at 35 weeks of postmenstrual age were generally less mature in their visual responses than those born at term, but there were significant differences only in ocular motility, fixation, and tracking on a black-and-white target. The overall comparison of the data collected for PT infants at 35 weeks, PT infants at term-equivalent age, and term-born infants 48 hours after delivery led the authors to broadly identify two groups of items: responses for the first group of items – comprising ocular movements (spontaneous or following a target) and tracking on a black-and-white target, vertically and in an arc – were more mature in the PT infants at both 35 and 40 weeks than in the term-born infants; the ability to fixate centrally and track horizontally did not differ between the three groups. Other responses were less mature in the PT infants at 35 weeks than in the PT infants at term-equivalent age or the term-born infants, including response to color contrast, attention at a distance, and discrimination of stripes – all aspects of visual function that are likely to require some cortical input and more mature subcortical/cortical connectivity.

These findings support the idea that more cortically-mediated aspects of early visual development are likely to depend more on postmenstrual age than on length of extrauterine life.

To investigate the respective contributions of visual experience and preprogrammed mechanisms to visual development, Bosworth and Dobkins (2009) studied chromatic (red/green) and luminance (light/dark) contrast sensitivity (CS) in full-term and PT infants. These two different types of CS are mediated respectively by the magnocellular and the parvocellular pathways, which seem to be affected differently by visual experience and/or differently susceptible to various developmental disorders (see Braddick *et al.*, 2003). Bosworth and Dobkins found that luminance CS was predicted by post-term age during the first few months, suggesting that preprogrammed development sufficed to account for luminance CS, while chromatic CS exceeded the predictions based on post-term age, which would suggest that time since birth has a beneficial effect on chromatic CS. These results indicate that chromatic CS is influenced by early postnatal visual experience more than luminance CS, and this may have implications for the development of the parvocellular and magnocellular pathways.

A similar result was described by Birtles *et al.* (2007), who used VEP to study orientation-specific cortical responses (mediated by the magnocellular pathway) and motion-specific responses (mediated by the parvocellular pathway). Orientation-specific cortical responses develop earlier in infancy than motion-specific responses, but direction-reversal responses across the age range were found smaller in the PT infants, suggesting a delayed maturation of motion processing.

So, PT babies with no major brain lesions seem to be more vulnerable in dorsal than in ventral stream development, but the question is, 'Is this deficit transient or persistent?'

Guzzetta *et al.* (2009) tested 26 school-aged children born preterm (at a GA below 34 weeks), 13 with and 13 without periventricular brain damage. Four different visual stimuli were used to assess perception of pure global motion (optic flow), global motion with some information on form (segregated translational motion), and static stimuli of defined form, comparing our results with a group of age-matched healthy term-born controls. The PT children with brain damage were significantly less sensitive than the term-born controls in all four tests, while the PT children without brain damage fared significantly worse than controls only for the pure motion stimuli. When information on the form was embedded in the stimulus, PT children with brain lesions scored significantly worse than did those without lesions. These results suggest that dorsal-stream-related functions are impaired in preterm children irrespective of any presence of brain damage, while ventral stream deficits are more related to the presence of periventricular brain damage.

This hypothesis was confirmed by studies on biological motion (BM), too. BM is the term used to describe motion patterns characteristic of living beings. Humans can efficiently detect other living beings within their visual environment, and retrieve many features from kinematics, such as identifying their gender (Barclay *et al.*, 1978; Troje, 2002), recognizing various action patterns (Dittrich, 1993), identifying individual persons (Barclay *et al.*, 1978), and even recognizing themselves. Perception of such motion patterns is a fundamental property of the human visual system and this is true even if the stimulus is degraded to only 12 light points attached to the body's joints, as demonstrated by Johansson (1973).

It is clear from the literature that BM contains different kinds of information on motion and form, and neuroimaging data (Giese & Poggio, 2003) provide evidence of BM processing in adults occurring in the posterior part of the superior temporal sulcus (pSTS) (Vaina *et al.*, 2001), an area that receives projections from the anterior parts of the dorsal stream, specializing in the analysis of complex motions, and from the ventral stream, which is crucial to object recognition. We can therefore hypothesize that only a deficit in motion perception tasks, linked to a deficit in form recognition tasks can explain a BM perception impairment.

Pavlova *et al.* (2006) recently studied BM perception in adolescents born prematurely (between 27 and 33 weeks) with and without brain lesions, and in controls matched for age. They found that even patients with only mild PVL were substantially less sensitive than either the PT cases without PVL or the term-born controls ($p < 0.003$ and $p < 0.005$, respectively).

Conclusions

Preterm birth is *per se* an established factor for high mortality and morbidity rates. Despite the considerable number of studies on healthy preterm children, further studies on larger samples are needed to describe their visuocognitive and visual phenotype and its neuroanatomic grounds. For the time being, the atypical perceptual, spatial and visuomotor performance pattern seen in children born preterm but neurologically healthy may be correlated with an atypical visual exposure. Preterm birth places infants in a visual environment at a time when their vision system is extremely immature. This may affect the set-up of their visual neural architecture, which is refined by later experience.

Subtle structural abnormalities identified by DTI may also contribute, however, to the differences observed in preterm children's visual perception and the development of their dorsal and ventral stream functions.

It would be advisable to follow-up preterm populations to identify their strengths and the challenges to their visual behaviour, and possibly to plan measures to maximize their daily adaptive functioning and academic success. Such a follow-up will also contribute to improving our understanding of the developmental pathways from preterm birth to later cognitive achievements.

Acknowledgments: Some of the research reported in this paper has been supported by Grant 2006 from the Mariani Foundation, Milan (to G.C. and D.R.) and by Grant STANIB 229445 (to F.T.).

References

Abercrombie, M.L.J. (1964): *Perceptual and Visuomotor Disorders in Cerebral Palsy: A Survey of the Literature.* Little Club Clinics in Developmental Medicine. No.11. London: Spastic International Medical Publications.

Atkinson, J. & Braddick, O. (2007): Visual and visuo-cognitive development in children born very prematurely. *Prog. Brain Res.* **164,** 123–149.

Barclay, C.D., Cutting, J.E. & Kozlowski, L.T. (1978): Temporal and spatial factors in gait perception that influence gender recognition. *Percept. Psychophys.* **23,** 145–152.

Bassi, L., Ricci, D., Volzone, A., Allsop, J. M., Srinivasan, L., Pai, A., *et al.* (2008): Probabilistic diffusion tractography of the optic radiations and visual function in preterm infants at term equivalent age. *Brain* **131,** 573–582.

Berman, J.I., Glass, H.C., Miller, S.P., Mukherjee, O., Ferriero, D.M., *et al.* (2009): Quantitative fiber tracking analysis of the optic radiation correlated with visual performance in premature newborns. *AJNR Am. J. Neuroradiol.* **30,** 120–124.

Birtles, D.B., Braddick, O.J., Wattam-Bell, J., Wilkinson, A.R. & Atkinson, J. (2007): Orientation and motion-specific visual cortex responses in infants born preterm. *NeuroReport* **18,** 1975–1979.

Bosworth, R.G. & Dobkins, K.R. (2009): Chromatic and luminance contrast sensitivity in fullterm and preterm infants. *J. Vis.* **9,** 15.1–16.

Braddick, O., Atkinson, J. & Wattam-Bell, J. (2003): Normal and anomalous development of visual motion processing: motion coherence and 'dorsal-stream vulnerability'. *Neuropsychologia* **41,** 1769–1784.

Buitendijk, S., Zeitlin, J., Cuttini, M., Langhoff -Roos, J. & Bottu, J. (2003): Indicators of fetal and infant health outcomes. *Eur. J. Obstet. Gynecol. Reprod. Biol.* **111,** S66–77.

Caravale, B., Tozzi, C., Albino, G. & Vicari, S. (2005): Cognitive development in low risk preterm infants at 3-4 months of life. *Arch. Dis. Child. Fetal Neonatal Ed.* **90,** F474–F479.

Cioni, G., Bertuccelli, B., Boldrini, A., Canapicchi, R., Fazzi, B., Guzzetta, A. & Mercuri, E. (2000): Correlation between visual function, neurodevelopmental outcome, and magnetic resonance imaging findings in infants with periventricular leucomalacia. *Arch. Dis. Child Fetal Neonatal Ed.* **82,** F134–140.

Counsell, S.J., Edwards, A.D., Chew, A.T.M., Anjari, M, Dyet L.E., Srinivasan, L., *et al.* (2008): Specific relations between neurodevelopmental abilities and white matter microstructure in children born preterm. *Brain* **131,** 3201–3208.

Dittrich, W.H. (1993): Action categories and the perception of biological motion. *Perception* **22,** 15–22.

Fazzi, E., Bova, S.M. & Uggetti, C. (2004): Visual-perceptual impairment in children with periventricular leukomalacia. *Brain Dev.* **26,** 506–512.

Fazzi, E., Bova, S., Giovenzana, A., Signorini, S., Uggetti, C. & Bianchi, P. (2009): Cognitive visual dysfunctions in preterm children with periventricular leukomalacia. *Dev. Med. Child Neurol.* **51,** 974–981.

Fedrizzi, E., Inverno, M., Botteon, G., Anderloni, A., Filippine, G. & Farinotti, M. (1993): The cognitive development of children born preterm and affected by spastic diplegia. *Brain Dev.* **15,** 428–432.

Fedrizzi, E., Inverno, M., Bruzzone, M.G. & Botteon, G. (1996): MRI features of cerebral lesions and cognitive function in preterm spastic diplegic children. *Pediatr. Neurol.* **15,** 207–212.

Fedrizzi, E., Anderloni, A., Bono, R., Bova, S., Farinotti, M., Inverno, M. & Savoiardo, S. (1998): Eye-movement disorders and visual-perceptual impairment in diplegic children born preterm: a clinical evaluation. *Dev. Med. Child Neurol.* **40,** 682–688.

Foreman, N., Fielder, A., Minshell, C., Hurrion, E. & Sergienko, E. (1997): Visual search, perception, and visuo-motor skill in healthy children born at 27-32 weeks' gestation. *J. Exp. Child Psychol.* **64,** 27–41.

Giese, M.A. & Poggio, T. (2003): Neural mechanism for the recognition of biological movements. *Nat. Rev. Neurosci.* **4,** 179–192.

Glass, H.C., Berman, J.I., Norcia A.M., Rogers, E.E., Henry, R.G., Hou, C., *et al.* (2010): Quantitative fiber tracking of the optic radiation is correlated with visual-evoked potential amplitude in preterm infants. *AJNR Am. J. Neuroradiol.* **31,** 1424–1429.

Goyen, T.A., Lui, K. & Woods, R. (1998): Visual-motor, visual-perceptual and fine motor outcomes in very-low-birthweight children at 5 years. *Dev. Med. Child Neurol.* **40,** 76–81.

Goldenberg, R.L., Culhane, J.F., Iams, J.D. & Romero, R (2008): Epidemiology and causes of preterm birth. *Lancet* **371,** 75–84.

Goodale, M.A. & Westwood, D.A. (2004): An evolving view of duplex vision: separate but interacting cortical pathways for perception and action. *Curr. Opin. Neurobiol.* **14,** 203–211.

Guzzetta, A., Tinelli, F., Del Viva, M.M., Bancale, A., Arrighi, R., Pascale, R.R. & Cioni G. (2009): Motion perception in preterm children: role of prematurity and brain damage. *NeuroReport* **20,** 1339–1343.

Jacobson, L. (1999): Visual dysfunction and ocular signs associated with periventricular leukomalacia in children born preterm. *Acta Ophthalmol. Scand.* **77,** 365–366.

Jacobson, L.K. & Dutton, G.N. (2000): Periventricular leukomalacia: an important cause of visual and ocular motility dysfunction in children. *Surv. Ophthalmol.* **45,** 1–13.

Johansson, G. (1973): Visual perception of biological motion and a model for its analysis. *Percept. Psychophys.* **14,** 201–211.

Lobmaier, J.S., Klaver, P., Loenneker T., Martin E. & Mast, F.W. (2008): Featural and configural face processing strategies: evidence from a functional magnetic resonance imaging study. *NeuroReport* **19,** 287–291.

Luoma, L., Herrgard, E. & Marticainen, A. (1998): Neuropsychological analyses of the visuo-motor problems in children born preterm at < 32 weeks of gestation: a 5 years prospective follow-up. *Dev. Med. Child Neurol.* **40,** 21–30.

MacKay, T.L., Jakobson, L.S., Ellemberg, D., Lewis, T.L., Maurer, D. & Casiro, O. (2005): Deficits in the processing of local and global motion in very low birthweight children. *Neuropsychologia* **43,** 1738–1748.

O'Reilly, M., Vollmer, B., Vargha-Khadem, F., Neville, B., Connelly, A., Wyatt, J., *et al.* (2010): Ophthalmological, cognitive, electrophysiological and MRI assessment of visual processing in preterm children without major neuromotor impairment. *Dev. Sci.* **13,** 692–705.

Pagliano, E., Fedrizzi, E., Erbetta, A., Bulgheroni, S., Solari, A., Bono, R., *et al.* (2007): Cognitive profiles and visuoperceptual abilities in preterm and term spastic diplegic children with periventricular leukomalacia. *J. Child Neurol.* **22,** 282–288.

Pavlova, M., Sokolov, A., Birbaumer, N. & Krägeloh-Mann, I. (2006): Biological motion processing in adolescents with early periventricular brain damage. *Neuropsychologia* **44,** 586–593.

Ramenghi, L.A., Ricci, D., Mercuri, E., Groppo, M., De Carli, A., Ometto, A., *et al.* (2010): Visual performance and brain structures in the developing brain of pre-term infants. *Early Hum. Dev.* **86,** (Suppl. 1), 73–75.

Ricci, D., Cesarini, L., Groppo, M., De Carli, A., Gallini, F., Serrao, F., *et al.* (2008): Early assessment of visual function in full term newborns. *Early Hum Dev.* **84,** 107–113.

Ricci, D., Cesarini, L., Gallini, F., Serrao, F., Leone, D., Baranello, G., *et al.* (2010): Cortical visual function in preterm infants in the first year. *J. Pediatr.* **156,** 550–555.

Santos, A., Duret, M., Mancini, J., Busuttil, M. & Deruelle, C. (2009a): Does preterm birth affect global and configural processing differently? *Dev. Med. Child Neurol.* **52,** 293–298.

Santos, A., Duret, M., Mancini, J., Gire, C. & Deruelle, C. (2009b): Preterm birth affects dorsal-stream functioning even after age 6. *Brain Cognit.* **69,** 490–494.

Stiers, P. (1998): *Impairments of a Visual Perceptual Nature in Pre-School Aged Children with Peri- or Neonatal Brain Lesions.* Unpublished PhD dissertation, Katholieke Universiteit Leuven, Leuven, Belgium.

Stiers, P., van den Hout, B.M., Haers, M., Vanderkelen, R., de Vries, L.S., van Nieuwenhuizen, O., *et al.* (2001): The variety of visual perceptual impairments in pre-school children with perinatal brain damage. *Brain Dev.* **23,** 333–348.

Taylor, N.M., Jakobson, L.S., Maurer, D. & Lewis, T.L. (2009): Differential vulnerability of global motion, global form, and biological motion processing in full-term and preterm children. *Neuropsychologia* **47,** 2766–2778.

Torrioli, M.G., Frisone, M.F., Bonvini, L., Luciano, R., Pasca, M.G., Lepori, R., *et al.* (2000): Perceptual-motor, visual and cognitive ability in very low birthweight preschool children without neonatal ultrasound abnormalities. *Brain Dev.* **22,** 163–168.

Troje, N.F. (2002): Decomposing biological motion: a framework for analysis and synthesis of human gait patterns. *J. Vis.* **2,** 371–387.

Vaina, L.M., Solomon, J., Chowdhury, S., Sinha, P. & Belliveau. J.W. (2001): Functional neuroanatomy of biological motion perception in human. *Proc. Natl. Acad. Sci. USA* **98,** 11656–11661.

Van den Hout, B.M., Stiers, P., Haers, M., van der Schouw, Y.T., Eken, P., Vandenbussche, E., *et al.* (2000): Relation between visual perceptual impairment and neonatal ultrasound diagnosis of haemorrhagic-ischaemic brain lesions in 5-years-old children. *Dev. Med. Child Neurol.* **42,** 376–386.

Van den Hout, B.M., de Vries, L.S., Meiners, L.C., Stiers, P., van der Schouw, Y.T., Jennekens-Schinkel, A., *et al.* (2004): Visual perceptual impairment in children at 5 years of age with perinatal haemorrhagic or ischaemic brain damage in relation to cerebral magnetic resonance imaging. *Brain Dev.* **26,** 251–261.

Mariani Foundation
Paediatric Neurology Series

1: Occipital Seizures and Epilepsies in Children
Edited by: *F. Andermann, A. Beaumanoir, L. Mira, J. Roger and C.A. Tassinari*
2: Motor Development in Children
Edited by: *E. Fedrizzi, G. Avanzini and P. Crenna*
3: Continuous Spikes and Waves during Slow Sleep – Electrical Status Epilepticus during Slow Sleep
Edited by: *A. Beaumanoir, M. Bureau, T. Deonna, L. Mira and C.A. Tassinari*
4: Metabolic Encephalopathies: Therapy and Prognosis
Edited by: *S. Di Donato, R. Parini and G. Uziel*
5: Neuromuscular Diseases during Development
Edited by: *F. Cornelio, G. Lanzi and E. Fedrizzi*
6: Falls in Epileptic and Non-Epileptic Seizures during Childhood
Edited by: *A. Beaumanoir, F. Andermann, G. Avanzini and L. Mira*
7: Abnormal Cortical Development and Epilepsy – From Basic to Clinical Science
Edited by: *R. Spreafico, G. Avanzini and F. Andermann*
8: Limbic Seizures in Children
Edited by: *G. Avanzini, A. Beaumanoir and L. Mira*
9: Localization of Brain Lesions and Developmental Functions
Edited by: *D. Riva and A. Benton*
10: Immune-Mediated Disorders of the Central Nervous System in Children
Edited by: *L. Angelini, M. Bardare and A. Martini*
11: Frontal Lobe Seizures and Epilepsies in Children
Edited by: *A. Beaumanoir, F. Andermann, P. Chauvel, L. Mira and B. Zifkin*
12: Hereditary Leukoencephalopathies and Demyelinating Neuropathies in Children
Edited by: *G. Uziel, F. Taroni*
13: Neurodevelopmental Disorders: Cognitive/Behavioural Phenotypes
Edited by: *D. Riva, U. Bellugi and M.B. Denckla*
14: Autistic Spectrum Disorders
Edited by: *D. Riva and I. Rapin*

15: Neurocutaneous Syndromes in Children
Edited by: *P. Curatolo and D. Riva*
16: Language: Normal and Pathological Development
Edited by: *D. Riva, I. Rapin and G. Zardini*
17: Movement Disorders in Children: a Clinical Update, with video recordings
Edited by: *N. Nardocci and E. Fernandez-Alvarez*
18: Mental Retardation
Edited by: *D. Riva, S. Bulgheroni and C. Pantaleoni*
19: Perinatal Brain Damage: From Pathogenesis to Neuroprotection
Edited by: *L.A. Ramenghi, P. Evrard and E. Mercuri*
20: Genetics of Epilepsy and Genetic Epilepsies
Edited by: *G. Avanzini and J. Noebels*
21: Neurology of the Infant
Edited by: *F. Guzzetta*
22: Brain Lesion Localization and Developmental Functions
Basal ganglia – Connecting systems – Cerebellum – Mirror neurons
Edited by: *D. Riva and C. Njiokiktjien*
23: Lysosomal Storage Diseases: Early Diagnosis and New Treatments
Edited by: *R. Parini, G. Andria*
24: New Diagnostic and Therapeutic Tools in Child Neurology
Edited by: *E. Mercuri, E. Fedrizzi and G. Cioni*

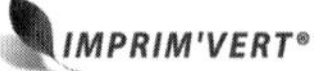

Achevé d'imprimer par Corlet, Imprimeur, S.A.
14110 Condé-sur-Noireau
N° d'Imprimeur : 142477 - Dépôt légal : janvier 2012
Imprimé en France